2023

ADVANCES IN
PSYCHIATRY AND BEHAVIORAL HEALTH

EDITOR-IN-CHIEF
Deepak Prabhakar

SECTION EDITORS
Claudia L. Reardon
Aryandokht Fotros
Eric A. Storch
Lauren M. Osborne
Lindsay Standeven
Andres G. Viana
Carly Johnco

ELSEVIER

Editor: Megan Ashdown
Developmental Editor: Hannah Almira Lopez

Editorial Office:
Elsevier, Inc.
1600 John F. Kennedy Blvd,
Suite 1800
Philadelphia, PA 19103-2899

International Standard Serial Number: 2667-3827
International Standard Book Number: 13: 978-0-443-18276-1

ADVANCES IN PSYCHIATRY AND BEHAVIORAL HEALTH

EDITOR IN CHIEF

DEEPAK PRABHAKAR, MD, MPH -
Education and Clinical Practice
Chief of Medical Staff
Sheppard Pratt
Associate Professor (Adjunct)
Department of Psychiatry
University of Maryland School of Medicine
Baltimore, MD, USA

SECTION EDITORS

CLAUDIA L. REARDON, MD - Sports Psychiatry
Professor, Department of Psychiatry
University of Wisconsin School of Medicine and
Public Health

ARYANDOKHT FOTROS MD, MSC -
Neurosciences
Assistant Professor of Psychiatry
Warren Alpert Medical School of Brown University

ERIC A. STORCH, PH.D. - Psychotherapeutics
McIngvale Presidential Endowed Chair & Professor
Vice Chair & Head of Psychology
Department of Psychiatry and Behavioral Sciences
Baylor College of Medicine

**LAUREN M. OSBORNE, MD - Women's Mental
Health**
Associate Professor of Obstetrics & Gynecology and of
Psychiatry Vice Chair for Clinical Research

Department of Obstetrics & Gynecology
Weill Cornell Medicine

**LINDSAY STANDEVEN, MD - Women's Mental
Health**
Assistant Professor of Psychiatry and Behavioral
Sciences
Clinical And Education Director, The Johns Hopkins
Center for Women's Reproductive Mental Health
Johns Hopkins School of Medicine

**ANDRES G. VIANA, PHD, ABPP - Child and
Adolescent**
Associate Professor of Psychology Department of
Psychology, University of Houston

CARLY JOHNCO, PHD - Geriatrics
Associate Professor, School of Psychological Sciences
Macquarie University

CONTRIBUTORS

ELIZABETH M. AARON, MA
Graduate Assistant, Department of Psychology, Miami University, Oxford, Ohio, USA

AFIFA ADIBA, MD
Attending Psychiatrist, Sheppard Pratt Health System, Towson, Maryland, USA; Assistant Professor (Adjunct) of Psychiatry, University of Maryland, Baltimore, Maryland, USA; Clinical Instructor (Adjunct) of Psychiatry, Yale School of Medicine, New Haven, Connecticut, USA

MALENE AHERN, BAppSc (Physiotherapy), PhD
Postdoctoral Fellow, School of Psychological Sciences, Centre for Emotional Health, Centre for Ageing, Cognition and Wellbeing, Macquarie University, Sydney, New South Wales, Australia

CINDY MILLER ARON, LCSW, CGP, FAGPA
Adjunct Professor, Department of Psychiatry, University of Wisconsin-Madison School of Medicine and Public Health, Madison, Wisconsin, USA; Ascend Consultation in Healthcare/Illinois Sports Performance Center, Chicago, Illinois, USA

GARRETT P. BANKS, MD
Department of Neurosurgery, Baylor College of Medicine, Houston, Texas, USA

KATHRYN E. BARBER, MS
Department of Psychology, Marquette University, Milwaukee, Wisconsin, USA

NICOLE M. BAUMGARTNER, MA
Graduate Assistant, Department of Psychology, Miami University, Oxford, Ohio, USA

MARISSA L. BEAL, DO
Assistant Professor, Department of Psychiatry and Behavioral Sciences, Johns Hopkins School of Medicine, Baltimore, Maryland, USA

RYAN BENOY, MD
Department of Psychiatry, University of Wisconsin-Madison School of Medicine and Public Health, Madison, Wisconsin, USA

OBIANUJU O. BERRY, MD, MPH
Hassenfeld Children's Hospital at NYU Langone, Department of Child and Adolescent Psychiatry, Child Study Center, New York, New York, USA

JONATHAN F. CAHILL, MD
Rhode Island Hospital, The Warren Alpert Medical School of Brown University, Providence, Rhode Island, USA

GREGORY S. CHASSON, PhD
Associate Professor, Department of Psychiatry and Behavioral Neuroscience, University of Chicago, Chicago, Illinois, USA

SOPHIA CHOUKAS-BRADLEY, PhD
Department of Psychology, University of Pittsburgh, Pittsburgh, Pennsylvania, USA

TEGAN CRUWYS, PhD/MClinPsy, PhB (Sci)(Hons), MAPS FCCLP
School of Medicine and Psychology, The Australian National University, Canberra, Australia

JOHN E. DONAHUE
Rhode Island Hospital, The Warren Alpert Medical School of Brown University, Providence, Rhode Island, USA

BRIAN DRAPER, MBBS (Hons), MD
Conjoint Professor, Discipline of Psychiatry and Mental Health, Faculty of Medicine and Health, UNSW Sydney, Eastern Suburbs Older Persons' Mental Health Service, Randwick, New South Wales, Australia

HINDA F. DUBIN, MD
Department of Psychiatry, University of Maryland School of Medicine, Baltimore, Maryland, USA

CARLA D. EDWARDS, MSc, MD, FRCPC
Assistant Clinical Professor, Department of Psychiatry and Behavioural Neurosciences, McMaster University, St. Joseph's Healthcare Hamilton, Hamilton, Ontario, Canada

MARK J. EHRENREICH, MD
Department of Psychiatry, University of Maryland School of Medicine, Baltimore, Maryland, USA

ELIZABETH M. FITELSON, MD
Psychiatry, NewYork-Presbyterian, Columbia University Irving Medical Center, New York, New York, USA

JULIA R. FREW, MD
Assistant Professor, Department of Psychiatry, Geisel School of Medicine, Dartmouth Health, Hanover, New Hampshire, USA

ARKA GHOSH, PhD
Department of Psychology, Stony Brook University, Stony Brook, New York, USA

NISHA GIRIDHARAN, MD
Department of Neurosurgery, Baylor College of Medicine, Houston, Texas, USA

WAYNE K. GOODMAN, MD
Menninger Department of Psychiatry and Behavioral Sciences, Baylor College of Medicine, Houston, USA

KELSEY HANNAN, BA
Department of Psychiatry and Behavioral Sciences, Johns Hopkins School of Medicine, Research Assistant, The Johns Hopkins Reproductive Mental Health Center (RMHC), Baltimore, Maryland, USA

LIISA HANTSOO, PhD
Assistant Professor, Department of Psychiatry and Behavioral Sciences, Johns Hopkins School of Medicine, Director of Research, The Johns Hopkins Reproductive Mental Health Center (RMHC), Baltimore, Maryland, USA

TIMOTHY P. HERZOG, EdD
Counselor and Mental Performance Consultant, Reaching Ahead LLC, Annapolis, Maryland, USA

MARY HITCHCOCK, MA, MS
Senior Academic Librarian, University of Wisconsin-Madison, Ebling Library for the Health Sciences, Madison, Wisconsin, USA

VEDRANA HODZIC, MD
Director of Fellowships, Mentorship and Medical Education, American Psychiatric Association Foundation, Washington, DC, USA; Adjunct Assistant Professor, University of Maryland School of Medicine, Department of Psychiatry, Baltimore, Maryland, USA

EMILY FEDERO HUNGRIA, MD
Rhode Island Hospital, The Warren Alpert Medical School of Brown University, Providence, Rhode Island, USA

VIRGINIA N. IANNONE, PhD
Professor of Psychology, Stevenson University, Owings Mills, Maryland, USA

NISHA JAGANNATHAN, MS
Department of Psychology, Illinois Institute of Technology, Chicago, Illinois, USA

SARAH E. JOHNSON, MD, JD
PGY-3 Resident, University of Maryland, Sheppard Pratt Psychiatry Residency Program, Baltimore, Maryland, USA

ABBAS KARIM, BS
The University of Texas Medical Branch (UTMB), John Sealy School of Medicine, Galveston, Texas, USA

MANAL KHAN, MD
Assistant Professor of Psychiatry, University of California, Los Angeles, Los Angeles, California, USA

ELIZABETH J. KIEL, PhD
Professor, Department of Psychology, Miami University, Oxford, Ohio, USA

ZELAL KILIC, BA
Department of Psychology, University of Pittsburgh, Pittsburgh, Pennsylvania, USA

MICHAEL KRITSELIS, DO
Rhode Island Hospital, The Warren Alpert Medical School of Brown University, Providence, Rhode Island, USA

LISA MACLEAN, MD
Chief Clinical Wellness Officer, Henry Ford Medical Group, Clinical Professor, Michigan State University, Department of Behavioral Services, Henry Ford Health, Detroit, Michigan, USA

DIANA MATOVIC, BPsych (Hons), PhD
Postdoctoral Fellow, School of Psychological Sciences, Centre for Emotional Health, Centre for Ageing, Cognition and Wellbeing, Macquarie University, Sydney, New South Wales, Australia

RILEY MCDANAL, MA
Department of Psychology, Stony Brook University, Stony Brook, New York, USA

DAVID R. MCDUFF, MD
Clinical Professor, University of Maryland School of Medicine, Baltimore, Maryland, USA

CHRISTOPHER W.T. MILLER, MD
Department of Psychiatry, University of Maryland School of Medicine, Baltimore, Maryland, USA

RICHARD P. MOSER, PhD
Training Director and Research Methods Coordinator, Behavioral Research Program, National Cancer Institute, Rockville, Maryland, USA

GAYATHIRI PATHMANATHAN, MBBS
Concord Centre for Mental Health, Concord West, New South Wales, Australia

BRANDON X. PITTS, BS
Department of Psychology, Marquette University, Milwaukee, Wisconsin, USA

NICOLE R. PROVENZA, PhD
Department of Neurosurgery, Baylor College of Medicine, Houston, Texas, USA

ZHEALA QAYYUM, MD, MMSc
Assistant Professor of Psychiatry, Harvard Medical School, Assistant Professor of Psychiatry (Adjunct), Yale School of Medicine, Boston, Massachusetts, USA

CLAUDIA L. REARDON, MD
Professor, Department of Psychiatry, University of Wisconsin-Madison School of Medicine and Public Health, Madison, Wisconsin, USA

MOHONA REZA, MD
Rhode Island Hospital, The Warren Alpert Medical School of Brown University, Providence, Rhode Island, USA

EMILY J. RICKETTS, PhD
Department of Psychiatry and Biobehavioral Sciences, University of California, Los Angeles, Los Angeles, California, USA

SAVANNAH R. ROBERTS, MA
Department of Psychology, University of Pittsburgh, Pittsburgh, Pennsylvania, USA

M. ZACHARY ROSENTHAL, PhD
Departments of Psychiatry and Behavioral Sciences, and Psychology and Neuroscience, Duke University, Durham, North Carolina, USA

ARMAAN A. ROWTHER, MD, PhD
JHU Medical Scientist Training Program, Department of International Health, Johns Hopkins Bloomberg School of Public Health, Baltimore, Maryland, USA

VICTORIA SANBORN, PhD
Rhode Island Hospital, The Warren Alpert Medical School of Brown University, Providence, Rhode Island, USA

JESSICA L. SCHLEIDER, PhD
Department of Psychology, Stony Brook University, Stony Brook, New York, USA

DEEPIKA SHALIGRAM, MD
Attending Psychiatrist, Boston Children's Hospital, Harvard Medical School, Waltham, Massachusetts, USA

YANYAN SHAN, MA
Departments of Psychiatry and Behavioral Sciences, and Psychology and Neuroscience, Duke University, Durham, North Carolina, USA

SAMEER A. SHETH, MD, PhD
Department of Neurosurgery, Baylor College of Medicine, Houston, Texas, USA

BEN SHOFTY, MD, PhD
Department of Neurosurgery, University of Utah, Salt Lake City, Utah, USA

SHAWN SINGH SIDHU, MD, DFAPA, DFAACAP
Associate Professor, Division of Child and Adolescent Psychiatry, Department of Psychiatry, University of California, San Diego Medical Center, Rady Children's Hospital of San Diego, Escondido, California, USA

BHUCHITRA SINGH, MD, MPH, MS, MBA
Clinical Research Program Manager, Department of Gynecology and Obstetrics, Division of Reproductive Sciences and Women's Health Research, Johns Hopkins School of Medicine, Baltimore, Maryland, USA

ORRI SMÁRASON, MA
Faculty of Psychology, University of Iceland,
Reykjavík, Iceland

LINDSAY R. STANDEVEN, MD
Department of Psychiatry and Behavioral
Sciences, Assistant Professor of Psychiatry and
Behavioral Sciences, Clinical and Education
Director, The Johns Hopkins Reproductive Mental
Health Center (RMHC), Johns Hopkins University
School of Medicine, Baltimore, Maryland,
USA

LAURA STANTON, MD
Rhode Island Hospital, The Warren Alpert Medical
School of Brown University, Providence, Rhode
Island, USA

JORDAN T. STIEDE, MS
Menninger Department of Psychiatry and Behavioral
Sciences, Baylor College of Medicine, Houston, Texas,
USA

ERIC A. STORCH, PhD
Menninger Department of Psychiatry and Behavioral
Sciences, Baylor College of Medicine, Houston,
USA

CLAIRE D. STOUT, BA
Department of Psychology, University of Pittsburgh,
Pittsburgh, Pennsylvania, USA

ERIKA S. TRENT, MA
Department of Psychology, University of Houston,
Houston, Texas, USA

JACQUELINE TRUMBULL, MA
Departments of Psychiatry and Behavioral Sciences,
and Psychology and Neuroscience, Duke University,
Durham, North Carolina, USA

ANDRES G. VIANA, PhD, ABPP
Department of Psychology, University of Houston,
Texas Institute of Measurement, Evaluation, and
Statistics, University of Houston, Houston, Texas, USA

ANNE WAND, MBBS(Hons), PhD
Conjoint Associate Professor, Specialty of Psychiatry,
Faculty of Medicine and Health, The University of
Sydney, Conjoint Senior Lecturer, Discipline of
Psychiatry and Mental Health, Faculty of Medicine and
Health, UNSW Sydney and Concord Centre for Mental
Health, Older Peoples Mental Health, Concord
Hospital, Concord, New South Wales, Australia

CHUANG-KUO WU, MD, PhD
Rhode Island Hospital, The Warren Alpert Medical
School of Brown University, Providence, Rhode
Island, USA

VIVIANA M. WUTHRICH, BPsych (Hons), MPsych
(Clin), PhD
Professor of Clinical Psychology, School of
Psychological Sciences, Centre for Emotional Health,
Centre for Ageing, Cognition and Wellbeing, Macquarie
University, Sydney, New South Wales, Australia

DANIEL M. ZIMET, PhD
Daniel M Zimet, LLC, Columbia, Maryland,
USA

CONTENTS

Psychotherapeutics
Psychotherapy for Treatment-Resistant Obsessive-Compulsive Disorder
Nisha Giridharan, Orri Smárason, Nicole R. Provenza, Garrett P. Banks, Ben Shofty, Wayne K. Goodman, Sameer A. Sheth, and Eric A. Storch

Obsessive-compulsive disorder is a neuropsychiatric illness associated with significant disability. The neurobiology of the disease is thought to be related to dysregulation of cortico-striato-thalamo-cortical loops that leads to overexcitation of the orbitofrontal cortex. Standard evidence-based therapies include exposure and response prevention and serotonin reuptake inhibitors, but 10% to 15% of patients fail to achieve response to these treatments. Treatment resistance has been defined by a lack of meaningful improvement in time spent on obsessions and compulsions and the distress associated with them. This article discusses intensive cognitive-behavioral therapy, alternative psychotherapy programs, and neurosurgery as therapeutic options for refractory cases.

Hoarding Disorder
Nisha Jagannathan and Gregory S. Chasson

Hoarding disorder (HD) was split from obsessive-compulsive disorder and categorized separately in the DSM-5, and since then research on its features has rapidly increased. To date, clinical and research studies have demonstrated that pathological hoarding can be characterized by unique diagnostic criteria, biopsychosocial features, and treatment responsivity. Evidence-based treatments for HD target various aspects of its symptomology, including cognitions, behaviors, and emotions (cognitive behavioral therapy) and associated brain chemistry (pharmacology). Given the medical and public health implications of pathological hoarding, further research on its etiology and treatment is warranted.

Behavioral Treatment of Tourette Disorder
Jordan T. Stiede, Brandon X. Pitts, Kathryn E. Barber, and Emily J. Ricketts

Tourette disorder is a childhood-onset neurological condition that can lead to impairment in social, school, occupational, and familial domains. The biobehavioral model of tics provides a strong theoretical foundation that helps inform effective treatment. Behavioral therapy, which includes habit reversal training, comprehensive behavioral intervention for tics (CBIT), and exposure and response prevention, is the gold standard treatment of tic disorders, with support from empirical evidence and practice guidelines. A case vignette that demonstrates CBIT in practice and ways to overcome challenges associated with treatment is also provided.

Treatment of Misophonia

M. Zachary Rosenthal, Yanyan Shan, and Jacqueline Trumbull

Misophonia is a newly defined sound intolerance disorder characterized by strong multi-modal emotional responses to aversive repetitive auditory cues and associated stimuli. This prototypically features highly unpleasant physiological, cognitive, and behavioral responses elicited by oral or facial cues (but can include other sounds) made by others (eg, chewing, throat-clearing). No specific treatments are recommended at this time for all people with misophonia. Instead, we recommend a multi-disciplinary treatment strategy with audiology, occupational therapy, and mental health clinicians.

Sports Psychiatry
Obsessive–Compulsive Disorder in Sports–Beyond Superstitions

Carla D. Edwards and Cindy Miller Aron

Obsessive-compulsive disorder (OCD) in elite athletes can hide in plain sight. Unique stressors and the culture of sport (including socially acceptable superstitions and rituals) can create adaptive and maladaptive behaviors, which may conceal the presence of an illness. Superstitions, routines, and peculiar behaviors in sports are distinguishable from the features of OCD. OCD is a distinct mental health condition with potentially debilitating consequences for those afflicted, including athletes. Common comorbidities with and overlapping features with eating disorders, body dysmorphic disorder, and perfectionism may complicate identification and treatment. Interference by OCD symptoms in the functioning of an athlete can result in physical danger to the athlete, significant disruption in the training environment, and negative performance outcomes. Early detection and a comprehensive approach to management may mitigate the development of more severe pathology.

Eating Disorders and Disordered Eating in Athletes During Times of Transition: A Narrative Systematic Review of the Literature
Claudia L. Reardon, Ryan Benoy, and Mary Hitchcock

Times of transition are known to be high risk periods for mental health symptoms and disorders in athletes, but disordered eating and eating disorders during these times have been relatively underresearched. This novel narrative systematic review summarizes the literature on the risk of disordered eating and eating disorders across a comprehensive set of transitions: retirement, injury, COVID-19 pandemic-related transitions, pregnancy, and the off-season. The review suggests the risk is high during these times. Psychoeducational and other prevention programming on and screening for disordered eating and eating

disorders during times of transition should be implemented for athletes, and further reserach must be undertaken.

Retirement from Elite Sport: Factors Associated with Adjustment and Holistic Health Outcomes
Daniel M. Zimet, David R. McDuff, Virginia N. Iannone, Timothy P. Herzog, and Richard P. Moser

Prior studies suggest that 16% to 20% of athletes experience difficulties transitioning out of competitive sports. Additionally, numerous variables have been reported to impact different outcomes during an athlete's adjustment. This article aimed to describe the impact of an elite athlete's transition out of sport from a holistic, multi-dimensional health perspective. Additionally, this article examined factors that prior research has associated with adjustment outcomes. Participants were 483 retired elite athletes who participated in the Athlete Transition Study. Results suggested that approximately half of the athletes experience significant concerns or difficulties with their cognitive, mental, physical, or social health, and about a third engaged in risky or harmful behaviors. Eight variables commonly associated with transition difficulties were analyzed using a holistic health questionnaire as the outcome variable, and qualitative data were collected. Experiencing a sudden retirement, such as when an athlete endures a career-ending injury or is deselected from a roster, accounted for 10.3% of the variance and was the most predictive variable assessed. Career satisfaction, athlete identity, the positivity of team atmosphere, and gender accounted for an additional 12% of variance. The lack of a comparison group, the over-representation of White women athletes, and the use of convenience sampling and retrospective data limited this study.

Women's Mental Health
Perinatal Cannabis Use: A Clinical Review
Marissa L. Beal and Julia R. Frew

Cannabis use is increasing throughout the United States, including for women during pregnancy and postpartum. Outcome data regarding cannabis use during pregnancy are limited due to confounding variables and poor methodology. Data thus far highlight an association with preterm birth, low birth weight, and long-term neuropsychiatric adverse outcomes in offspring. Providers should discuss cannabis use with patients, identify reasons for use, treat co-occurring substance or psychiatric disorders, and discuss known and unknown risks of cannabis use to mother and baby. Further research into outcomes related to perinatal cannabis use, treatment of cannabis use disorder, and public health initiatives is necessary.

Polycystic Ovary Syndrome: A Guide for Psychiatric Providers
Lindsay R. Standeven, Kelsey Hannan, Bhuchitra Singh, and Liisa Hantsoo

Polycystic ovary syndrome (PCOS) is the most common endocrine disorder affecting reproductive-age women and is associated with increased rates of comorbid psychiatric illnesses. Studies evaluating the biological etiology of psychiatric symptoms in women with PCOS remain limited. This review presents an overview of recent research on the prevalence of comorbid psychiatric conditions and the effectiveness of current treatments in targeting psychiatric symptoms among PCOS women, as well as areas for future research.

Intimate Partner Violence and Women's Mental Health Across the Life Course: A Clinical Review
Armaan A. Rowther, Obianuju O. Berry, and Elizabeth M. Fitelson

Intimate partner violence (IPV) is a highly prevalent and traumatic exposure that contributes significantly to the overall burden of psychological distress and mental health disorders among women. IPV can occur across stages of the life course, both collectively among women survivors and through repeated or multimodal abuse for individual women. Because the negative sequelae of IPV on mental health similarly spans generations, helping survivors move toward safety and recovery requires not only effective safety screenings in mental health care settings but also innovative interventions that address unique risk factors for women by life stage and their structural barriers to care.

Child and Adolescent

Alcohol Use Among Latino Adolescents: Current State and Directions for Future Research and Practice
Erika S. Trent, Abbas Karim, and Andres G. Viana

Latino youth are the largest and fastest-growing ethnic minority group in the United States, and they face unique stressors that heighten their vulnerability to problematic alcohol use. This narrative review synthesizes the recent literature on problematic alcohol use in Latino adolescents in the US. Consistent with the ecodevelopmental framework, alcohol use among Latino adolescents is influenced by risk and protective factors across multiple contexts, including individual, family, peer, school, community, and sociocultural contexts. Although treatment efforts for alcohol use in Latino adolescents have made strides in the past two decades, they still lag behind efforts for other ethnic groups.

Digital Single-Session Interventions for Child and Adolescent Mental Health: Evidence and Potential for Dissemination Across Low- and Middle-Income Countries
Arka Ghosh, Riley McDanal, and Jessica L. Schleider

Over 70% of the youth population does not receive adequate treatment for their mental health problems. Long-waiting lists, social stigma, high costs, and rigid treatment delivery approaches contribute to this treatment gap. Single-session interventions (SSIs) are a form of low-intensity treatments that are designed to deliver maximum therapeutic impact in one session. SSIs have been shown to be effective in reducing multiple mental health problems. In this article, we discuss the evidence base for

SSIs, digital SSIs, and their potential for widespread dissemination. We also discuss the development of two SSIs which were created around evidence-informed principles for SSI design.

Temperament, Parenting, and Child Anxiety

Elizabeth M. Aaron, Nicole M. Baumgartner, and Elizabeth J. Kiel

Temperament and parenting remain commonly studied constructs in relation to anxiety development. Inhibited temperament continues to be one of the most robust predictors of anxiety. Avoidance-promoting and overcontrolling parenting behaviors have emerged as specific correlates and predictors of child anxiety. This review highlights recent advances in the understanding of these constructs, their complex interplay in the etiology of anxiety, and how etiological factors must be understood within cultural context. Research must continue to acknowledge multiple levels of influence, including biological underpinnings of emotion and behavior, child-driven effects on parenting, diverse caregivers, and societal values that shape parental perceptions and behavior.

Perfect Storms and Double-Edged Swords: Recent Advances in Research on Adolescent Social Media Use and Mental Health

Sophia Choukas-Bradley, Zelal Kilic, Claire D. Stout, and Savannah R. Roberts

Because adolescents' mental health concerns have increased in recent years, researchers have investigated the role of social media. Initial study focused on screen-time but recent methodological and conceptual advances have led to a more nuanced place as a field: recognizing that social media offers risks and opportunities that are as diverse as the adolescents experiencing them, with complex implications for mental health. We summarize recent research advances regarding specific positive and negative social media experiences, across 3 major research areas: body image and disordered eating, depressive symptoms and suicidality, and social media experiences among sexual and gender minority youth.

Geriatrics
The Next Steps in Reducing Risk for Dementia

Diana Matovic, Malene Ahern, and
Viviana M. Wuthrich

Without a cure for dementia, the focus is currently aimed at reducing modifiable lifestyle risk factors for dementia, including depression, social isolation, diabetes, smoking, midlife obesity, hypertension, physical inactivity, and alcohol overconsumption among others. Several multidomain dementia risk reduction interventions have shown promise in reducing cognitive decline and dementia risk in at-risk individuals. This review summarizes the evidence and discusses the barriers and facilitators to screening for and treating personalized risk factors in clinical settings. Psychology and psychiatry can improve current dementia risk reduction approaches through the application of motivation and behavior change principles.

Recent Trends and Developments in Suicide Prevention for Older Adults

Gayathiri Pathmanathan, Anne Wand, and
Brian Draper

Suicide rates peak in late life but few suicide prevention interventions have been adequately evaluated. Most evaluated interventions involve education and training, follow-up and aftercare, and psychological therapies with limited evidence of benefit. The positive impact of telephone support on suicide rates has not been replicated but efforts to improve social connection in lonely older adults are essential. Interventions with a suicide prevention focus that address ageism, coping mechanisms for aging men, the impact of declining physical health on well-being, post-dementia diagnosis support, and the stresses upon caregivers need to be formally evaluated. Linked multi-layered multicomponent interventions are required.

Future Directions in Addressing Loneliness Among Older Adults
Tegan Cruwys

This review begins by tackling myths about loneliness in older people, specifically that it is widespread, an inevitable symptom of health decline, or readily cured through the availability of technology. Instead, it is when older people experience rapid social change, are denied opportunities for meaningful contribution, or are subject to discrimination or disadvantage that loneliness is most likely. Recent advances in loneliness theorizing and interventions are reviewed, with a focus on social prescribing, social identity-building programs, and universal social cohesion initiatives. These breakthroughs speak to the need to look beyond the lonely person and consider their social context.

Education and Clinical Practice
Advances in Child Psychiatry Education and Training
Afifa Adiba, Shawn Singh Sidhu, Deepika Shaligram, Manal Khan, and Zheala Qayyum

The article provides a comprehensive overview of the current state of child and adolescent psychiatry, including historical background and the impact of the COVID-19 pandemic. It discusses recent advances in theoretical frameworks related to physician burnout, prevention, access to care, diversity, equity, and inclusion, and trauma-informed care. The authors conclude by emphasizing the importance of education and training in improving the lives of youth and families and encourage their colleagues to push the boundaries of education and training for a better today and brighter tomorrow, while honoring and doing justice to those they serve.

Clinician Well-Being: Addressing Distress and Burnout

Lisa MacLean

Regardless of the role played, clinicians in medicine continue to face the challenge of delivering high-quality care that is increasingly patient-centered while also keeping pace with rapidly changing technology and regulatory requirements. New reimbursement models, increasing patient demands, and advancing health care delivery models (eg, minute clinics) are creating increased pressure on clinicians (medical students, trainees, and faculty) and their well-being. This article seeks to understand how these factors impact clinician well-being, the consequences to individuals personally and professionally and what organizations should consider when addressing this national crisis within their own organization.

Current Landscape, Obstacles, and Opportunities in the Teaching of Psychotherapy in Psychiatric Residency

Christopher W.T. Miller, Hinda F. Dubin, and Mark J. Ehrenreich

Psychotherapy is a required and essential component of psychiatry residency training. There is, however, a tremendous amount of variability in the amount, quality, and type of training that is provided in programs. The challenges in offering comprehensive psychotherapy training include a predominant focus on acute care management, differential priorities of academic psychiatry departments, uneven presence of faculty with content expertise, and lack of supervisors in various modalities of therapy.

Crisis Management in Psychiatry: Overview and Training

Vedrana Hodzic and Sarah E. Johnson

Competently managing a psychiatric emergency demands the effective utilization of complex skills, which must be learned and honed during residency training. Psychiatrists must assess patients in crisis for serious psychiatric concerns, exclude medical causes, manage behavioral emergencies through verbal de-escalation and pharmacological means, foster a positive therapeutic alliance, deliver trauma-informed care, and engage in safety and disposition planning. Managing violence and safety risk are areas that are crucial to the safe delivery of emergency care and especially ripe for the enhancement of resident training.

Neurosciences
Neuropsychiatric Manifestations of Multiple Sclerosis and the Effects of Modern Disease-Modifying Therapies

Mohona Reza, Jonathan F. Cahill,
Emily Federo Hungria, Laura Stanton,
Michael Kritselis, John E. Donahue, Victoria Sanborn,
and Chuang-Kuo Wu

The recent advance in disease-modifying therapies (DMTs) continues to improve the quality of life in patients with multiple sclerosis (MS) by controlling central nervous system inflammation and preventing neurodegeneration. Although DMTs have reduced the burden of neuropsychiatric symptoms in MS, persistent cognitive impairment of MS can still affect daily living. Therefore, proper intervention and therapies can be provided by the specialists; the concerning caregivers will be informed in time of the complicated comorbidity situation so that they can prepare for the care plan.

Preface

Advances: The Three Sisters

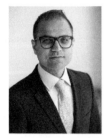

Deepak Prabhakar, MD, MPH

Editor

It is with great pleasure that I introduce the third issue of *Advances in Psychiatry and Behavioral Health*. As the editor-in-chief, I am honored to present the collection of outstanding contributions from leading scholars in our discipline. The emphasis of this issue is on recent advances in our field, building on the momentum from the first two issues.

As work began on this issue, I took the opportunity to look back while charting our future course. Launched in 2021, thus far, all three issues have been impacted by the pandemic. As we deal with the lingering aftereffects including the burgeoning mental health crisis in our communities, it's pertinent that we reflect on the broader themes that have emerged and lessons that we have learned. A sense of community, coexistence, and shared growth is one such theme that merits recognition to help us chart the future course. Leaning on indigenous knowledge, this potential accelerant effect reminds me of the wisdom drawn from centuries of Native American agricultural tradition of planting the three sisters—corn, beans, and squash, together. These three crops, planted together, have provided nutrition to populations for centuries while nurturing each other and the environment. Corn provides the stalk for the beans to rise, ensuring sunshine exposure and space to grow. Beans provide a rich nitrogen source to naturally fertilize the soil while also supporting the corn during high winds. Squash leaves cover the ground, helping retain moisture and preventing weeds. As if taking a cue from the three sisters, the sections in this issue work synergistically—nurturing the discussion while advancing knowledge. As is true with all scholarly work, the *Advances in Psychiatry and Behavioral Health* series leans on the wisdom gained from the past while laying new foundations.

The articles in the third issue cover a wide range of topics, including management of difficult-to-treat obsessive-compulsive disorder, misophonia, Tourette disorder, eating disorders in athletes, retirement from elite sports, crisis management, intimate partner violence, clinician well-being, substance use in Latino youth, adolescent social media use, suicide prevention in older adults, and interventions to address the risk of dementia, among several others. These articles not

https://doi.org/10.1016/j.ypsc.2023.05.001
2667-3827/23/ © 2023 Published by Elsevier Inc.

only contribute to the advancement of knowledge in these areas but also provide important insights into current issues and challenges facing the field. These reviews will be particularly useful for learners, and clinicians who are looking to gain a deeper understanding and access to practical tools while navigating the current practice landscape.

I would like to express my sincere gratitude to the section editors, authors, and editorial staff who have contributed to this issue. Their dedication to advancing knowledge and promoting excellence is truly inspiring.

I hope that you will find this issue illuminating, practical, and engaging.

Deepak Prabhakar, MD, MPH
Sheppard Pratt
Baltimore, MD 21204, USA

E-mail address: dprabhakar@sheppardpratt.org

Psychotherapeutics

Advances in Psychiatry and Behavioral Health 3 (2023) 1–10

ADVANCES IN PSYCHIATRY AND BEHAVIORAL HEALTH

Psychotherapy for Treatment-Resistant Obsessive-Compulsive Disorder

Nisha Giridharan, MD[a], Orri Smárason, MA[b], Nicole R. Provenza, PhD[a], Garrett P. Banks, MD[a], Ben Shofty, MD, PhD[c], Wayne K. Goodman, MD[d], Sameer A. Sheth, MD, PhD[a], Eric A. Storch, PhD[d,*]

[a]Department of Neurosurgery, Baylor College of Medicine, 1 Baylor Plaza, Suite S100, Houston, TX, USA; [b]Faculty of Psychology, University of Iceland, Nýi Garður Sæmundargata 12, Reykjavík 102, Iceland; [c]Department of Neurosurgery, University of Utah, 175 North Medical Drive East, Salt Lake City, UT, USA; [d]Menninger Department of Psychiatry and Behavioral Sciences, Baylor College of Medicine, 1977 Butler Boulevard, Houston, TX 77030, USA

KEYWORDS
- Cognitive-behavioral therapy • Exposure and response prevention • Neurosurgery
- Obsessive-compulsive disorder • Psychotherapy • Treatment-resistance

KEY POINTS
- Evidence-based therapies for obsessive-compulsive disorder (OCD) include exposure and response prevention and serotonin reuptake inhibitors, however, 10% to 15% of patients fail these standard treatments.
- Treatment-resistance is the failure to achieve at least a 25% reduction in the Yale-Brown Obsessive Compulsive Scale with first-line therapies.
- Intensive cognitive-behavioral therapy is a therapeutic option for patients with treatment-resistant OCD.
- Neurosurgical treatments such as stereotactic ablation and deep brain stimulation are also available for patients with severe, refractory OCD.

INTRODUCTION

Obsessive-compulsive disorder (OCD) is a debilitating neuropsychiatric illness with a lifetime prevalence of 2.3% [1]. The disorder is marked by intrusive, unwanted thoughts (obsessions) and repetitive, ritualized behaviors (compulsions) [2]. Compulsions are acts or mental rituals that patients perform to minimize the distress caused by obsessions [3]. OCD is associated with significant disability and without effective intervention, it runs a chronic course [4].

Evidence-based treatments are available and include a specific form of cognitive behavioral therapy (CBT) called exposure and response prevention (ERP) and serotonin reuptake inhibitors (SRIs). Approximately 65% to 80% of adults with OCD respond to ERP alone and 50% to 60% respond to SRI monotherapies. About 65% to 85% of individuals benefit from combined treatment [5]. Treatment outcome is typically assessed with the Yale-Brown Obsessive-Compulsive Scale (YBOCS), the gold standard clinical measure of OCD symptom severity [6]. Full therapeutic response to psychotherapy, pharmacotherapy or surgery is defined by at least a 35% reduction in YBOCS. Most individuals who achieve response are still symptomatic. The scale was later revised to increase sensitivity to symptom changes in patients with severe OCD, among other updates [7].

*Corresponding author. Menninger Department of Psychiatry and Behavioral Sciences, Baylor College of Medicine, 1977 Butler Boulevard, Suite 4-400, Houston, TX 77030, USA. *E-mail address:* Eric.Storch@bcm.edu

https://doi.org/10.1016/j.ypsc.2023.03.010
2667-3827/23/

Despite the availability of effective interventions, many individuals do not respond completely and 10% to 15% fail to achieve any meaningful response [8]. Treatment resistance has been characterized by an insufficient improvement in obsessive-compulsive symptoms following adequate courses of standard therapies. This article will focus on intervention strategies for those who fail to achieve benefit from first-line therapies. The article starts by discussing the neurobiological basis of OCD, conventional first-line therapies, and the definition of treatment resistance. Thereafter, several options with a significant evidence-base for treating refractory cases are presented, including intensive treatment programs (ie, intensive outpatient programs, day treatment programs, and residential programs), other nonintensive psychotherapeutic options (ie, acceptance and commitment therapy [ACT]), and neurosurgery.

Neurobiological Basis of Obsessive-Compulsive Disorder

OCD is understood to be a circuit disorder involving several cortical and subcortical regions. The prevailing model of OCD pathophysiology is dysregulation of cortico-striato-thalamo-cortical (CSTC) loops [9]. Cortical regions such as the orbitofrontal (OFC), dorsolateral prefrontal cortex (dlPFC), ventromedial prefrontal cortex, and dorsal anterior cingulate cortex (dACC) send projections to the striatum. Excitation of the striatum initiates a cascade of events, leading to either excitatory (direct pathway) or inhibitory (indirect pathway) feedback to the cortex (Fig. 1) [10]. In healthy subjects, there is a balance between the direct and indirect pathways. In patients with OCD, an excessive activation of the OFC direct pathway leads to persistent attentiveness to a perceived danger and performance of ritualistic behaviors to neutralize the threat [10]. Hypoactivity in a second CSTC loop between the dlPFC and caudate has been linked to deficits in executive function and the repetitive behaviors of OCD [9].

Understanding of OCD through the framework of cortico-striatal dysfunction has evolved over time. Early PET studies implicated the OFC in the neurobiological basis of OCD but did not appreciate the distinct roles of its subregions [9]. Subsequent neuroimaging studies have shown hyperactivation of the lateral OFC in response to symptom provocation, supporting its function in threat response, whereas the medial OFC, thought to regulate emotion and reward processing, is hypoactive [11–13]. The dACC, which is involved in resolving cognitive conflict, may also play a central

role in the pathophysiology of OCD [14,15]. The control signal theory postulates that dACC dysfunction leads to impaired fear extinction and the inability to adapt behaviors to changes in stimuli [15]. In the original CTSC hypothesis, the role of the amygdala and hippocampus was not included in the mechanisms underlying fear expression. Studies have shown hyperactivation of the amygdala and parahippocampal cortex in response to emotional faces and symptom-provoking stimuli in patients with OCD when compared with healthy controls [16,17]. Thus, further exploration of the role of amplified amygdala responses in the underlying pathophysiology of OCD is needed.

Standard Evidence-Based Therapies

OCD is a heterogenous disorder and response to conventional treatment may depend, in part, on patient-specific symptom dimensions, which are beyond the scope of this review. Standard evidence-based treatments for OCD include psychotherapy and pharmacotherapy.

Exposure and response prevention

CBT is the most efficacious and well-studied psychotherapy for OCD and has been shown to be significantly more successful than medication alone [18]. Treatment consists primarily of ERP, which was first described in the 1960s. Patients with OCD suffer from recurrent, intrusive thoughts that are perceived as threatening. To alleviate the distress caused by these obsessions, patients carry out acts or mental rituals (compulsions) to avoid a negative outcome. The performance of these compulsions, however, negatively reinforces the behavior and patients fail to develop effective coping mechanisms [3]. In ERP, clinicians expose patients to progressively more distressing stimuli and instruct them not to perform palliative rituals. The goal of ERP is to disrupt the association between certain stimuli/thoughts and ritualistic behaviors that reduce anxiety [19].

Numerous studies have demonstrated the efficacy of ERP compared with SRI treatment alone, as well as active control conditions such as relaxation training [20–22]. However, approximately 15% to 25% of individuals do not respond to treatment and many responders only partially benefit. Treatment can be dosed in terms of content, as will be discussed later. Patient characteristics thought to predict poor response to CBT treatment in OCD include higher symptom severity, comorbid depressive symptoms, a comorbid personality disorder, and hoarding symptoms [23–27]. For children and adolescents, a family history of OCD, less insight, younger age, greater functional

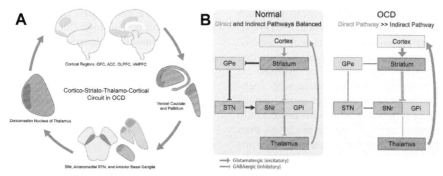

FIG. 1 Cortico-striato-thalamo-cortical (CSTC) circuit dysfunction in OCD. (**A**) OCD is associated with dysfunction in multiple CSTC loops, spanning both cortical and subcortical regions including the orbitofrontal cortex (OFC), dorsolateral prefrontal cortex (dlPFC), dorsal anterior cingulate cortex (dACC), ventromedial prefrontal cortex (vmPFC), striatum, globus pallidus internus (GPi), globus pallidus externus (GPe), substantia nigra pars reticulata (SNr), and thalamus. (**B**) Coordinated activity from these structures provides feedback to the thalamus both directly and indirectly. During normal functioning, the direct and indirect pathways provide excitatory and inhibitory cortical feedback in a balanced manner. In OCD, the direct pathway is overactivated relative to the indirect pathway, leading to pathological excitation of cortex. (*Adapted from* Karas et al., 2019; with permission.)

impairment, higher comorbid externalizing and internalizing symptoms, as well as more family accommodation predict poorer treatment response [28,29].

Pharmacotherapy

First-line medications for OCD are selective serotonin reuptake inhibitors (SSRIs) due to their efficacy and tolerability [30]. Clinical practice guidelines recommend prescribing SSRIs at a maximum tolerated dose for at least 8 to 12 weeks and continuing the medications for at least 6 to 12 months after treatment response [30]. Blinded, placebo-controlled trials have not shown any significant differences in efficacy between SSRIs [31]. Although SSRIs are first-line pharmacotherapy, clomipramine remains the gold standard for treatment [32]. Clomipramine, which is a nonselective SRI, was the first drug on the market with demonstrated efficacy for OCD; however, due to substantial side effects (ie, anticholinergic), it has become a more appropriate second-line treatment [32]. Multiple randomized controlled trials have demonstrated that SRIs (both SSRIs and clomipramine) are superior to placebo in the treatment of OCD [33–37]. Several randomized controlled trials have also shown SRIs are superior to antidepressants (eg, desipramine) that lack potent effects on serotonin reuptake [33].

When patients have failed to achieve response with SRIs, augmentation with an antipsychotic may be appropriate especially in patients with comorbid tic disorders. At present, augmentation with low-dose antipsychotics such as risperidone represents the only established medication combination strategy for OCD. Based on growing interest in the role of the glutamatergic system in OCD, medications that modulate glutamate have been evaluated as potential third-line treatment choices including ketamine, riluzole, N-acetylcysteine, memantine, and d-cycloserine [32]. Although preliminary studies suggested these agents were promising in reducing OCD symptoms, the evidence from randomized controlled trials is inconclusive [38–42]. Patients who have tried standard CBT and medications without success are eligible for additional psychotherapeutic and neurosurgical options if they meet criteria of treatment resistance.

Definition of Treatment Resistance

Three key features establish treatment resistance in psychiatric disorders: an appropriate diagnosis, an adequate course of treatment, and an insufficient response [43]. In OCD, several published consensus statements have categorized the stages of disease as response, remission, recovery, and relapse [44,45]. A full treatment response is defined by a clinically significant reduction in obsessions and compulsions, or at least a 35% reduction in YBOCS. A Clinical Global Impression scale of 1 or 2, "very much improved" or "much improved" has also been included in the definition of response due to the scale's greater sensitivity in detecting subtle changes in symptomatology. Alternatively, a 25% to 35% reduction in YBOCS is considered a partial response. Although these guidelines use symptom severity as a surrogate marker of response, there has not been an established correlation between symptom severity and level of disability or distress in OCD [45].

Although several definitions of treatment resistance or refractory status have been proposed, sustained obsessive-compulsive symptomology as assessed by the YBOCS following adequate treatment with high-fidelity CBT, first-line medications, and augmentation with atypical antipsychotic medication is generally used [45–47]. Operationally, clinicians use a less than 25% decrease in YBOCS to define treatment refractoriness [44,45].

Approach to Treatment Resistant Cases
Combination therapies
Nonresponse to first-line evidence-based OCD treatment is well documented, and thus a few combination psychotherapeutic-medication approaches have been developed to improve response levels. When the initial treatment with an SSRI or clomipramine fails to demonstrate an adequate response, augmenting treatment with CBT has been shown to be effective in both pediatric and adult patients. Franklin and colleagues [48] showed that adding weekly CBT sessions for children on stable antidepressant doses was associated with significantly improved response rates (67%), relative to children who received brief instructional CBT together with continued antidepressant treatment (34%) or continued antidepressant treatment alone (30%). In an adult sample, nonresponders to SRI treatment kept on stable dosages benefitted significantly more from 17 sessions of CBT with ERP than they did from an equal number of sessions of stress management training [49].

When a course of CBT is ineffective, expert guidelines generally recommend SRI augmentation. However, while this is generally accepted as standard of care, there is currently little evidence available to support this approach [50]. A randomized controlled trial in adults indicated that nonresponders to ERP-based therapy benefitted more by switching to an SRI (fluvoxamine) than by undergoing a 12-week course of cognitive therapy without ERP [51]. A large trial of children and adolescents, however, showed no statistically significant difference between CBT nonresponders who were randomized to receive SRI treatment (sertraline) for 16 weeks or an additional 10 sessions of CBT-ERP during 16 weeks [52]. In at least some cases, a longer course of high-fidelity CBT is sufficient to elicit a response from previously refractory children and adolescents. Krebs and colleagues [53] treated a group of 43 adolescents, classified as having severe, treatment-resistant OCD (all had a CY-BOCS score of 30 or

higher), with a manualized CBT protocol at a specialized OCD clinic. This high-fidelity treatment produced a significant and durable reduction in OCD symptoms. At 3-month follow-up, 58% of participants showed a meaningful clinical response. A subset of participants completed a semistructured interview assessing the quality of their previous CBT treatment. In 96% of cases, previous treatment was rated as inadequate, with a lack of exposure techniques being the most common drawback.

Intensive treatment programs
Intensive formats of CBT, where treatment sessions are often conducted several times per week during a short time period, have been suggested as potentially more effective for severe OCD than weekly single treatment sessions [54]. These protocols have similar components as traditional outpatient treatment (ie, exposure-response prevention, psychoeducation, and so forth) but rather manipulate the "dose" of psychotherapy by providing significantly "more" of putative ingredients of symptom change.

Intensive formats can be a practical and, in some instances, a more accessible option than traditional one-session-per-week formats. Intensive treatment might often be the preferred option for students, employed patients, parents, and children who have to travel to attend sessions, as well as in cases when immediate clinical improvement is crucial [55]. Patient motivation is also often enhanced when treatment becomes the primary focus during the short-term duration of an intensive program [56]. Furthermore, for patients with high-emotional reactivity, poor insight, or difficulty comprehending the rationale of the treatment procedures, intensive CBT has been recommended [57,58]. The National Institute for Health and Care Excellence and the American Psychological Association recommend intensive CBT for patients that have not responded to more traditional formats of cognitive therapy.

There is growing evidence for intensive treatment regimens as first-line therapy. In a meta-analysis of OCD therapy in children and adults, intensive CBT was found to be initially superior to regular CBT in reducing obsessive-compulsive symptoms, although this difference was no longer present at 3-month follow-up [55]. A more recent study found that intensive treatment formats achieved comparable results to traditional CBT formats in less time, as well as having a larger effect on comorbid depressive symptoms [59]. It is worth noting that these meta-analyses did not include a number of open, uncontrolled studies and smaller waitlist (or self-help) controlled trials of intensive OCD treatments for adults and children. In general, these smaller studies have yielded response and remission rates comparable or superior to those reported in studies of traditional CBT formats, both at posttreatment and follow-up, in adult and pediatric samples [60–66].

Intensive approaches have also been examined specifically for those not fully responsive to initial traditional treatment. In adult populations, inpatient treatment incorporating intensive CBT and medication management has shown benefits for severe patients, resistant to SRIs. A meta-analysis examining inpatient with OCD and residential treatments for refractory patients found a large effect for intensive treatment, although there was considerable heterogeneity between studies [67]. In a more recent study, 58 adult patients received comprehensive inpatient treatment, combining pharmacotherapy and intensive CBT [68]. Thirty-five participants (60%) met the prespecified criteria for response and 19 (33%) for remission. There was a significant reduction in YBOCS scores at discharge (24%) and follow-up (29%) as compared with baseline ($P < .01$).

For children and adolescents, there are less data available regarding intensive treatments for nonresponders. Storch and colleagues [69] applied an intensive form of CBT treatment (14 daily sessions) to children and adolescents deemed partial responders or nonresponders to medication (n = 30) in an open clinical trial. Eighty percent of the sample had a 30% or greater reduction in YBOCS at posttreatment and at 3-month follow-up; overall, they experienced a 54% mean reduction in symptoms. Moreover, 57% were deemed in remission at posttreatment and 53% remained remitters at follow-up. Björgvinsson and colleagues [70] reported on 23 adolescents that did not respond to outpatient treatment and were treated in an intensive inpatient program, emphasizing ERP with multidisciplinary support (ie, nursing, psychopharmacology). At discharge, 70% of participants were judged to meet criteria for clinically significant change. In a study of residential treatment, Leonard and colleagues [71] found that complex, highly comorbid and treatment refractory adolescents with OCD achieved significant decreases in both OCD and depression severity with intensive exposure-based therapy and medication management. All participants (n = 172) had a history of pharmacological treatment and 90% had previously also attempted outpatient psychotherapy.

Beyond efficacy data in support of intensive programs, cost effectiveness has been evaluated. Gregory and colleagues [72] examined the cost-effectiveness of 7 treatment strategies for adults with treatment-refractory OCD. Higher levels of care represented specialty placements for OCD treatment. Partial hospitalization (ie, day treatment programs) with step-down to an intensive outpatient treatment program was the most cost-effective intervention strategy. This was followed the combination of expert outpatient CBT and antidepressant treatment, intensive outpatient treatment, and partial hospitalization treatment, all which were equally effective. Antidepressant monotherapy and antipsychotic augmentation were found to be the least effective. These findings were generally replicated among children with treatment refractory OCD except that intensive outpatient program was the most cost-effective strategy followed by partial hospitalization, and then high-fidelity outpatient CBT and antidepressant treatment [73].

Alternative psychotherapy programs

In recent years, alternative formats of cognitive and behavioral approaches have become more widespread. Among those, ACT has perhaps the strongest evidence base in OCD treatment although randomized controlled trials are limited and tend to focus on treatment-naive cases [74]. Although it has strong similarities to traditional CBT and utilizes ERP principles, ACT is associated with theoretically different mechanisms of change. A preliminary meta-analysis of 5 studies (only one of which was an RCT), concluded that ACT has modest research support as an acceptable and efficacious treatment of adult OCD [75]. A randomized controlled trial showed no difference between ERP alone and a combination of ERP plus ACT with both interventions proving highly effective [76]. No differences emerged in main outcomes for the treatment groups as both interventions proved highly effective [76]. Only 2 studies have examined ACT for children and adolescents with OCD, showing preliminarily promising results [77]. Additionally, the efficacy of ACT has yet to be studied specifically in nonresponders to other psychotherapies.

Inference-based CBT is a specialized treatment model for OCD, which is an alternative to prolonged and repeated ERP exercises. It instead focuses on correcting the dysfunctional reasoning giving rise to erroneous obsessional doubts and ideas. Research has supported its use in adults with OCD but the technique has not been studied in pediatric cohorts or in those not responding to first-line treatment [78].

Telehealth delivery formats of CBT for OCD have been extensively studied in recent years. Evidence generally suggests that Telehealth delivery of CBT with ERP is just as efficacious and acceptable for patients as in-person delivery [79,80]. Telehealth delivery of intensive CBT for adult patients with severe OCD symptoms has also been shown to be just as effective as in-person intensive CBT when used in partial hospitalizations and intensive outpatient therapy [81].

Nonsurgical neuromodulation. Nonsurgical neuromodulation techniques such as electroconvulsive therapy and transcranial magnetic stimulation (TMS) have been used in patients with treatment-resistant OCD [82,83]. In a multicenter, randomized controlled trial, patients receiving high-frequency deep TMS over the medial prefrontal cortex and anterior cingulate cortex showed significantly greater reductions in YBOCS compared with patients receiving sham treatment [84]. The results from this trial led to FDA approval of deep TMS for OCD.

Neurosurgery

Psychosurgery has been historically stigmatized due to ethical concerns harkening back to the days of indiscriminate frontal lobotomies. Advances in stereotactic neurosurgery in the midtwentieth century ushered in a new era in the surgical treatment of psychiatric disease. Stereotaxy allows clinicians to localize an anatomic structure within a standardized three-dimensional coordinate system and plan coordinate-based trajectories to reach the target structure. Two main stereotactic procedures emerged to treat severe, refractory psychiatric disorders: surgical lesioning and deep brain stimulation (DBS).

The anterior capsulotomy and anterior cingulotomy were among the first lesioning procedures and initially performed using radiofrequency ablation [85]. In time, modalities such as stereotactic radiosurgery, laser interstitial thermal therapy, and MRI-guided focused ultrasound have eclipsed its use [86–88]. When all techniques of ablation are considered, the anterior capsulotomy has been shown to have an overall response rate of 59% [89]. Alternatively, the anterior cingulotomy has also been shown to be a safe and effective procedure with long-term follow-up studies demonstrating a 47% response rate [90].

The lessons from decades of stereotactic lesioning led to development of DBS in the late 1980s. In 1999, a group in Belgium first used DBS of the anterior limb of the internal capsule for patients with treatment-resistant OCD [91]. Encouraging results from this small study led to a successful multicenter trial and a humanitarian device exemption (HDE) approval by the US FDA in 2009 [92]. Since the HDE approval of DBS for OCD, there have been 34 studies published demonstrating an overall response rate of 66% [93]. Surgery for psychiatric disorders has experienced a renaissance in the last few decades with innovation in minimally invasive ablative approaches and the advent of DBS as an adjustable and reversible therapy.

Surgical candidacy

Patients being considered for neurosurgical treatment of OCD should be discussed in a multidisciplinary conference with a psychiatrist, psychologist, and neurosurgeon to determine candidacy [86]. Candidates include adults (aged 18–75 years) with a primary diagnosis of OCD, and severe symptoms (YBOCS >28) that have been significantly impairing their daily functioning for at least 5 years. A multidisciplinary team must also decide whether a patient has tried and failed adequate trials of CBT and medication. If possible, verification of a patient's nonresponse to standard therapies with a treating provider can help guide appropriateness for surgery. A recent suicide attempt, substance abuse disorder, or comorbid psychiatric disorder interfering with treatment is exclusionary criteria. Other important considerations should include the ability to medically tolerate surgery, the patient's social support system, accessibility to the treatment site, and resources for long-term follow-up.

SUMMARY

Several novel therapeutic options exist for patients with OCD who fail standard CBT and SRI treatment. Intensive psychotherapy, acceptance and commitment therapy, and interference-based CBT are among the psychotherapeutic options. Neurosurgical approaches including stereotactic ablation and DBS procedures have also demonstrated high levels of efficacy for patients otherwise refractory to conventional treatment. As our understanding of the pathophysiology of treatment resistance grows, new biomarkers may help identify patients who are likely to be treatment resistant and who may benefit from more intensive intervention early on.

CLINICS CARE POINTS

- Obsessive-compulsive disorder is a neuropsychiatric illness marked by intrusive, unwanted thoughts (obsessions) and repetitive, ritualized behaviors (compulsions).

- Standard, evidence-based treatments for obsessive-compulsive disorder are exposure and response prevention and serotonin reuptake inhibitors.
- Some patients may be classified as treatment resistant, meaning they have sustained obsessive-compulsive symptoms despite adequate treatment with high-fidelity cognitive-behavioral therapy, first-line medications, and augmentation with atypical antipsychotics.
- For treatment refractory cases, intensive outpatient programs, day treatment programs, residential programs, other non-intensive psychotherapeutic options, nonsurgical neuromodulation, and neurosurgery may be options.

DISCLOSURES

E.A. Storch receives grant support from NIH, United States, the REAM Foundation, United States, Greater Houston Community Foundation, United States, International OCD Foundation, United States, and Texas Higher Education Coordinating Board, United States. He receives book royalties from Elsevier, Springer, American Psychological Association, Jessica Kingsley, Oxford, and Lawrence Erlbaum. He holds stock in NView, where he serves on the clinical advisory board. He was a consultant for Levo Therapeutics and is currently a consultant for Biohaven Pharmaceuticals and Brainsway. He cofounded and receives payment from Rethinking Behavioral Health, which is a consulting firm that provides support for implementing evidence-based psychological treatment strategies. S.A. Sheth is a consultant for Boston Scientific, Neuropace, Koh Young, Abbott, Zimmer Biomet, and cofounder of Motif Neurotech. W.K. Goodman is a consultant for Biohaven Pharmaceuticals and receives royalties from Nview, LLC, and OCDscales, LLC.

REFERENCES

[1] Ruscio AM, Stein DJ, Chiu WT, et al. The epidemiology of obsessive-compulsive disorder in the National Comorbidity Survey Replication. Mol Psychiatry 2010; 15(1):53–63.

[2] American Psychiatric Association. Diagnostic and statistical manual of mental disorders (DSM-5 (R)). 5th edition. Washington, DC: American Psychiatric Association Publishing; 2013.

[3] Goodman WK, Storch EA, Sheth SA. Harmonizing the neurobiology and treatment of obsessive-compulsive disorder. Am J Psychiatry 2021;178(1):17–29.

[4] Fineberg NA, Dell'Osso B, Albert U, et al. Early intervention for obsessive compulsive disorder: an expert consensus statement. Eur Neuropsychopharmacol 2019; 29(4):549–65.

[5] Foa EB, Liebowitz MR, Kozak MJ, et al. Randomized, placebo-controlled trial of exposure and ritual prevention, clomipramine, and their combination in the treatment of obsessive-compulsive disorder. Am J Psychiatry 2005;162(1):151–61.

[6] Goodman WK, Price LH, Rasmussen SA, et al. The yale-brown obsessive compulsive scale. I. Development, use, and reliability. Arch Gen Psychiatry 1989;46(11): 1006–11.

[7] Storch EA, Rasmussen SA, Price LH, et al. Development and psychometric evaluation of the Yale-Brown Obsessive-Compulsive Scale–Second Edition. Psychol Assess 2010;22(2):223–32.

[8] Denys D. Pharmacotherapy of obsessive-compulsive disorder and obsessive-compulsive spectrum disorders. Psychiatr Clin North Am 2006;29(2):553–84, xi.

[9] Saxena S, Rauch SL. Functional neuroimaging and the neuroanatomy of obsessive-compulsive disorder. Psychiatr Clin North Am 2000;23(3):563–86.

[10] Karas PJ, Lee S, Jimenez-Shahed J, et al. Deep brain stimulation for obsessive compulsive disorder: Evolution of surgical stimulation target parallels changing model of dysfunctional brain circuits. Front Neurosci 2018;12: 998.

[11] Adler CM, McDonough-Ryan P, Sax KW, et al. fMRI of neuronal activation with symptom provocation in unmedicated patients with obsessive compulsive disorder. J Psychiatr Res 2000;34(4–5):317–24.

[12] Breiter HC, Rauch SL, Kwong KK, et al. Functional magnetic resonance imaging of symptom provocation in obsessive-compulsive disorder. Arch Gen Psychiatry 1996;53(7):595–606.

[13] Yücel M, Harrison BJ, Wood SJ, et al. Functional and biochemical alterations of the medial frontal cortex in obsessive-compulsive disorder. Arch Gen Psychiatry 2007;64(8):946–55.

[14] Sheth SA, Mian MK, Patel SR, et al. Human dorsal anterior cingulate cortex neurons mediate ongoing behavioural adaptation. Nature 2012;488(7410):218–21.

[15] McGovern RA, Sheth SA. Role of the dorsal anterior cingulate cortex in obsessive-compulsive disorder: converging evidence from cognitive neuroscience and psychiatric neurosurgery. J Neurosurg 2017;126(1):132–47.

[16] Cardoner N, Harrison BJ, Pujol J, et al. Enhanced brain responsiveness during active emotional face processing in obsessive compulsive disorder. World J Biol Psychiatry 2011;12(5):349–63.

[17] Simon D, Kaufmann C, Müsch K, et al. Fronto-striato-limbic hyperactivation in obsessive-compulsive disorder during individually tailored symptom provocation. Psychophysiology 2010;47(4):728–38.

[18] Öst LG, Havnen A, Hansen B, et al. Cognitive behavioral treatments of obsessive-compulsive disorder. A systematic review and meta-analysis of studies published 1993-2014. Clin Psychol Rev 2015;40:156–69.

[19] Kozak MJ, Foa EB. Mastery of obsessive- compulsive disorder. Academic Press; 1999.

[20] Christensen H, Hadzi-Pavlovic D, Andrews G, et al. Behavior therapy and tricyclic medication in the treatment of obsessive-compulsive disorder: a quantitative review. J Consult Clin Psychol 1987;55(5):701–11.

[21] Abramowitz JS. Effectiveness of psychological and pharmacological treatments for obsessive-compulsive disorder: a quantitative review. In: Hyman SE, editor. The science of mental Health. New York, NY: Routledge; 2022. p. 246–54.

[22] Ferrando C, Selai C. A systematic review and meta-analysis on the effectiveness of exposure and response prevention therapy in the treatment of Obsessive-Compulsive Disorder. J Obsessive Compuls Relat Disord 2021;31(100684):100684.

[23] Brennan BP, Lee C, Elias JA, et al. Intensive residential treatment for severe obsessive-compulsive disorder: characterizing treatment course and predictors of response. J Psychiatr Res 2014;56:98–105.

[24] Keeley ML, Storch EA, Merlo LJ, et al. Clinical predictors of response to cognitive-behavioral therapy for obsessive–compulsive disorder. Clin Psychol Rev 2008;28(1): 118–30.

[25] Knopp J, Knowles S, Bee P, et al. A systematic review of predictors and moderators of response to psychological therapies in OCD: do we have enough empirical evidence to target treatment? Clin Psychol Rev 2013; 33(8):1067–81.

[26] Sharma E, Thennarasu K, Reddy YCJ. Long-term outcome of obsessive-compulsive disorder in adults. J Clin Psychiatry 2014;75(09):1019–27.

[27] Steketee G, Siev J, Fama JM, et al. Predictors of treatment outcome in modular cognitive therapy for obsessive-compulsive disorder. Depress Anxiety 2011;28(4): 333–41.

[28] Garcia AM, Sapyta JJ, Moore PS, et al. Predictors and moderators of treatment outcome in the pediatric obsessive compulsive treatment study (POTS I). J Am Acad Child Adolesc Psychiatry 2010;49(10):1024–33.

[29] Torp NC, Dahl K, Skarphedinsson G, et al. Predictors associated with improved cognitive-behavioral therapy outcome in pediatric obsessive-compulsive disorder. J Am Acad Child Adolesc Psychiatry 2015;54(3): 200–7.e1.

[30] Koran LM, Hanna GL, Hollander E, et al, American Psychiatric Association. Practice guideline for the treatment of patients with obsessive-compulsive disorder. Am J Psychiatry 2007;164(7 Suppl):5–53.

[31] Skapinakis P, Caldwell DM, Hollingworth W, et al. Pharmacological and psychotherapeutic interventions for management of obsessive-compulsive disorder in adults: a systematic review and network meta-analysis. Focus 2021;19(4):457–67.

[32] Hirschtritt ME, Bloch MH, Mathews CA. Obsessive-compulsive disorder: advances in diagnosis and treatment. JAMA 2017;317(13):1358–67.

[33] Goodman WK, Price LH, Delgado PL, et al. Specificity of serotonin reuptake inhibitors in the treatment of obsessive-compulsive disorder. Comparison of fluvoxamine and desipramine. Arch Gen Psychiatry 1990; 47(6):577–85.

[34] Pittenger C, Bloch MH. Pharmacological treatment of obsessive-compulsive disorder. Psychiatr Clin North Am 2014;37(3):375–91.

[35] Katz RJ, DeVeaugh-Geiss J, Landau P. Clomipramine in obsessive-compulsive disorder. Biol Psychiatry 1990; 28(5):401–14.

[36] Goodman WK, Price LH, Rasmussen SA, et al. Efficacy of fluvoxamine in obsessive-compulsive disorder. A double-blind comparison with placebo. Arch Gen Psychiatry 1989;46(1):36–44.

[37] Perse TL, Greist JH, Jefferson JW, et al. Fluvoxamine treatment of obsessive-compulsive disorder. Am J Psychiatry 1987;144(12):1543–8.

[38] Pittenger C, Bloch MH, Wasylink S, et al. Riluzole augmentation in treatment-refractory obsessive-compulsive disorder: a pilot randomized placebo-controlled trial. J Clin Psychiatry 2015;76(8):1075–84.

[39] Andrade C. Augmentation with memantine in obsessive-compulsive disorder. J Clin Psychiatry 2019;80(6). https://doi.org/10.4088/JCP.19f13163.

[40] Bloch MH, Wasylink S, Landeros-Weisenberger A, et al. Effects of ketamine in treatment-refractory obsessive-compulsive disorder. Biol Psychiatry 2012;72(11): 964–70.

[41] Costa DLC, Diniz JB, Requena G, et al. Randomized, double-blind, placebo-controlled trial of N-acetylcysteine augmentation for treatment-resistant obsessive-compulsive disorder. J Clin Psychiatry 2017;78(7):e766–73.

[42] Storch EA, Wilhelm S, Sprich S, et al. Efficacy of augmentation of cognitive behavior therapy with weight-adjusted d-cycloserine vs placebo in pediatric obsessive-compulsive disorder: a randomized clinical trial. JAMA Psychiatr 2016;73(8):779–88.

[43] Howes OD, Thase ME, Pillinger T. Treatment resistance in psychiatry: state of the art and new directions. Mol Psychiatry 2022;27(1):58–72.

[44] Mataix-Cols D, de la Cruz LF, Nordsletten AE, et al. Towards an international expert consensus for defining treatment response, remission, recovery and relapse in obsessive-compulsive disorder. World Psychiatr 2016; 15(1):80–1.

[45] Pallanti S, Hollander E, Bienstock C, et al. Treatment non-response in OCD: methodological issues and operational definitions. Int J Neuropsychopharmacol 2002; 5(02). https://doi.org/10.1017/s1461145702002900.

[46] Kühne F, Ay DS, Marschner L, et al. The heterogeneous course of OCD - A scoping review on the variety of definitions. Psychiatry Res 2020;285(112821):112821.

[47] Pallanti S, Quercioli L. Treatment-refractory obsessive-compulsive disorder: methodological issues, operational definitions and therapeutic lines. Prog Neuro Psychopharmacol Biol Psychiatry 2006;30(3):400–12.

[48] Franklin ME, Sapyta J, Freeman JB, et al. Cognitive behavior therapy augmentation of pharmacotherapy in pediatric obsessive-compulsive disorder: the Pediatric OCD Treatment Study II (POTS II) randomized controlled trial. JAMA 2011;306(11):1224–32.

[49] Simpson HB, Foa EB, Liebowitz MR, et al. A randomized, controlled trial of cognitive-behavioral therapy for augmenting pharmacotherapy in obsessive-compulsive disorder. Am J Psychiatry 2008;165(5):621–30.

[50] Marazziti D, Pozza A, Avella MT, et al. What is the impact of pharmacotherapy on psychotherapy for obsessive-compulsive disorder? Expert Opin Pharmacother 2020; 21(14):1651–4.

[51] van Balkom AJLM, Emmelkamp PMG, Eikelenboom M, et al. Cognitive therapy versus fluvoxamine as a second-step treatment in obsessive-compulsive disorder nonresponsive to first-step behavior therapy. Psychother Psychosom 2012;81(6):366–74.

[52] Skarphedinsson G, Weidle B, Thomsen PH, et al. Continued cognitive-behavior therapy versus sertraline for children and adolescents with obsessive-compulsive disorder that were non-responders to cognitive-behavior therapy: a randomized controlled trial. Eur Child Adolesc Psychiatry 2015;24(5):591–602.

[53] Krebs G, Isomura K, Lang K, et al. How resistant is "treatment-resistant" obsessive-compulsive disorder in youth? Br J Clin Psychol 2015;54(1):63–75.

[54] Foa EB. Steketee behavioral treatment of phobics and obsessive-compulsives. Psychotherapists in clinical practice: cognitive and behavioral perspectives. New York, NY: Guilford Press; 1987. p. 78–120.

[55] Jónsson H, Kristensen M, Arendt M. Intensive cognitive behavioural therapy for obsessive-compulsive disorder: a systematic review and meta-analysis. J Obsessive Compuls Relat Disord 2015;6:83–96.

[56] Storch EA, Gelfand KM, Geffken GR, et al. An intensive outpatient approach to the treatment of: obsessive-compulsive disorder. Ann Am Psychother Assoc 2003; 6(4):14–9.

[57] Ben-Arush O, Wexler JB, Zohar J. Intensive outpatient treatment for obsessive-compulsive spectrum disorders. Isr J Psychiatry Relat Sci 2008;45(3):193–200.

[58] Available at: https://www.sciencedirect.com/science/ article/pii/S2211364915000408?casa_token=LgD7puC G1DoAAAAA:FyyYU5ZH7-Jk4BUSoSrUbanX-_jDhircaQ bAJdYkFVI243wKWkml55A8p1NgOkYS8tIl7iCY0M.

[59] Remmerswaal KCP, Lans L, Seldenrijk A, et al. Effectiveness and feasibility of intensive versus regular cognitive behaviour therapy in patients with anxiety and obsessive-compulsive disorders: a meta-analysis. J Affect Disord Rep 2021;6(100267):100267.

[60] Hansen B, Kvale G, Hagen K, et al. The Bergen 4-day treatment for OCD: four years follow-up of concentrated ERP in a clinical mental health setting. Cogn Behav Ther 2019;48(2):89–105.

[61] Launes G, Hagen K, Sunde T, et al. A randomized controlled trial of concentrated ERP, self-help and

[62] Davíðsdóttir SD, Sigurjónsdóttir Ó, Ludvigsdóttir SJ, et al. Implementation of the Bergen 4-day treatment for obsessive compulsive disorder in Iceland. Clin Neuropsychiatry 2019;16(1):33–8.

[63] Whiteside SPH, McKay D, De Nadai AS, et al. A baseline controlled examination of a 5-day intensive treatment for pediatric obsessive-compulsive disorder. Psychiatry Res 2014;220(1–2):441–6.

[64] Farrell LJ, Oar EL, Waters AM, et al. Brief intensive CBT for pediatric OCD with E-therapy maintenance. J Anxiety Disord 2016;42:85–94.

[65] Wolters LH, Ball J, Brezinka V, et al. Brief intensive cognitive behavioral therapy for children and adolescents with OCD: two international pilot studies. J Obsessive Compuls Relat Disord 2021;29(100645):100645.

[66] Riise EN, Kvale G, Öst LG, et al. Concentrated exposure and response prevention for adolescents with obsessive-compulsive disorder: an effectiveness study. J Obsessive Compuls Relat Disord 2016;11:13–21.

[67] Veale D, Naismith I, Miles S, et al. Hodsoll Outcomes for residential or inpatient intensive treatment of obsessive-compulsive disorder: a systematic review and meta-analysis. Journal of Obsessive-Compulsive and Related Disorders 2016;8:38–49.

[68] Nanjundaswamy MH, Arumugham SS, Narayanaswamy JC. A prospective study of intensive inpatient treatment for obsessive-compulsive disorder. Psychiatry Res 2020;291(113303). https://doi.org/10.1016/ j.psychres.2020.113303.

[69] Storch EA, Lehmkuhl HD, Ricketts E, et al. An Open trial of intensive family based cognitivebehavioral therapy in youth with obsessive-compulsive disorder who are medication partial responders or nonresponders. J Clin Child Adolesc Psychol 2010;39(2):260–8.

[70] Björgvinsson T, Wetterneck CT, Powell DM, et al. Treatment outcome for adolescent obsessive-compulsive disorder in a specialized hospital setting. J Psychiatr Pract 2008;14(3):137–45.

[71] Leonard RC, Franklin ME, Wetterneck CT, et al. Residential treatment outcomes for adolescents with obsessive-compulsive disorder. Psychother Res 2016;26(6):727–36.

[72] Gregory ST, Kay B, Smith J, et al. Treatment-refractory obsessive-compulsive disorder in adults: a cost-effectiveness analysis of treatment strategies. J Clin Psychiatry 2018;79(2). https://doi.org/10.4088/JCP.17m11552.

[73] Gregory ST, Kay B, Riemann BC, et al. Cost-effectiveness of treatment alternatives for treatment-refractory pediatric obsessive-compulsive disorder. J Anxiety Disord 2020;69(102151):102151.

[74] Abramowitz JS, Blakey SM, Reuman L, et al. New directions in the cognitive-behavioral treatment of OCD: Theory, research, and practice. Behav Ther 2018;49(3): 311–22.

[75] Bluett EJ, Homan KJ, Morrison KL, et al. Acceptance and commitment therapy for anxiety and OCD spectrum

disorders: an empirical review. J Anxiety Disord 2014; 28(6):612–24.

[76] Twohig MP, Abramowitz JS, Smith BM, et al. Adding acceptance and commitment therapy to exposure and response prevention for obsessive-compulsive disorder: a randomized controlled trial. Behav Res Ther 2018; 108:1–9.

[77] Armstrong AB, Morrison KL, Twohig MP. A preliminary investigation of acceptance and commitment therapy for adolescent obsessive-compulsive disorder. J Cogn Psychother 2013;27(2):175–90.

[78] Aardema F, Bouchard S, Koszycki D, et al. Evaluation of inference-based cognitive-behavioral therapy for obsessive-compulsive disorder: a multicenter randomized controlled trial with three treatment modalities. Psychother Psychosom 2022;91(5):348–59.

[79] Orsolini L, Pompili S, Salvi V, et al. A systematic review on TeleMental health in youth mental health: Focus on anxiety, depression and obsessive-compulsive disorder. Medicina (Kaunas) 2021;57(8):793.

[80] Hiranandani S, Ipek SI, Wilhelm S, et al. Digital mental health interventions for obsessive compulsive and related disorders: a brief review of evidence-based interventions and future directions. J Obsessive Compuls Relat Disord 2023;36(100765):100765.

[81] Pinciotti CM, Bulkes NZ, Horvath G, et al. Efficacy of intensive CBT telehealth for obsessive-compulsive disorder during the COVID-19 pandemic. J Obsessive Compuls Relat Disord 2022;32(100705):100705.

[82] Trevizol AP, Shiozawa P, Cook IA, et al. Transcranial magnetic stimulation for obsessive-compulsive disorder: an updated systematic review and meta-analysis. J ECT 2016;32(4):262–6.

[83] Fontenelle LF, Coutinho ESF, Lins-Martins NM, et al. Electroconvulsive therapy for obsessive-compulsive disorder: a systematic review. J Clin Psychiatry 2015; 76(7):949–57.

[84] Carmi L, Tendler A, Bystritsky A, et al. Efficacy and safety of deep transcranial magnetic stimulation for obsessive-compulsive disorder: a prospective multicenter randomized double-blind placebo-controlled trial. Am J Psychiatry 2019;176(11):931–8.

[85] Ballantine HT Jr, Cassidy WL, Flanagan NB, et al. Stereotaxic anterior cingulotomy for neuropsychiatric illness and intractable pain. J Neurosurg 1967;26(5):488–95.

[86] Miguel EC, Lopes AC, McLaughlin NCR, et al. Evolution of gamma knife capsulotomy for intractable obsessive-compulsive disorder. Mol Psychiatry 2019;24(2): 218–40.

[87] McLaughlin NCR, Lauro PM, Patrick MT, et al. Magnetic resonance imaging-guided laser thermal ventral capsulotomy for intractable obsessive-compulsive disorder. Neurosurgery 2021;88(6):1128–35.

[88] Chang JG, Jung HH, Kim SJ, et al. Bilateral thermal capsulotomy with magnetic resonance-guided focused ultrasound for patients with treatment-resistant depression: a proof-of-concept study. Bipolar Disord 2020;22(7): 771–4.

[89] Lai Y, Wang T, Zhang C, et al. Effectiveness and safety of neuroablation for severe and treatment-resistant obsessive-compulsive disorder: a systematic review and meta-analysis. J Psychiatry Neurosci 2020;45(5):356–69.

[90] Sheth SA, Neal J, Tangherlini F, et al. Limbic system surgery for treatment-refractory obsessive-compulsive disorder: a prospective long-term follow-up of 64 patients. J Neurosurg 2013;118(3):491–7.

[91] Nuttin B, Cosyns P, Demeulemeester H, et al. Electrical stimulation in anterior limbs of internal capsules in patients with obsessive-compulsive disorder. Lancet 1999; 354(9189):1526.

[92] Greenberg BD, Gabriels LA, Malone DA Jr, et al. Deep brain stimulation of the ventral internal capsule/ventral striatum for obsessive-compulsive disorder: worldwide experience. Mol Psychiatry 2010;15(1):64–79.

[93] R. Gadot, R. Najera, S. Hirani, et al., Efficacy of deep brain stimulation for treatment-resistant obsessive-compulsive disorder: systematic review and meta-analysis, J Neurol Neurosurg Psychiatry 93 (11) (2022) jnnp-2021-328738.

Advances in Psychiatry and Behavioral Health 3 (2023) 11–22

ADVANCES IN PSYCHIATRY AND BEHAVIORAL HEALTH

Hoarding Disorder

Nisha Jagannathan, MS[a,1], Gregory S. Chasson, PhD[b,*]

[a]Department of Psychology, Illinois Institute of Technology, 201 Tech Central, 3242 South State Street, Chicago, IL 60616, USA;
[b]Department of Psychiatry and Behavioral Neuroscience, University of Chicago, 5841 South Maryland Avenue, MC3077, Chicago, IL 60637-1470, USA

KEYWORDS

- Hoarding disorder • Clutter • Saving • Difficulty discarding • Acquiring • Cognitive behavioral therapy
- Medication • Pharmacotherapy

KEY POINTS

- Pathological hoarding is distinct from normative collecting, disorganization, or messiness and is characterized by a unique confluence of etiological factors and behavioral reinforcement mechanisms.
- Per the DSM-5, hoarding disorder (HD) is principally characterized by difficulty discarding items due to distress and/or a perceived need to save; a majority of individuals also present with excessive aquisition of items, but this is not a necessary diagnostic feature.
- Difficulty discarding and excessive acquisition result in clutter that impedes the intended use of primary living areas.
- Empirically tested treatments for HD thus far include a number of hoarding-specific cognitive behavioral therapy protocols, as well as pharmacotherapy.
- Individuals with HD commonly present with treatment ambivalence and limited insight, causing motivational barriers to treatment engagement.

INTRODUCTION

The acquisition and accumulation of possessions is a longstanding human behavior, one that has arguably become more accessible and prevalent because mass production of goods has advanced. During the past 2 decades, however, mounting evidence has indicated that some presentations of these behaviors can be pathological and reflective of specific biological, psychological, and environmental aberrations [1]. With an estimated 30% of the general population engaging in various forms of collecting [2], what factors differentiate the normative behaviors from those that may be pathological? Moreover, what assessments and interventions exist to treat this pathologic condition once it has been identified? To help answer these questions, the present article will outline the key diagnostic features of hoarding disorder (HD), recent findings regarding its cause, and updated developments in evidence-based treatment protocols.

Diagnostic Criteria

Previously categorized as a subtype of obsessive-compulsive disorder, pathological hoarding was reconceptualized for DSM-5 and is now classified as 1 of the 5 obsessive-compulsive and related disorders [1,3]. HD is chiefly characterized by difficulty discarding possessions due to distress and beliefs about needing to save the items, as well as the resultant clutter that impedes or prevents the use of key living spaces (Fig. 1) [3]. Additionally, 80% to 90% of individuals with HD also display pathological acquisition behavior, such as excessive shopping (ie, active acquisition) or collection

---

[1] Present address: 5415 Arrowhead Drive, San Antonio, TX 78228.

*Corresponding author, *E-mail address:* gchasson@uchicago.edu

https://doi.org/10.1016/j.ypsc.2023.03.011
2667-3827/23/ © 2023 Elsevier Inc. All rights reserved.

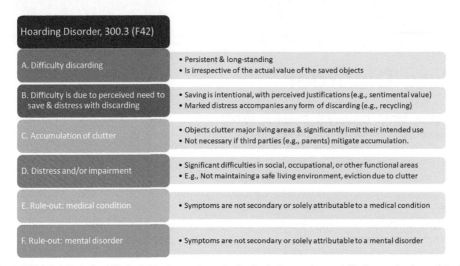

FIG. 1 DSM-5 criteria for HD. Individuals must meet all criteria to receive an HD diagnosis. Associated specifiers include (1) with excessive acquisition, (2) with good or fair insight, (3) with poor insight, or (4) with absent insight/delusional beliefs.

of free items (ie, passive acquisition) [3]. Importantly, difficulty discarding persists regardless of the value of the saved objects, such that many individuals with HD accumulate items that have little to no monetary or functional value (eg, empty bottles, trash) [3–5]. Of note, it is not the acquisition of objects itself that constitutes pathological hoarding but rather the persistent difficulty with discarding objects and the resultant clutter and impairment [1,3]. Additionally, clutter is not necessary for an HD diagnosis if the accumulation is prevented or mitigated by a third party (eg, a parent). These caveats can function as a key distinction between normative and pathological object accumulation. An avid coin collector, for instance, could acquire and store large numbers of coins without displaying clinically significant difficulties with discarding or clutter. An individual with HD, however, will generally display a significantly less focused, intentional, and organized collection of items, as well as present with clutter causing functional impairment and marked distress at discarding any of these items [6].

In addition to these core features, individuals with HD also frequently display limited insight related to their symptoms and associated consequences. Although individuals with HD may experience significant distress and impairment due to their hoarding symptoms, beliefs regarding object acquisition, object utility, and fear of discarding may make it difficult for them to recognize HD as the cause of distress [7]. This poor insight and the overall ego-syntonic nature of symptoms in HD are thought to contribute to reduced

treatment-seeking behaviors, as well as contribute to difficulty adhering to—and high treatment attrition from—treatment [4,7,8]. In addition to poor insight, individuals with HD also display unique beliefs related to the self, object attachment, and saving. Specifically, beliefs about objects and anthropomorphization (eg, that the object may be useful, that it has particular feelings), beliefs about the self (eg, that one's memory is flawed, that objects represent an extension of oneself), and beliefs about others (eg, that others cannot be trusted with one's possessions) are all thought to contribute to the development and maintenance of HD symptoms [5,7,8]. Such beliefs and cognitive patterns (and their associated emotions) are thought to underlie subsequent HD behaviors—namely, the excessive acquisition of objects and difficulty discarding.

In addition to differentiating between normative collecting and pathological hoarding behaviors, accurate differential diagnosis of HD amid the various other conditions involving pathological hoarding is essential (Fig. 2). Pathological hoarding is secondary to a number of medical conditions, including injury to the brain, infections affecting the brain and/or spinal cord, and genetic disorders affecting brain development and functioning [3]. Hoarding behaviors may also occur secondary to neurodevelopmental disorders (eg, autism) or neurocognitive disorders (eg, dementia) [2,3]. Finally, pathological hoarding has been observed in other forms of psychopathology, such as obsessive-compulsive disorder (ie, compulsive saving of objects in direct response to obsessions), psychotic spectrum disorders (eg, object

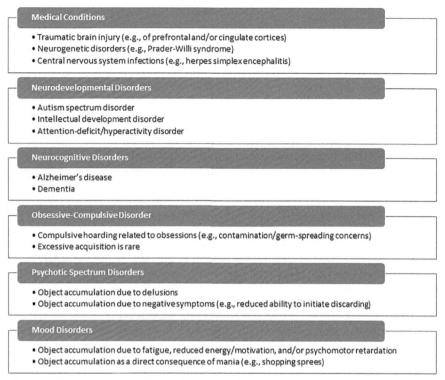

FIG. 2 Rule-out disorders and conditions relevant for differential diagnosis of HD. As pathological hoarding can emerge as a secondary feature of these rule-outs, HD would not be an appropriate diagnosis for these cases.

accumulation as part of a delusion), and mood disorders (eg, the difficulty discarding that can accompany the low energy/fatigue of a major depressive episode) [3].

Adverse consequences due to pathological hoarding are numerous and can be life-threatening [9]. Individuals with HD are at risk of developing health issues due to poor sanitation and clutter-related dust, as well as injuries or death resulting from falls and fires [10,11]. Importantly, the risks associated with HD are not isolated to the individual alone; rather, they can affect third parties such as neighbors, codwelling family, and emergency responders [12]. Interpersonal rejection is therefore common in HD, as well as decreased physical and mental well-being in codwelling family members [13]. Finally, HD is associated with significant economic burden, such as costs associated with eviction, emergency cleanouts, emergency fire response, and associated legal proceedings [12].

Epidemiology

Prevalence of HD is currently estimated to be between 1.5% and 5.8%, with some community-based and epidemiological studies reporting a higher incidence among men. Clinical HD samples, however, have been overrepresented by women, which possibly reflects the increased likelihood of treatment-seeking behavior in women relative to men across mental health conditions [14]. Notably, HD prevalence in older populations (aged 70+) is 6%, and HD prevalence has been found to increase by 20% with every 5-year increase in age [15]. In fact, several studies have observed a near linear increase in HD symptoms with age, with the physical and cognitive decline in older adults being directly associated with HD severity. Finally, although the bulk of HD research has centered on American and European (ie, Caucasian) samples, pathological hoarding seems to be ubiquitous across cultures and has thus far been documented in Asian, South American, and Turkish populations as well [4,16].

Age of onset for HD is generally in early to midadolescence (ages 11–15 years), with onset in early childhood (ie, <10 years) being an indicator of greater symptom severity and poorer prognosis [3]. Of note, collecting or saving behaviors are normative and developmentally appropriate in early childhood (ie, until around 6 years of age), and hoarding symptoms occurring in childhood may not persist into adulthood [17]. Symptoms gradually and persistently increase and tend to become increasingly problematic in middle age (ie, ages 40–55 years) [4,5]. This chronic pattern is distinct from courses observed in other disorders such as OCD, body dysmorphic disorder, and body-focused repetitive behaviors, where symptoms are chronic without treatment but tend to wax and wane throughout an individual's lifetime [1,4,5,18]. It is worth noting, however, that several of the key symptoms associated with HD (eg, object accumulation) are contingent on time, such that it may take decades before enough possessions have accumulated to cause notable distress and impairment.

Psychiatric comorbidity is the norm and not the exception among individuals with HD. Mood disorders are highly co-occurring with HD, with nearly 75% of individuals with HD reporting mood and/or anxiety symptoms [3]. Major depressive disorder, social anxiety disorder, generalized anxiety disorder are the most common comorbidities, with roughly 20% of individuals with HD also reporting comorbid OCD [4,7,11]. Attention-deficit/hyperactivity disorder (ADHD) is also highly comorbid with HD, with a particular link to symptoms of inattention [19,20]. Medical comorbidities are also prevalent in HD, with a number of studies implicating an increased number of medical conditions and overall poorer physical health in HD populations, independent of age and other demographic factors (eg, higher rates of diabetes, hypertension, stroke, obesity) [2,21].

DISCUSSION

Etiology

Recent research has uncovered several pathophysiological mechanisms involved in the development and maintenance of HD. These biological, psychological, and environmental factors are consolidated in Fig. 3, as well as elucidated in the subsequent text. The heritability and genetic basis of pathological hoarding has been investigated in several family and multivariate twin studies. Up to 50% of the variance in HD has been attributed to genetic factors, with 50% of individuals with HD endorsing having a biological relative who also engages in pathological hoarding [8,22]. HD has also displayed genetic correlations with related forms of psychopathology, including OCD (41%) and tics (35%) [8,21–24].

Although neuroimaging research on HD remains scarce, several important studies have highlighted unique neural correlates specific to pathological hoarding. Neuroanatomically, one study examining structural features found significantly increased gray matter volume in the right frontal pole of the prefrontal cortex in HD compared with both OCD and healthy controls [25]. No significant associations were found, however, between this structural abnormality and clinical features such as hoarding symptom severity, suggesting that this abnormality may function more as a neural marker of HD than a maintenance factor. Another recent study found white matter abnormalities in the frontothalamic circuit, frontoparietal network, and frontolimbic pathway in HD relative to healthy controls, further highlighting the role that frontal regions may have in pathological hoarding [26]. Finally, activation studies have found increased error-related negativity in HD on probabilistic learning tasks [27], as well as increased activation in the dorsolateral prefrontal cortex and anterior cingulate cortex on response inhibition tasks [28]. Considered together, these structural and functional findings suggest that the neural areas involved several higher order functions are abnormal in HD relative to healthy controls. Specifically, the abnormal reward and salience processing observed in HD may reflect these neural abnormalities and underlie its key features (eg, exaggerated appraisals of an object's value, pleasure associated with obtaining an item) [4,5,8]. Indeed, Tolin [29] proposed a biopsychosocial model of HD that emphasizes *biphasic abnormalities* based on context-dependent hyperactivation and hypoactivation of the salience network—a brain system involved in self-awareness, as well as selective attention to, and appraisal of, relevant stimuli. Individuals with HD demonstrate *hyperactivation* of the salience network relative to non-HD controls, but only in HD-relevant contexts, such as being asked to discard possessions (ie, salient tasks). Conversely, those with HD show *hypoactivation* in the salience network compared with non-HD controls in contexts that are not relevant to HD (ie, nonsalient tasks) [29].

Drawing from these biological underpinnings, research has identified a number of psychological factors associated with HD. Deficits in emotion regulation have been identified in HD, along with higher levels of anxiety sensitivity, greater intolerance of uncertainty, and reduced distress tolerance [1,4,30,31]. Perfectionism and heightened indecision are also associated with many HD presentations [5,7]. Finally, cognitive and executive functioning deficits have been identified, including issues with memory recall, risk and error processing, visual memory and categorization, and decision-making [5,7,11,32,33]. Given the aforementioned abnormalities in frontal regions of the HD brain, these neurocognitive and

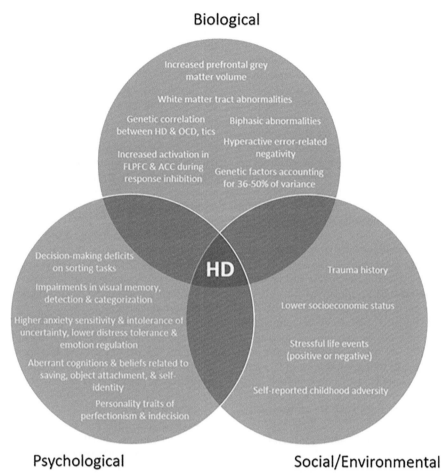

Biological

Increased prefrontal grey matter volume

White matter tract abnormalities

Genetic correlation between HD & OCD, tics

Biphasic abnormalities

Hyperactive error-related negativity

Increased activation in FLPFC & ACC during response inhibition

Genetic factors accounting for 36-50% of variance

Decision-making deficits on sorting tasks

Impairments in visual memory, detection & categorization

Higher anxiety sensitivity & intolerance of uncertainty, lower distress tolerance & emotion regulation

Aberrant cognitions & beliefs related to saving, object attachment, & self-identity

Personality traits of perfectionism & indecision

HD

Trauma history

Lower socioeconomic status

Stressful life events (positive or negative)

Self-reported childhood adversity

Psychological

Social/Environmental

FIG. 3 Key etiological features of HD. These biological (*green*), psychological (*orange*), and environmental (*pink*) factors give rise to hoarding disorder, as well as contribute to the course and development of pathological hoarding. ACC, anterior cingulate cortex; FLPFC, frontolateral prefrontal cortex; HD, hoarding disorder; OCD, obsessive-compulsive disorder.

processing deficits seem consistent. Of note, a recent meta-analysis found deficits only in the categorization skills of HD populations relative to healthy controls, with no differences observed in attention, memory, information processing, response inhibition, cognitive flexibility, visuospatial skills, language, or planning [34]. Because HD populations have also displayed higher levels of self-perceived memory and attention impairment (which has positively associated with degree of object saving), it is possible that this self-perception functions as a key maintenance variable for HD, even in the absence of an actual neurocognitive deficits [35]. For instance, an individual with HD who displays no actual memory deficits may engage in object saving as a compensatory strategy to mitigate the memory issues they perhaps erroneously perceive themselves as having. In addition—as part of a self-fulfilling prophecy of sorts—aging, subsequent clutter, related medical comorbidities, and psychosocial stress (eg, stigma, eviction) may eventually instigate the very memory deficits they had originally thought themselves as having. This process may explain the variations in research findings, as well as the unique role of advanced age in HD compared with other disorders such as OCD. Furthermore, this cycle may also be exacerbated by the variable levels of insight [7] and abnormal beliefs regarding saving, object attachment, and the self frequently observed in HD populations [1]. Further neuropsychological study of HD seems warranted given these contradictions and the unclear role of beliefs and perceived deficits on HD symptoms.

In conjunction with these biological and psychological mechanisms, several social and environmental factors have been linked to HD and are hypothesized to contribute to its cause. As with most psychopathology, these factors likely fuel a cascade of diathesis–stress interactions that increase the likelihood of HD development (as well as subsequent symptom severity). A history of trauma, self-reported childhood adversity, stressful life events, and lower socioeconomic status have all associated with the development of HD [1,7,23]. Given that these environmental risk factors have been found to associate with most (if not all) psychopathology, their role in the development of HD is unsurprising and warrants further investigation. Social factors in particular may influence HD course and prognosis, given that individuals with HD are particularly prone to social issues such as eviction and expenses related to mandated clean-outs and health code violations [36]. These social consequences could, in turn, fuel further stress and hoarding behaviors. As mentioned, HD populations are also especially susceptible to general health issues related to hoarding and self-neglect (eg, food contamination, poor hygiene). In fact, a recent analysis of autopsy reports found an increased risk of accidental death and/or being found in a state of decomposition in HD individuals within the Chicagoland area [37].

General Case Conceptualization of Hoarding Disorder

First proposed by Frost and Hartl [38] and later expanded by Frost and Steketee [11], the cognitive behavioral model of HD involves 4 core components: vulnerability factors, beliefs and attachment processes, emotions, and hoarding behaviors. Updated case conceptualizations have also highlighted the role of positive and negative reinforcement as a cornerstone of HD symptomology [5]. Specifically, the etiological factors associated with HD (ie, biopsychosocial elements such as genetic predisposition, neural abnormalities, environmental factors, and personality features) underlie a persistent pattern of beliefs and cognitive distortions related to possessions, such as the perceived usefulness of an object, the anthropomorphizing of objects, and object attachment. These distortions then give rise to emotional processes and experiences, such as pleasure, pride, anxiety, and sadness. Through these emotional experiences, hoarding behavior can be positively reinforced (eg, feelings of elation at acquiring a new object or viewing one's collection) and negatively reinforced (eg, mitigation of sadness through object acquisition, reduction of fear associated with avoiding discarding) [5]. Considered together, these cycles of reinforcement maintain HD symptoms (ie, acquisition, difficulty discarding, and clutter), as well as feedback into their underlying cognitive components [5,11].

Assessment

Evidence-based assessment of HD currently includes diagnostic interviews, severity assessments, and tailored measures assessing various facets of pathological hoarding (eg, impairment, saving beliefs). DSM-5-based diagnostic protocols include the Structured Interview for Hoarding Disorder and the Diagnostic Interview for Anxiety, Mood, and OCD and Related Neuropsychiatric Disorders [39,40]. Clinician and self-report measures of symptom severity include the Hoarding Rating Scale-Interview (HRS-I), the UCLA Hoarding Severity Scale, the Clutter Image Rating Scale (CI-R), the Saving Inventory-Revised (SI-R), and the self-report version of the HRS (HRS-SR) [41–45]. Other assessments include the Home Environment Index (for squalor), the HOMES Hoarding Risk Assessment (for hoarding-related harm potential), the Activities of Daily Living-Hoarding scale (for functional impairment), and the Saving Cognitions Inventory (for hoarding beliefs) [46–48]. Finally, HD assessments tailored to youth include the Child Saving Inventory [49], with the HRS-SR also demonstrating good psychometric properties in adolescents [22].

Treatment

As evidence regarding the clinical features and maintenance mechanisms of HD accumulates, creating and refining treatment protocols specific to pathological hoarding has become increasingly possible. Given the severity of functional impairment that can result from untreated HD, tailored interventions are of the utmost importance. Nevertheless, treatment-seeking in HD populations remains low, treatment efficacy is somewhat variable, and full remission is rare [50]. Treatment types that have been investigated in the literature thus far are consolidated in Fig. 4 and outlined below. Generally, 4 categories of mental health treatment have been explored in HD: individual and group psychotherapy, self-help interventions, and pharmacotherapy. For both individual and group psychotherapy, cognitive behavioral therapy (CBT) has been considered the gold standard and is recommended as a first-line treatment, both for clinician and peer-led interventions [50,51]. Other interventions with varying levels of empirical support include motivational interviewing [52], harm reduction [53], family-based approaches [54,55], cognitive remediation [56], and bibliotherapy [57,58]. Pharmacological treatment of HD remains in its infancy and has displayed some

Treatment Component	Number of Sessions (Approx.)	Locations of Sessions	Description of Activities
Assessment	2	Office & Home	Office: Administer self-report measures of hoarding and clinical correlates; Conducting interviews of hoarding symptoms and comorbidity Home: Assess and photograph clutter; assessment of daily functioning; identification of a family member who could serve as a coach
Psychoeducation & Case Formulation	2	Office	Provide psychoeducation on hoarding; develop a personalized cognitive-behavioral model of hoarding with the patient; include vulnerability factors, beliefs about possessions, information processing and learning styles, emotional responses, the identified function of the hoarding behavior; develop and discuss a treatment plan; troubleshoot anticipated barriers to hoarding treatment plan
Acquisition Limiting (ERP)	3	Office & Community	Exposure and Response Prevention (ERP): provide psychoeducation on and rationale for ERP; Develop plan for systematic, gradual, prolonged acquiring ERP; initiate ERP by having patient carry out acquiring exercises
Skills Training	2	Office	Provide psychoeducation on skills; practice skills required for effective sorting and discarding of possessions, making decisions, managing attentional difficulties, and increasing organization
Sorting and Discarding (ERP) & Cognitive Therapy	15	Office & Home	Sorting and discarding: develop plan for systematic, gradual, prolonged sorting and discarding ERP; initiate ERP by having patient carry out sorting and discarding exercises Cognitive therapy: address maladaptive hoarding thought patterns using techniques such as Socratic questioning, downward arrow approach, thought records, behavioral experiments
Relapse Prevention	2	Office	Review treatment techniques; summarize treatment progress; develop plan for identifying indicators of relapse and how to address return of maladaptive symptoms

FIG. 4 Key components and features of cognitive behavioral therapy for HD. (Reprinted with permission from Hoarding Disorder by Gregory S. Chasson and Jedidiah Siev, ISBN 9780889374072 ©2019 by Hogrefe Publishing www.hogrefe.com, http://doi.org/10.1027/00407-000.)

positive results [59,60], particularly for HD individuals who display ADHD-like symptomatology such as inattentiveness and planning deficits [61,62]. Finally, professional organization services may complement evidence-based pharmacological and/or psychotherapeutic interventions. Efficacy of all of these treatments has varied, with an overall symptom reduction rate of 14% to 40% and most participants remaining in the clinically significant range of HD posttreatment [50]. Nevertheless, it seems that psychotherapy tailored to HD features and pharmacological interventions focused on mood, anxiety, and/or attentional difficulties are helpful starting points for future development.

Individual cognitive behavioral therapy
Drawing from the aforementioned cognitive behavioral conceptualization of HD, individual CBT tailored to HD symptoms has been developed and refined during the past decade (see Fig. 4). The cognitive components of CBT for HD chiefly involve restructuring of thinking patterns (ie, maladaptive thoughts and beliefs related to the self and/or objects, such as anthropomorphizing), whereas the behavioral components primarily involve graded exposure to discarding of existing items and nonacquiring of new items [7,11,51,63]. This foundational protocol has been enhanced with additional evidence-based components such as motivational interviewing (to increase treatment adherence and decrease ambivalence), harm reduction (to reduce functional impairment and improve quality of life), family accommodation reduction, and structured organizational/skills training (eg, practicing appropriate sorting and storing of items to minimize clutter; Fig. 5) [7,63]. Home visits conducted by the clinician are common during treatment, both for accurate assessment of symptom presentation as well as development of more tailored behavioral interventions.

Group cognitive behavioral therapy
In addition to the individual protocol outlined above, CBT for HD administered in a group format (G-CBT) has proven efficacious [7,63,64]. G-CBT for HD has been linked to improved outcomes even in the absence of clinician home visits [65], and meta analyses have

Treatment Component	Intervention Goals
Motivational Interviewing	• To reduce treatment ambivalence and facilitate treatment engagement • To clearly identify areas of impairment (e.g., interpersonal problems) and benefits of symptom improvement (e.g., family being able to visit)
Harm Reduction	• To promote a more acceptable and less judgmental approach to encourage change • To reduce harm/impairment caused by hoarding symptoms (e.g., health issues due to clutter) • To improve overall quality of life irrespective of complete symptom remission
Family Accommodation Reduction	• To provide psychoeducation and tools for helping family members reduce and eliminate their behaviors that maintain a loved one's hoarding behaviors • To reduce negative impact of hoarding symptoms on family & improve the health and well-being of family members
Structured Organizational, Skills Training, Cognitive Rehabilitation	• To provide training on decision-making and problem-solving skills related to sorting, organizing, and discarding possessions • To provide coping strategies for executive function difficulties (e.g., attentional problems)

FIG. 5 Evidence-based interventions that comprise and/or supplement cognitive behavioral therapy for HD.

not revealed any moderating effects of group format (vs individual) on treatment outcomes [66]. Additionally, social support among members has been identified as a key benefit of the group format [64,65]. Considered together, these data highlight the capability of CBT for HD to be administered in a group setting without detrimental effects on treatment efficacy. Nevertheless, such protocols are still limited by the need for mental health professionals trained in CBT and necessary access to care for individuals with HD. To address these limitations, community-based, peer-led groups such as Buried in Treasures (BITs) have emerged as viable alternatives to clinician-led G-CBT [58].

Using the same CBT-oriented principles and interventions utilized in clinician-led HD treatment protocols, BITs workshops involve working through a 13-week self-help manual in a weekly group setting [58]. The facilitators of BIT workshops frequently endorse their own lived experiences with HD symptoms, and the groups accordingly aim to provide a less stigmatizing, more accessible alternative to traditional group or individual CBT [7,67]. Notably, such peer-led groups have been found to be as effective as clinician-led groups [58,67,68], highlighting this form of treatment as particularly useful in the many areas with a paucity of mental health professionals. Additionally, early data prompted by the recent COVID-19 pandemic have supported the efficacy of virtual BIT groups using teleconferencing platforms [69].

Cognitive rehabilitation

Although clinician and peer-led forms of CBT for HD have demonstrated symptom reduction, many individuals continue to display clinically significant HD symptoms posttreatment [50,70]. For this reason, CBT supplemented with additional cognitive interventions may be efficacious. Given the deficits in executive functioning (eg, in attention, decision-making, and memory) often observed in HD, treatment protocols involving forms of cognitive remediation and rehabilitation have been tested and proved promising. Group cognitive rehabilitation and exposure/sorting therapy has demonstrated improvements in inhibition and cognitive flexibility in HD individuals, as well as notable reductions in HD symptom severity and comorbid anxiety and depression [70–72]. Similarly, a pilot program involving repeated task and strategy training resulted in improved attention in HD individuals, although no changes in memory, executive functioning, or HD severity were observed [56]. Considered together, these data suggest that interventions targeting the neurocognitive deficits in HD can improve individuals' functioning in these domains, and therefore may serve as a helpful supplement to CBT.

Psychopharmacology

To date, structured randomized clinical trials of medication for HD are few, and medication response in HD has generally been mixed. Nevertheless, several pharmacological interventions have shown early promise in addressing symptoms of HD, as well as the neurocognitive deficits that frequently accompany these symptoms (eg, attentional difficulties). Selective serotonin reuptake inhibitors (SSRIs; ie, paroxetine) and serotonin-norepinephrine reuptake inhibitors (SNRIs; ie, venlafaxine) have both been administered to HD populations and shown clinically significant improvements in HD symptoms [59,60]. Stimulants such as methylphenidate and atomoxetine have also been administered to HD individuals, with subsequent improvements in attention and modest reductions in HD symptoms [61]. Despite these initial findings, small sample sizes, mixed diagnoses in the samples (eg, hoarding symptoms in OCD vs HD) and poor tolerance of medication doses among participants make definitive conclusions difficult. Further research is therefore warranted and can shed further light on the utility of pharmacotherapy (also in conjunction with CBT) in treating HD symptomology [73].

Addressing barriers to treatment engagement

As previously mentioned, lack of insight and difficulties with motivation pose significant barriers to treatment seeking behavior and engagement in treatment of HD populations. To this end, interventions that target these barriers could be invaluable in maximizing treatment efficacy. Specifically, having individuals with HD navigate a virtual reality rendition of rooms in their own home sans clutter was found to increase motivation and openness to change [74]. Similarly, it may be possible to involve family members of individuals with HD by developing their motivational interviewing and coping skills in an effort to facilitate readiness for change and promote treatment-seeking in their loved ones with HD individuals [54]. Finally, reducing the societal stigma associated with pathological hoarding [75,76] could help minimize shame and thereby encourage more treatment-seeking behavior in HD populations.

SUMMARY

Overall, HD has emerged as a unique form of psychopathology characterized by difficulty discarding possessions due to distress and a perceived need to save items, as well as resultant clutter affecting the use of primary living spaces. Due to its chronic course and associations with medical comorbidities, low quality of life, and public health concerns, pathological hoarding warrants targeted clinical and research attention. Thus far, CBT-based interventions and some forms of pharmacotherapy have delivered promising reductions in HD symptoms and associated impairment. In conjunction with interventions enhancing motivation and mitigating the effects of treatment barriers, these treatments could reduce HD severity and significantly improve outcomes. Future research would therefore benefit from further investigation of HD treatment motivation, outcomes, and plausible mechanisms of change, as well as the role of various etiological factors (eg, comorbidities) on symptom onset, maintenance, and severity. Methods such as longitudinal treatment studies, further neuroimaging, and mapping trajectories of HD symptom

development could all serve to refine current conceptualizations of HD and elucidate best practices for treatment.

CLINICS CARE POINTS

- Hoarding mitigation often necessitates a multidisciplinary team approach, for example, services from psychiatrists, cognitive behavioral therapists, social workers, professional organizers, attorneys, housing authorities, and inspectors.

- Individuals with hoarding often present with treatment ambivalence or refusal. This may be driven by poor insight and/or low motivation to change hoarding behavior.

- CBT approaches are the gold standard psychosocial intervention for hoarding and include individual and group CBT, as well as peer-facilitated or professional-facilitated self-help groups.

- CBT interventions emphasize exposure and response prevention techniques, which challenge the individual to accept distress from sorting and discarding possessions and not acquiring new belongings.

- Other CBT elements include psychoeducation, skill development for categorizing and decision-making, cognitive restructuring, motivation-enhancement, and relapse prevention.

- Evidence for effectiveness of pharmacotherapy for HD is mixed. Some evidence highlights benefits from serotonin reuptake inhibitors, and stimulants may help in individuals with comorbid ADHD symptoms.

DISCLOSURE

G.S. Chasson receives annual royalties from Hogrefe publishing.

REFERENCES

[1] Mataix-Cols D, Frost RO, Pertusa A, et al. Hoarding disorder: a new diagnosis for DSM-V? Depress Anxiety 2010;27(6):556–72.

[2] Bates S, Chang WC, Hamilton CE, et al. Hoarding disorder and co-occurring medical conditions: A systematic review. J Obsessive-Compuls Relat Disord 2021;30: 100661.

[3] APA AP. Diagnostic and statistical manual of mental disorders. 5th edition. Washington, DC: American Psychiatric Publishing; 2013.

[4] Davidson EJ, Dozier ME, Pittman JOE, et al. Recent Advances in Research on Hoarding. Curr Psychiatry Rep 2019;21(9):91.

[5] Timpano KR, Muroff J, Steketee G. A Review of the Diagnosis and Management of Hoarding Disorder. Curr Treat Options Psychiatry 2016;3(4):394–410.

[6] Stumpf BP. Hoarding disorder: a review.

[7] Mathews CA. Hoarding Disorder: More than just a problem of too much stuff. J Clin Psychiatry 2014;75(8):893–4.

[8] Dozier ME, Ayers CR. The Etiology of Hoarding Disorder: A Review. Psychopathology 2017;50(5):291–6.

[9] Steketee G, Frost R. Compulsive hoarding: Current status of the research. Clin Psychol Rev 2003;23(7):905–27.

[10] Monk I.M., Lucini G.L., Szlatenyi C.S., An Analysis of Fire Incidents Involving Hoarding Households.

[11] Steketee G, Frost RO. Compulsive hoarding and acquiring. New York, NY: Oxford University Press; 2006.

[12] Tolin DF, Frost RO, Steketee G, et al. The economic and social burden of compulsive hoarding. Psychiatry Res 2008;160(2):200–11.

[13] Tolin DF, Frost RO, Steketee G, et al. Family burden of compulsive hoarding: results of an internet survey. Behav Res Ther 2008;46(3):334–44.

[14] Bristow K, Patten S. Treatment-Seeking Rates and Associated Mediating Factors among Individuals with Depression. Can J Psychiatry 2002;47(7):660–5.

[15] Cath DC, Nizar K, Boomsma D, et al. Age-Specific Prevalence of Hoarding and Obsessive Compulsive Disorder: A Population-Based Study. Am J Geriatr Psychiatry Off J Am Assoc Geriatr Psychiatry 2017;25(3):245–55.

[16] Timpano KR, Çek D, Fu ZF, et al. A consideration of hoarding disorder symptoms in China. Compr Psychiatry 2015;57:36–45.

[17] Morris SH, Jaffee SR, Goodwin GP, et al. Hoarding in Children and Adolescents: A Review. Child Psychiatry Hum Dev 2016;47(5):740–50.

[18] Ayers CR. Age-Specific Prevalence of Hoarding and Obsessive Compulsive Disorder: A Population-Based Study. Am J Geriatr Psychiatry 2017;25(3):256–7.

[19] Morein-Zamir S, Kasese M, Chamberlain SR, et al. Elevated levels of hoarding in ADHD: A special link with inattention. J Psychiatr Res 2021;145:167–74.

[20] Frost RO, Steketee G, Tolin DF. Comorbidity in hoarding disorder. Depress Anxiety 2011;28(10):876–84.

[21] Nordsletten AE, Reichenberg A, Hatch SL, et al. Epidemiology of hoarding disorder. Br J Psychiatry J Ment Sci 2013;203(6):445–52.

[22] Ivanov VZ, Nordsletten A, Mataix-Cols D, et al. Heritability of hoarding symptoms across adolescence and young adulthood: A longitudinal twin study. PLoS One 2017; 12(6):e0179541.

[23] Mathews CA, Delucchi K, Cath DC, et al. Partitioning the etiology of hoarding and obsessive–compulsive symptoms. Psychol Med 2014;44(13):2867–76.

[24] Zilhão NR, Smit DJ, Boomsma DI, et al. Cross-Disorder Genetic Analysis of Tic Disorders, Obsessive–Compulsive, and Hoarding Symptoms. Front Psychiatry 2016;7. https://www.frontiersin.org/articles/10.3389/fpsyt.2016.00120. Accessed 30 September, 2022.

[25] Yamada S, Nakao T, Ikari K, et al. A unique increase in prefrontal gray matter volume in hoarding disorder compared to obsessive-compulsive disorder. PLoS One 2018;13(7):e0200814.

[26] Mizobe T, Ikari K, Tomiyama H, et al. Abnormal white matter structure in hoarding disorder. J Psychiatr Res 2022;148:1–8.

[27] Mathews CA, Perez VB, Roach BJ, et al. Error-related brain activity dissociates hoarding disorder from obsessive-compulsive disorder. Psychol Med 2016;46(2):367–79.

[28] Hough CM, Luks TL, Lai K, et al. Comparison of brain activation patterns during executive function tasks in hoarding disorder and non-hoarding OCD. Psychiatry Res Neuroimaging 2016;255:50–9.

[29] Tolin DF. Toward a biopsychosocial model of hoarding disorder. J Obsessive-Compuls Relat Disord 2023;36: 100775.

[30] Hillman SR, Lomax CL, Khaleel N, et al. The roles of intolerance of uncertainty, anxiety sensitivity and distress tolerance in hoarding disorder compared with OCD and healthy controls. Behav Cogn Psychother 2022;50(4): 392–403.

[31] Akbari M, Seydavi M, Mohammadkhani S, et al. Emotion dysregulation and hoarding symptoms: A systematic review and meta-analysis. J Clin Psychol 2022;78(7): 1341–53.

[32] Grisham JR, Brown TA, Savage CR, et al. Neuropsychological impairment associated with compulsive hoarding. Behav Res Ther 2007;45(7):1471–83.

[33] Woody SR, Kellman-McFarlane K, Welsted A. Review of cognitive performance in hoarding disorder. Clin Psychol Rev 2014;34(4):324–36.

[34] Stumpf BP, de Souza LC, Mourão MSF, et al. Cognitive impairment in hoarding disorder: a systematic review. CNS Spectr 2022;1–13. https://doi.org/10.1017/S1092852922000153, Published online April 28.

[35] Zakrzewski JJ, Henderson R, Archer C, et al. Subjective cognitive complaints and objective cognitive impairment in hoarding disorder. Psychiatry Res 2022;307:114331.

[36] Frost RO, Steketee G, Williams L. Hoarding: a community health problem. Health Soc Care Community 2000;8(4):229–34.

[37] Waters DM, Eckhardt M, Eason EA. Characteristics of Deaths With Evidence of Pathological Hoarding in Cook County 2017 to 2018. Am J Forensic Med Pathol 2022;43(1):2–6.

[38] Frost RO, Hartl TL. A cognitive-behavioral model of compulsive hoarding. Behav Res Ther 1996;34(4): 341–50.

[39] Tolin DF, Christina G, Wootton BM, et al. Psychometric Properties of a Structured Diagnostic Interview for DSM-5 Anxiety, Mood, and Obsessive-Compulsive and Related Disorders. Assessment 2018;25(1):3–13. https://journals.sagepub.com/doi/abs/10.1177/1073191116638410. Accessed 30 November, 2022.

[40] Nordsletten AE, Fernández de la Cruz L, Pertusa A, et al. The Structured Interview for Hoarding Disorder (SIHD): Development, usage and further validation. J Obsessive-Compuls Relat Disord 2013;2(3):346–50.

[41] Norberg MM, Chasson GS, Tolin DF. A Standardized Approach to Calculating Clinically Significant Change in Hoarding Disorder Using the Saving Inventory-Revised. J Obsessive-Compuls Relat Disord 2021;28: 100609.

[42] Tolin DF, Frost RO, Steketee G. A brief interview for assessing compulsive hoarding: The Hoarding Rating Scale-Interview. Psychiatry Res 2010;178(1):147–52.

[43] Frost RO, Steketee G, Tolin DF, et al. Development and Validation of the Clutter Image Rating. J Psychopathol Behav Assess 2008;30(3):193–203.

[44] Frost RO, Steketee G, Grisham J. Measurement of compulsive hoarding: saving inventory-revised. Behav Res Ther 2004;42(10):1163–82.

[45] Saxena S, Ayers CR, Dozier ME, et al. The UCLA Hoarding Severity Scale: Development and validation. J Affect Disord 2015;175:488–93.

[46] Steketee G, Frost RO, Kyrios M. Cognitive Aspects of Compulsive Hoarding. Cogn Ther Res 2003;27(4): 463–79.

[47] Rasmussen JL, Steketee G, Frost RO, et al. Assessing Squalor in Hoarding: The Home Environment Index. Community Ment Health J 2014;50(5):591–6.

[48] Frost RO, Hristova V, Steketee G, et al. Activities of Daily Living Scale in Hoarding Disorder. J Obsessive-Compuls Relat Disord 2013;2(2):85–90.

[49] Storch EA, Muroff J, Lewin AB, et al. Development and Preliminary Psychometric Evaluation of the Children's Saving Inventory. Child Psychiatry Hum Dev 2011; 42(2):166–82.

[50] Thompson C, Fernández de la Cruz L, Mataix-Cols D, et al. A systematic review and quality assessment of psychological, pharmacological, and family-based interventions for hoarding disorder. Asian J Psychiatry 2017;27: 53–66.

[51] Muroff J, Steketee G, Frost RO, et al. Cognitive Behavior Therapy for Hoarding Disorder: Follow-up Findings and Predictors of Outcome. Depress Anxiety 2014;31(12): 964–71.

[52] Meyer E, Shavitt RG, Leukefeld C, et al. Adding motivational interviewing and thought mapping to cognitive-behavioral group therapy: results from a randomized clinical trial. Braz J Psychiatry 2010;32:20–9. https://doi.org/10.1590/S1516-44462010000100006.

[53] Tompkins MA. Working with families of people who hoard: A harm reduction approach. J Clin Psychol 2011;67(5):497–506.

[54] Chasson GS, Carpenter A, Ewing J, et al. Empowering families to help a loved one with Hoarding Disorder: Pilot study of Family-As-Motivators training. Behav Res Ther 2014;63:9–16.

[55] Thompson C, Fernández de la Cruz L, Mataix-Cols D, et al. Development of a brief psychoeducational group intervention for carers of people with hoarding disorder: A proof-of-concept study. J Obsessive-Compuls Relat Disord 2016;9:66–72.

[56] DiMauro J, Genova M, Tolin DF, et al. Cognitive remediation for neuropsychological impairment in hoarding disorder: A pilot study. J Obsessive-Compuls Relat Disord 2014;3(2):132–8.

[57] Frost RO, Pekareva-Kochergina A, Maxner S. The effectiveness of a biblio-based support group for hoarding disorder. Behav Res Ther 2011;49(10):628–34.

[58] Frost RO, Ruby D, Shuer LJ. The buried in treasures workshop: Waitlist control trial of facilitated support groups for hoarding. Behav Res Ther 2012;50(11):661–7.

[59] Saxena S, Brody AL, Maidment KM, et al. Paroxetine treatment of compulsive hoarding. J Psychiatr Res 2007;41(6):481–7.

[60] Saxena S, Sumner J. Venlafaxine Extended-Release Treatment of Hoarding Disorder. Int Clin Psychopharmacol 2014;29(5):266–73.

[61] Rodriguez CI, Bender J, Morrison S, et al. Does Extended Release Methylphenidate Help Adults with Hoarding Disorder? A Case Series. J Clin Psychopharmacol 2013; 33(3):444–7.

[62] Grassi G, Micheli L, Di Cesare Mannelli L, et al. Atomoxetine for hoarding disorder: A pre-clinical and clinical investigation. J Psychiatr Res 2016;83:240–8.

[63] Tolin DF, Frost RO, Steketee G, et al. Cognitive Behavioral Therapy For Hoarding Disorder: A Meta-Analysis. Focus Am Psychiatr Publ 2021;19(4):468–76.

[64] Bodryzlova Y, Audet JS, Bergeron K, et al. Group cognitive-behavioural therapy for hoarding disorder: Systematic review and meta-analysis. Health Soc Care Community 2019;27(3):517–30.

[65] Gilliam CM, Norberg MM, Villavicencio A, et al. Group cognitive-behavioral therapy for hoarding disorder: An open trial. Behav Res Ther 2011;49(11):802–7.

[66] Rodgers N, McDonald S, Wootton BM. Cognitive behavioral therapy for hoarding disorder: An updated meta-analysis. J Affect Disord 2021;290:128–35.

[67] Mathews CA, Mackin RS, Chou CY, et al. Randomised clinical trial of community-based peer-led and psychologist-led group treatment for hoarding disorder. BJPsych Open 2018;4(4):285–93.

[68] Mathews CA, Uhm S, Chan J, et al. Treating Hoarding Disorder in a real-world setting: Results from the Mental Health Association of San Francisco. Psychiatry Res 2016; 237:331–8.

[69] Yap K, Chen W, Wong SF, et al. Is it as good as being in person? The effectiveness of a modified clinician facilitated buried in treasures group for hoarding disorder using video teleconferencing. Psychiatry Res 2022;314: 114631.

[70] Ayers CR, Dozier ME, Taylor CT, et al. Group Cognitive Rehabilitation and Exposure/Sorting Therapy: A Pilot Program. Cogn Ther Res 2017;42:315–27.

[71] Ayers CR, Davidson EJ, Dozier ME, et al. Cognitive Rehabilitation and Exposure/Sorting Therapy for Late-Life

Hoarding: Effects on Neuropsychological Performance. J Gerontol B Psychol Sci Soc Sci 2020;75(6):1193–8.

[72] Ayers CR, Dozier ME, Twamley EW, et al. Cognitive Rehabilitation and Exposure/Sorting Therapy (CREST) for Hoarding Disorder in Older Adults: A Randomized Clinical Trial. J Clin Psychiatry 2018;79(2):16m11072.

[73] Saxena S. Pharmacotherapy of compulsive hoarding. J Clin Psychol 2011;67(5):477–84.

[74] Chasson GS, Elizabeth Hamilton C, Luxon AM, et al. Rendering promise: Enhancing motivation for change

in hoarding disorder using virtual reality. J Obsessive-Compuls Relat Disord 2020;25:100519.

[75] Bates S, De Leonardis AJ, Corrigan PW, et al. Buried in stigma: Experimental investigation of the impact of hoarding depictions in reality television on public perception. J Obsessive-Compuls Relat Disord 2020;26:100538.

[76] Chasson GS, Guy AA, Bates S, et al. They aren't like me, they are bad, and they are to blame: A theoretically-informed study of stigma of hoarding disorder and obsessive-compulsive disorder. J Obsessive-Compuls Relat Disord 2018;16:56–65.

Advances in Psychiatry and Behavioral Health 3 (2023) 23–32

ADVANCES IN PSYCHIATRY AND BEHAVIORAL HEALTH

Behavioral Treatment of Tourette Disorder

Jordan T. Stiede, MS[a],*, Brandon X. Pitts, BS[b], Kathryn E. Barber, MS[b], Emily J. Ricketts, PhD[c]

[a]Menninger Department of Psychiatry and Behavioral Sciences, Baylor College of Medicine, One Baylor Plaza, MS:350, Houston, TX 77030, USA; [b]Department of Psychology, Marquette University, 307 Cramer Hall, Milwaukee, WI 53201, USA; [c]Department of Psychiatry and Biobehavioral Sciences, University of California Los Angeles, 760 Westwood Plaza, Los Angeles, CA 90095, USA

KEYWORDS

- Tourette disorder (TD) • Tics • Behavioral therapy • Comprehensive behavioral intervention for tics (CBIT)
- Habit reversal training (HRT) • Exposure and response prevention (ERP) • Case vignette

KEY POINTS

- Behavioral therapy for tics, encompassing habit reversal training, comprehensive behavioral intervention for tics, and exposure and response prevention, is an empirically supported treatment of individuals with tic disorders.
- Behavioral treatments for tics also involve teaching patients skills to modify antecedents and consequences that influence and maintain tics.
- Clinicians should assess for clinical complexities that may interfere with the behavioral therapy protocol and personalize treatment accordingly.

Tourette disorder (TD) is a child-onset neuropsychiatric condition defined by the presence of several motor and one or more vocal tics persisting beyond 1 year [1]. Tics, which are rapid, nonrhythmic motor movements or vocalizations, can be categorized as simple or complex. Simple tics are brief, repetitive, and seemingly purposeless in nature and typically involve a single muscle group (eg, eye blinking, nose scrunching) or simple sounds (eg, throat clearing, grunting), whereas complex tics seem more purposeful and entail coordinated action of multiple muscle groups, such as gestures, grooming behaviors, evening up, elaborate limb movements, or combinations of sounds or words (ie, syllables, words, phrases, sentences, echolalia—repeating others words or phrases, coprolalia—rude words or phrases). Tics may be voluntarily suppressed for brief periods [2], and they are often preceded by premonitory urges, most commonly referring to uncomfortable physical sensations typically temporarily relieved by tic expression [3–5].

TD affects between 0.5% and 1.0% of youth and is more prevalent in men, with a male to female prevalence ratio of 3 to 4:1 [5]. Tics commonly onset between 4 and 8 years [6] and peak in severity around ages 10 to 12 years [7]. For many individuals, tics decline in frequency and severity during the course of adolescence, with most individuals reporting none to minimal levels of tics by young adulthood [8]. Tics typically wax and wane in occurrence, intensity, and manifestation. Many youth with TD experience tic-related impairment, which can impede social, academic, and home functioning [9,10]. TD has also been linked to lower quality of life, and tic-related impairment can extend into adulthood [11,12]. Psychiatric comorbidity is the norm in TD because approximately 85% of individuals with TD have a co-occurring psychiatric diagnosis, with

*Corresponding author, *E-mail address:* jordan.stiede@bcm.edu

https://doi.org/10.1016/j.ypsc.2023.03.012
2667-3827/23/

attention-deficit/hyperactivity disorder (ADHD) and obsessive-compulsive disorder (OCD), and anxiety being most common [6,13].

BIOBEHAVIORAL MODEL OF TICS

The biobehavioral model of tics suggests there are 3 primary factors contributing to tic occurrence and maintenance. First, tics have a neurobiological basis, and TD is a heritable condition that stems from structural and functional abnormalities within the basal ganglia and cortico-striatal-thalamo-cortical (CSTC) loops [14–16]. Second, aversive premonitory urges are associated with tic expression and suppression [17,18]. Finally, contextual factors, such as antecedent stimuli and tic-contingent consequences, play an important role in tic fluctuation [19]. The evidence supporting these 3 factors is described below.

Biological basis of Tics. Tic emergence is associated with failed inhibition within CSTC pathways [14–16]. Clusters of striatal neurons within the basal ganglia of individuals with TD become abnormally active, leading to the inhibition of globus pallidus pars interna and substantia nigra pars reticulata neurons [14,16]. Tic occurrence is related to inhibition of these neurons, which disinhibits thalamocortical circuits; and tic topography depends on which striatal neuronal clusters are overactivated [16]. Chemical systems within the CSTC also contribute to tic expression. Tics have been linked to dopaminergic dysfunction in the CSTC, which leads to overactivation of "Go" pathways connected to the execution of actions and the underactivation of "NoGo" pathways connected to the inhibition of unwanted actions [15]. Glutamatergic, histaminergic, cholinergic, and GABA systems are also purported to play a role in tic expression [20].

Additionally, research supports a strong genetic component in TD, with high concordance rates for tic disorders demonstrated in monozygotic twin studies [21]. However, studies have not found major susceptibility genes for TD due to the complex association between genetic and environmental factors, genetic diversity in populations, and the impact of comorbid conditions [22].

Premonitory Urges and Tics. Premonitory urges are often described as uncomfortable physical sensations that precede tics. These urges may be localized to the body region associated with a given tic but may also involve nonlocalized physical sensations or *not-just-right* feelings [17,18]. Premonitory urges are reported by approximately 90% of individuals with tic disorders [17]. Individuals typically begin to identify these urges around the age of 8 to 10 years, and tic suppression has been associated with premonitory urge exacerbation [17,18,23]. Matsuda and colleagues [24] also demonstrated that urge awareness is positively related to an individual's ability to suppress tics.

Descriptive studies have indicated that aversive premonitory urges decrease on tic occurrence [17,18,25]. This clinical finding led to the negative reinforcement hypothesis, which suggests that a reduction in aversive premonitory urges following tic occurrence maintains tics. Several experimental studies have supported this claim, demonstrating that premonitory urge severity is higher during tic suppression relative to free-to-tic intervals [3,23]. However, future studies should continue to examine this hypothesis as other experimental studies have shown no difference in premonitory urge ratings between the 2 conditions [26,27].

Impact of Contextual Variables on Tic Expression. Contextual variables, such as internal (eg, anxiety, boredom) and external (eg, settings, activities) antecedents and tic-contingent consequences, impact the likelihood of tic occurrence [19]. Activities such as watching television (TV), playing video games, and completing homework are commonly linked to tic exacerbation [28,29], whereas physical activity, listening to or performing music, and artistic activities have been linked to reduced tic expression [28,30,31]. Internal antecedents, such as boredom and fatigue, have also been directly associated with tic exacerbation [31,32]. There is a complicated relationship between stress and tics as descriptive studies show that stress is related to increases in tics [28,31,32], whereas experimental studies demonstrate no increases in tics during periods of high stress [26,33]. However, Conelea and colleagues [26] found that stress may interfere with tic suppressibility.

Additionally, tic-contingent consequences influence tic expression. Descriptive and experimental research demonstrate that aversive (eg, teasing), attention (eg, physical comfort after tics), and escape-based (eg, individual does not complete schoolwork because of tics) consequences are associated with tic exacerbation [29,34]. Studies have also shown that rewards delivered contingent on tic-free intervals can lead to short-term tic suppression [34,35].

BEHAVIORAL TREATMENTS

Behavioral treatments for tics include habit reversal training (HRT), comprehensive behavioral intervention for tics (CBIT), and exposure and response prevention (ERP). CBIT, in particular, is considered a first-line intervention for TD per practice guidelines from the

American Academy of Neurology (AAN) [36]. This section details the protocols of these interventions.

Habit Reversal Training. HRT originally consisted of self-monitoring, awareness training (AT), competing response training (CRT), social support, motivational enhancement procedures, and generalization training [37]. However, dismantling studies demonstrated that AT, CRT, and social support are the primary components involved in the intervention's effectiveness [38]. In HRT, treatment elements are administered for every tic, with one tic targeted per session. AT involves training patients to generate a detailed description of the target tic (response description) and to practice noticing tics and pre-tic warning signs (response detection). The goal of AT is to improve patient perceptual awareness of the target tic and increase their ability to predict when the tic will occur. In CRT, patients develop a competing response for the target tic, which should be used as soon as they feel the urge to tic, or immediately after the tic occurs. The competing response is an alternative action that should adhere to several rules: incompatible with the tic, able to be held for a minute or until the urge to tic diminishes—whichever is longer, less noticeable than the tic, and able to be performed in most everyday situations. Finally, a social support person is selected to regularly prompt and reinforce the child's use of competing responses.

Comprehensive Behavioral Intervention for Tics. CBIT is a structured 10-week treatment protocol including psychoeducation, HRT, function-based assessment and intervention, behavioral rewards, relaxation training, and relapse prevention [39]. Psychoeducation serves to increase patient understanding of tic disorders, correct common misconceptions about tics and therapy, and reduce stigma and blame, while laying the groundwork for understanding the rationale of CBIT. Functional assessment involves a clinician-administered interview to assess antecedents and consequences that exacerbate tics. Information from the assessment is used to develop function-based interventions to eliminate or modify antecedents that increase tic frequency and remove tic-contingent consequences (ie, attention and escape-based consequences). Next, HRT is administered, targeting one tic each session. A behavioral reward program is also used in CBIT to incentivize patient engagement, homework completion, and session attendance. As muscle tension and anxiety are associated with tics [19], CBIT also includes relaxation techniques, such as diaphragmatic breathing and progressive muscle relaxation [39]. Finally, therapists discuss relapse prevention in the final 2 sessions of treatment.

Exposure and Response Prevention. ERP treatment focuses on habituation to premonitory urges [40]. It entails response prevention, in which patients practice suppression of all tics, and premonitory urge exposure, which involves gradually exposing patients to contexts that increase intensity of premonitory urges during response prevention. In treatment, patients suppress all tics for successively increasing durations each session. Clinicians take on a "coach" role, encouraging patients to concentrate on the premonitory sensations and reminding them of gains associated with tic suppression. Patients also practice tic suppression outside of sessions to promote generalization.

RESEARCH SUPPORT FOR BEHAVIORAL TREATMENTS

Habit Reversal Training. Several studies have examined the efficacy of HRT. Azrin and Nunn [37] used an open, uncontrolled design to examine the effectiveness of HRT in 12 participants with nervous habits or tics. Following a 2-hour HRT session, tics and nervous habits decreased, with gains maintained at 5-month follow-up. Further, in the first controlled HRT trial of 10 participants with TD, Azrin and Peterson [41] found that those administered HRT experienced a significant reduction in tics compared with waitlist control (WLC). Wilhelm and colleagues [42] and Deckersbach and colleagues [43] completed randomized controlled trials (RCTs) that compared HRT to a supportive psychotherapy control in 32 and 30 participants with TD, respectively. The studies used the Yale Global Tic Severity Scale (YGTSS) [44], a clinician-rated and psychometrically valid outcome measure, to assess tic severity. Results of both studies showed greater tic reduction on the YGTSS for those receiving HRT relative to supportive psychotherapy [42,43]. Overall, empirical findings support the efficacy of HRT for decreasing tic severity and impairment.

Comprehensive Behavioral Intervention for Tics. CBIT is the first-line intervention for tics per AAN recommendations [36] and is considered a first-line intervention among behavioral treatments for TD in multiple countries [40,45]. Piacentini and colleagues [46] conducted an RCT of CBIT in 126 children with TD or persistent tic disorders (PTDs). Participants were randomly assigned to 8 sessions of CBIT or psychoeducation and supportive therapy (PST). At posttreatment, YGTSS tic severity scores were significantly lower in the CBIT group compared with PST. Further, 52.5% of CBIT participants were clinical responders compared with 18.5% of the PST group, and tic-related impairment decreased significantly more in CBIT participants. Treatment gains were maintained at 6-month follow-up, and youth also demonstrated decreases in overall behavior problems, anxiety, depression, and disruptive behavior [47]. Further, a long-term follow-up study of this trial found that improvements in tic severity were maintained after 11 years, supporting the durability of CBIT treatment effects [48].

Wilhelm and colleagues [49] adopted a similar study design, randomizing 122 adults with TD or PTDs into CBIT or PST. Participants administered CBIT experienced significantly greater reductions in tic severity than those who received PST. Moreover, 38% of participants in the CBIT group were responders at posttreatment, compared with 6.8% of those in the PST condition. Further, 80% of initial CBIT treatment responders still met responder status at 6-month follow-up. Other studies have also shown that CBIT can reduce tic severity in clinic settings outside of controlled trials [50,51].

Exposure and Response Prevention. Compared with HRT and CBIT, there is less research to support the efficacy of ERP. Hoogduin and colleagues [52] administered ERP to 4 participants with tics more than 10 2-hour treatment sessions. Results showed that 3 of 4 participants experienced reductions in tics. Additionally, Verdellen and colleagues [53] compared HRT and ERP in 43 participants with TD, with those in HRT receiving 10 60-minute sessions and those in ERP receiving 12 120-minute sessions. Both groups experienced significant reductions in tics, with no differences between groups; however, participants administered ERP received more than twice as many treatment hours. Treatment gains in both groups were maintained at 3-month follow-up.

Mixed Behavioral Therapy Studies. Recent research has combined these therapeutic approaches to test the broad impact of behavioral interventions for tics. Nissen and colleagues [54] randomized 59 children with PTDs to receive HRT or ERP treatment through either individual or group therapy. No between-group differences emerged; participants in both conditions experienced significant tic severity reductions. Further, Rizzo and colleagues [55] compared the efficacy of behavioral therapy (participants were randomly assigned to HRT or ERP), antipsychotic medication, and a psychoeducation control in 110 individuals with TD. Participants in the behavioral therapy and medication groups experienced significantly greater reductions in tics compared with those in the control condition. There were no differences between behavioral therapy and antipsychotic medication, suggesting that HRT and ERP may be as effective as medication [55]. Finally, in a naturalistic clinical setting, Andén and colleagues [56] found that children administered HRT or ERP experienced significant reductions in tics, with no between-group differences in tic severity scores at posttreatment.

Predictors of Treatment Outcome. Recent research has begun to identify moderators and predictors of behavioral treatment outcomes for children and adults with TD. A study examining data from the child [46] and adult [49] CBIT RCTs showed that higher tic severity and positive expectancy for treatment predicted greater improvements in tic symptoms [57]. However, higher premonitory urge severity and the presence of co-occurring anxiety disorders were associated with lower tic reductions [57]. In a study of children who received combined HRT and ERP, the presence of obsessive-compulsive symptoms was associated with a larger decrease in tics [58]. Moreover, a meta-analysis of behavioral therapy RCTs for TD found that higher number of treatment sessions and older age of participants were associated with larger treatment effect sizes, whereas trials with more participants with co-occurring ADHD showed attenuated treatment effects [59]. Further research is needed to continue delineating factors that might influence behavioral treatment response in patients with TD.

Alternative Delivery Formats. Despite empirical support for behavioral treatments for tics, these interventions are underutilized. Barriers to standard forms of treatment include lack of trained professionals and the time/cost of treatment [60]. In response to these limitations, pilot studies on alternative forms of treatment (eg, online, intensive, self-help) have been developed. For instance, Ricketts and colleagues [61] demonstrated that participants provided telehealth CBIT showed better treatment outcomes than WLC participants, while Himle and colleagues [62] found no differences in tic severity outcomes between telehealth and in-person CBIT. Additionally, Blount and colleagues [63] found that intensive CBIT, which included 8 sessions delivered over 4 days, led to significant decreases in tic severity in 4 of 5 participants. Studies have also examined the efficacy of Internet-based, self-help behavioral treatment programs with minimal therapist support. Findings showed that children in self-help programs demonstrated significantly greater decreases in tic severity than children in control conditions, with gains maintained at 6-month follow-up [64,65]. Preliminary evidence of these alternative delivery formats is encouraging; however, future studies with larger sample sizes are needed.

CASE VIGNETTE

Jason is an 11-year-old Caucasian boy who presented for treatment with his mother due to struggles with motor and vocal tics.[a] Jason's most bothersome tic is a complex motor tic, in which he jerks his head back and stretches his arms to the side simultaneously. This tic occurs approximately every 15 minutes, and the intensity of the tic has led to pain in Jason's neck. He also reported eye rolling and shoulder shrugging tics occurring approximately hourly. Further, Jason's vocal tics include sniffing in and coughing. Jason reported that peers at school make fun of his tics and mimic his complex motor tic. Several teachers have also reacted to his eye rolling tic due to perceiving it as intentional and disrespectful. Additionally, he noted that his sister becomes frustrated when his sniffing tic occurs as they watch TV.

The intake appointment involved the assessment of tic history (onset, diagnosis), course, topography, triggers, tic-related impairment (ie, home, school, social, family, and physical domains) and psychiatric comorbidity, and administration of a gold-standard clinical interview measure (ie, YGTSS) to assess motor and vocal tic severity and degree of tic-related impairment. Jason's total score on the YGTSS was 29 with a motor tic total of 16, vocal tic total of 13, and YGTSS tic impairment total of 30, indicating marked tic severity [66]. He also met criteria for ADHD—inattentive type—although his ADHD symptoms were secondary to his tics. Finally, during the intake appointment, the clinician explained the rationale for CBIT treatment and discussed treatment goals.

In the first session, Jason and his mother were provided with psychoeducation about tic disorders to decrease blame and stigma associated with tics. The clinician also completed a tic hierarchy, during which Jason ranked his tics from most to least bothersome on a 0 to 10 scale. Jason's highest rated tic was his head jerk with arm movement, which was rated on a 9 out of 10 scale. Further, an inconvenience review was completed in which Jason rated the distress level of inconveniences related to his tics on a 0 to 10 scale. His most bothersome tic-related inconvenience was being teased by other children at school. Finally, a behavioral reward program was implemented to increase Jason's motivation and adherence with treatment protocols. Jason had the opportunity to earn 3 tokens per

[a]This case is based on a combination of several patients with TD that have been treated in our clinical work. It is intended to demonstrate how CBIT is administered in practice. The case is not a reflection of one individual patient.

session for attending session, completing homework, and actively participating in session.

In the second session, the clinician conducted a functional assessment to assess the environmental variables that affect Jason's tic worsening. Several settings, such as his school classroom, recess, and watching TV, were associated with tic exacerbation. Jason indicated that in school, peers mimicked his tics, and frequently told him to stop his tics. Further, when Jason became sweaty while playing basketball at recess, his tics would also increase. Although watching TV at home, Jason's sister yelled at him for having his sniffing tic, and Jason's mother would occasionally give him neck massages after school if his neck hurt from engaging in his complex head jerk with arm movement tic.

In session 3, the clinician provided Jason and his mother with several function-based interventions to aid tic management in relevant tic exacerbating settings and decrease tic-contingent reactions. Table 1 shows the function-based interventions that were implemented. These tic management strategies were also discussed in subsequent sessions to ensure adherence and troubleshoot potential complications. Then, the clinician completed HRT for Jason's head jerk with arm movement tic, which was the most bothersome tic on his hierarchy. During AT, Jason discovered that his head jerk occurs slightly before his arm movement begins. He also indicated that the premonitory urge for this tic involves muscle tension in the back of his neck. During response detection, Jason was aware of every tic occurrence, and toward the end of the session, he was able to raise his finger before he engaged in the tic, indicating awareness. The competing response focused on the first muscle movement involved in the tic, which included Jason putting his chin and shoulders slightly down while slightly tensing his neck. As this movement alone did not block the remainder of his tic (ie, extending his arms), he also crossed his arm as a competing behavior for the arm movements. Jason's mother was the social support person, and she was instructed to praise Jason for correctly using his competing response and gently remind him to engage in the competing response if he missed a tic occurrence or did not use the exercise correctly.

In the subsequent sessions, HRT was implemented for each of the successive tics on Jason's tic hierarchy. Table 2 shows the competing responses for each tic. Jason struggled with awareness of his eye rolling tic, so a whole session was dedicated to practicing awareness of the tic before a competing response was introduced. Further, during sessions 5 and 6, the clinician taught diaphragmatic breathing and progressive muscle

TABLE 1
Jason's Functional Interventions

Tic Contextual Variables	Functional Interventions
Tendency to tic while in class	• Jason and his teacher provided tic education to his class to help them learn about tics and the importance of not reacting to them • Jason's seat was moved closer to the back of the class to decrease likelihood of others reacting to his tics • Jason was provided with short breaks during class that were not contingent on his tics
Tendency to tic while at recess	• Jason brought a cold washcloth or ice pack to recess because the heat was associated with increases in tics • Jason and his clinician practiced a phrase Jason could use if other kids asked about his tics at recess. He would say: "I have tics, which means I sometimes do movements and sounds that I cannot control. It would really help me if you just ignored them."
Tendency to tic while watching TV	• Limited daily TV time • Instead of sitting next to his sister on the couch, Jason moved to the chair in the living room • Jason's mother talked with his sister about the importance of not reacting to tics • Before watching TV, Jason's mother helped remind him to practice his competing response exercises

to practice his competing responses outside of session. In the final 2 sessions, relapse prevention was discussed. The clinician reviewed the steps of HRT with Jason and his mother in case additional tics emerge. They also discussed helpful functional interventions that Jason can continue to use. The clinician emphasized that Jason and his mother should monitor potential tic triggers and implement additional functional interventions if needed. At the last session, the clinician administered the YGTSS. Jason's total tic score was a 13 with a motor tic total of 7, vocal tic total of 6, and YGTSS tic-related impairment total of 5.

DISCUSSION

TD is a childhood-onset neurological condition that can exact impairment in a range of life domains [67]. Behavioral therapy for tics, including HRT, CBIT, and ERP, is a gold standard treatment of TD, with support from clinical trials and practice guidelines [36,56]. Behavioral treatment of tics leads to reductions in tic severity and tic-related impairment and has shown effectiveness across various real-world settings. The section below reviews several key components regarding the delivery of behavioral therapy and offers ways to overcome challenges associated with treatment.

Challenges in Behavioral Therapy for TD. There are several challenges that can develop when implementing behavioral therapy protocols for TD. For instance, patients with stronger premonitory urges may have more

TABLE 2
Jason's Competing Responses

Tic	Competing Response
Head jerk with arm movement	• Chin and shoulders pressed slightly down • Subtly draw neck inward with slight tension • Press arms into sides of abdomen or cross arms
Eye roll	• Slow, controlled eye blink • Focus eyes on a stationary object
Shoulder shrug	• Slightly press shoulders downward
Sniff in	• Breathe in through mouth and out through nose
Cough	• Breathe in through mouth and out through nose

relaxation so Jason could use these skills in anxiety-provoking situations.

During the course of treatment, tic frequency and intensity gradually decreased. Following implementation of the function-based interventions, Jason encountered fewer reactions to tics at home and school. Jason reported less teasing from peers at school, and pain from his tics decreased after implementation of competing responses. The final 2 sessions were spaced 2 weeks apart to provide Jason with additional time

difficulty using competing responses to manage tics [57]. Therefore, additional sessions focused on competing response practice could be helpful for these individuals. Clinicians could also implement mindfulness-based techniques, such as the use of breathing exercises while mindfully noticing the urge to tic. Indeed, Reese and colleagues [68] found that 8 sessions of mindfulness-based techniques led to significant decreases in tic severity and impairment.

Additionally, depending on findings from the functional assessment, some patients may require more in-depth functional interventions that include discussions with school staff or other family members. For example, children may have classmates that respond to tics by teasing, laughing, or telling them to stop performing tics. Should this be the case, the clinician, parents, or child could provide psychoeducation to teachers and peers to help them understand the importance of creating a tic-neutral environment. Family members may also think they are helping children by comforting them after a tic or relieving them from activities in which they experience heightened tics, such as homework. In such cases, clinicians can explain to family members how tic-contingent attention can reinforce tic expression and provide family members with ways to comfort the child independent of tics. Children should also not be allowed to skip homework or avoid chores or other tasks because of tics. For example, if homework exacerbates tics, clinicians can suggest implementing 5-minute homework breaks that are not contingent on tics, during which children can practice tic management strategies.

Poor tic awareness is another barrier that may impede treatment success. If patients struggle with AT, full sessions can be dedicated to increasing awareness. For difficulties with response description, clinicians could use mirrors or video recordings to help patients improve tic description accuracy. Response detection can also be completed in front of a mirror to assist with patient awareness. If patients continue to struggle with response detection, clinicians can perform the patient's tics themselves and ask the patient to point out when the clinician engages in the target tic. Once patients can acknowledge the clinician's simulated tics, then standard response detection can be implemented. If patients do not tic during AT, clinicians can ask for the patient's assent to use triggers identified from the functional assessment to evoke tics. For example, if watching TV exacerbates tics, the clinician and patient may watch TV while practicing response detection.

Several challenges can also develop during CRT. For example, patients may feel uncomfortable engaging in the competing response. There are multiple options for competing responses for most tics, so clinicians could suggest a different action to physically prevent the tic. Additionally, patients may indicate that competing responses are not preventing all components of complex tics. Typically, clinicians implement a competing response that targets the first movement of a complex tic but in such cases, clinicians can add other elements to the competing response. Further, poor competing response adherence is another factor that can impede treatment progress. Clinicians could use a reward program to reinforce correct competing response use both in and between sessions. Social support individuals could also remind patients to engage in competing responses before entering situations that exacerbate tics (eg, while watching TV, during homework).

Addressing Clinical Complexities. Individuals with tic disorders typically present with comorbid conditions, such as ADHD and OCD [6]. Döpfner and Rothenberger [69] indicated that ADHD symptoms that are more impairing than tics should be treated before beginning behavioral therapy for TD. Clinicians can also incorporate ADHD-related interventions into CBIT, such as organizational skills and task prioritization [70]. Further, children with comorbid ADHD tend to struggle with competing response homework adherence, so a reward program that focuses on competing response adherence could be useful. Additionally, for patients with comorbid OCD, it may be difficult to differentiate complex motor tics (eg, touching an object) from compulsions. In such cases, clinicians should assess whether patients feel an uncomfortable physical sensation (ie, premonitory urge) or an increase in anxiety before the movement. Treatment could also be modified to treat both tics and compulsions by including CRT and ERP. Finally, studies have shown that high anxiety may lead to less improvement in tic severity and impairment following treatment [54,57]. Relaxation techniques and cognitive restructuring may help reduce anxiety symptoms and improve treatment outcomes for these individuals.

Recommendations for Clinicians. Behavioral therapy is a well-established treatment of individuals with tic disorders, and several international professional groups recommend it as a first-line intervention for those with tics [36,40,45]. Based on the research presented above, the following recommendations are offered for treating patients with tic disorders.
- Flexibly implement behavioral therapy protocols and emphasize the importance of practicing competing responses outside of session

- Conduct a functional assessment and tailor function-based interventions to target a patient's specific tic-exacerbating antecedents and consequences
- Assess for possible clinical complexities that may interfere with behavioral therapy and personalize treatment accordingly

CLINICS CARE POINTS

- During AT, allow the patient to develop a detailed description of each target tic; avoid describing the tics to them.
- During CRT, implement a competing response that is incompatible with the first muscle movement of the target tic; avoid missing the first movement due to increased focus on secondary movements.
- When implementing function-based interventions for tics, tailor the interventions to target the patient's specific tic-exacerbating antecedents and consequences; avoid providing the same function-based interventions to each patient.

DISCLOSURE

J.T. Stiede, Brandon Pitts, and Kathryn Barber have no disclosures to report.

Dr E.J. Ricketts reports grants from the Tourette Association of America (TAA), United States, TLC Foundation for Body-Focused Repetitive Behaviors (BFRBs), United States: BFRB Precision Medicine Initiative, National Institute of Mental Health, United States, and Brain and Behavior Research Foundation, United States. She also reports honoraria from the TAA, Centers for Disease Control and Prevention, and Springer Nature, and service on the Tourette Association of America Diversity Committee.

REFERENCES

[1] American Psychiatric Association. Diagnostic and statistical manual of mental disorders. In: Text revision (DSM-5-TR). Fifth Edition. Arlington, VA: American Psychiatric Association; 2022.

[2] Banaschewski T, Woerner W, Rothenberger A. Premonitory sensory phenomena and suppressibility of tics in Tourette syndrome: developmental aspects in children and adolescents. Dev Med Child Neurol 2007;45(10): 700–3.

[3] Brandt VC, Beck C, Sajin V, et al. Temporal relationship between premonitory urges and tics in Gilles de la Tourette syndrome. Cortex 2016;77:24–37.

[4] Capriotti MR, Brandt BC, Turkel JE, et al. Negative reinforcement and premonitory urges in youth with Tourette Syndrome: an experimental evaluation. Behav Modif 2014;38(2):276–96.

[5] Freeman RD, Fast DK, Burd L, et al. An international perspective on Tourette syndrome: selected findings from 3,500 individuals in 22 countries. Dev Med Child Neurol 2000;42(7):436–47.

[6] Hirschtritt ME, Lee PC, Pauls DL, et al. Lifetime prevalence, age of risk, and genetic relationships of comorbid psychiatric disorders in Tourette Syndrome. JAMA Psychiatr 2015;72(4):325–33.

[7] Bloch MH, Peterson BS, Scahill L, et al. Adulthood outcome of tic and obsessive-compulsive symptom severity in children with Tourette syndrome. Arch Pediatr Adolesc Med 2006;160(1):65–9.

[8] Bloch MH, Leckman JF. Clinical course of Tourette syndrome. J Psychosom Res 2009;67(6):497–501.

[9] Claussen AH, Bitsko RH, Holbrook JR, et al. Impact of Tourette Syndrome on school measures in a nationally representative sample. J Dev Behav Pediatr 2018;39(4): 335–42.

[10] McGuire JF, Hanks C, Lewin AB, et al. Social deficits in children with chronic tic disorders: phenomenology, clinical correlates and quality of life. Compr Psychiatry 2013;54(7):1023–31.

[11] Conelea CA, Woods DW, Zinner SH, et al. The impact of tourette syndrome in adults: results from the tourette syndrome impact survey. Community Ment Health J 2013;49(1):110–20.

[12] Malaty I, Shineman D, Himle M. Tourette syndrome has substantial impact in childhood and adulthood as well. J Dev Behav Pediatr 2019;40(6):468–9.

[13] Wolicki SB, Bitsko RH, Danielson ML, et al. Children with tourette syndrome in the united states: parent-reported diagnosis, co-occurring disorders, severity, and influence of activities on tics. J Dev Behav Pediatr 2019;40(6):407–14.

[14] Ganos C, Roessner V, Münchau A. The functional anatomy of Gilles de la Tourette syndrome. Neurosci Biobehav Rev 2013;37(6):1050–62.

[15] Maia TV, Frank MJ. From reinforcement learning models to psychiatric and neurological disorders. Nat Neurosci 2011;14(2):154–62.

[16] Mink JW. Neurobiology of basal ganglia circuits in Tourette syndrome: faulty inhibition of unwanted motor patterns? Adv Neurol 2001;85:113–22.

[17] Leckman JF, Walker DE, Cohen DJ. Premonitory urges in Tourette's syndrome. Am J Psychiatry 1993;150(1):98–102.

[18] Woods DW, Piacentini J, Himle MB, et al. Premonitory Urge for Tics Scale (PUTS): Initial psychometric results and examination of the premonitory urge phenomenon in youths with Tic disorders. J Dev Behav Pediatr 2005; 26(6):397–403.

[19] Conelea CA, Woods DW. The influence of contextual factors on tic expression in Tourette's syndrome: a review. J Psychosom Res 2008;65(5):487–96.

[20] Kanaan AS, Gerasch S, García-García I, et al. Pathological glutamatergic neurotransmission in Gilles de la Tourette syndrome. Brain 2017;140(1):218–34.

[21] O'Rourke JA, Scharf JM, Yu D, et al. The genetics of Tourette syndrome: a review. J Psychosom Res 2009;67(6):533–45.

[22] Levy AM, Paschou P, Tümer Z. Candidate genes and pathways associated with gilles de la tourette syndrome—where are we? Genes 2021;12(9):1321.

[23] Himle MB, Woods DW, Conelea CA, et al. Investigating the effects of tic suppression on premonitory urge ratings in children and adolescents with Tourette's syndrome. Behav Res Ther 2007;45(12):2964–76.

[24] Matsuda N, Nonaka M, Kono T, et al. Premonitory awareness facilitates tic suppression: subscales of the premonitory urge for tics scale and a new self-report questionnaire for tic-associated sensations. Front Psychiatr 2020;11. https://doi.org/10.3389/fpsyt.2020.00592.

[25] Crossley E, Seri S, Stern JS, et al. Premonitory urges for tics in adult patients with Tourette syndrome. Brain & Dev 2014;36(1):45–50.

[26] Conelea CA, Woods DW, Brandt BC. The impact of a stress induction task on tic frequencies in youth with Tourette Syndrome. Behav Res Ther 2011;49(8):492–7.

[27] Specht MW, Woods DW, Nicotra CM, et al. Effects of tic suppression: ability to suppress, rebound, negative reinforcement, and habituation to the premonitory urge. Behav Res Ther 2013;51(1):24–30.

[28] Caurín B, Serrano M, Fernández-Alvarez E, et al. Environmental circumstances influencing tic expression in children. Europ J Paediatr Neurol 2014;18(2):157–62.

[29] Himle MB, Capriotti MR, Hayes LP, et al. Variables associated with tic exacerbation in children with chronic tic disorders. Behav Modif 2014;38(2):163–83.

[30] Bodeck S, Lappe C, Evers S. Tic-reducing effects of music in patients with Tourette's syndrome: self-reported and objective analysis. J Neurol Sci 2015;352(1):41–7.

[31] Silva RR, Munoz DM, Barickman J, et al. Environmental factors and related fluctuation of symptoms in children and adolescents with tourette's disorder. J Child Psychol Psychiatry 1995;36(2):305–12.

[32] Eapen V, Fox-Hiley P, Banerjee S, et al. Clinical features and associated psychopathology in a Tourette syndrome cohort. Acta Neurol Scand 2004;109(4):255–60.

[33] Conelea CA, Ramanujam K, Walther MR, et al. Is there a relationship between tic frequency and physiological arousal? Examination in a sample of children with co-occurring tic and anxiety disorders. Behav Modif 2014;38(2):217–34.

[34] Capriotti MR, Piacentini JC, Himle MB, et al. Assessing environmental consequences of ticcing in youth with chronic tic disorders: the tic accommodation and reactions scale. Child Health Care 2015;44(3):205–20.

[35] Himle MB, Woods DW. An experimental evaluation of tic suppression and the tic rebound effect. Behav Res Ther 2005;43(11):1443–51.

[36] Pringsheim T, Holler-Managan Y, Okun MS, et al. Comprehensive systematic review summary: treatment of tics in people with Tourette syndrome and chronic tic disorders. Neurology 2019;92(19):907–15.

[37] Azrin NH, Nunn RG. Habit-reversal: a method of eliminating nervous habits and tics. Behav Res Ther 1973;11(4):619–28.

[38] Woods DW, Miltenberger RG, Lumley VA. Sequential application of major habit-reversal components to treat motor tics in children. J Appl Behav Anal 1996;29:483–93.

[39] Woods DW, Piacentini J, Chang S, et al. Managing tourette syndrome: a behavioral intervention for children and adults therapist guide. New York, NY: Oxford University Press; 2008.

[40] Verdellen C, van de Griendt J, Hartmann A, et al. European clinical guidelines for Tourette Syndrome and other tic disorders. Part III: behavioural and psychosocial interventions. Eur Child Adolesc Psychiatry 2011;20(4):197–207.

[41] Azrin NH, Peterson AL. Treatment of tourette syndrome by habit reversal: a waiting-list control group comparison. Behav Ther 1990;21(3):305–18.

[42] Wilhelm S, Deckersbach T, Coffey BJ, et al. Habit reversal versus supportive psychotherapy for tourette's disorder: a randomized controlled trial. Am J Psychiatry 2003;160(6):1175–7.

[43] Deckersbach T, Rauch S, Buhlmann U, et al. Habit reversal versus supportive psychotherapy in Tourette's disorder: a randomized controlled trial and predictors of treatment response. Behav Res Ther 2006;44(8):1079–90.

[44] Leckman JF, Riddle MA, Hardin MT, et al. The yale global tic severity scale: initial testing of a clinician-rated scale of tic severity. J Am Acad Child Adolesc Psychiatry 1989;28(4):566–73.

[45] Steeves T, McKinlay BD, Gorman D, et al. Canadian guidelines for the evidence-based treatment of tic disorders: behavioural therapy, deep brain stimulation, and transcranial magnetic stimulation. Can J Psychiatry 2012;57(3):144–51.

[46] Piacentini J, Woods DW, Scahill L, et al. Behavior therapy for children with Tourette disorder: a randomized controlled trial. JAMA 2010;303(19):1929–37.

[47] Woods DW, Piacentini JC, Scahill L, et al. Behavior therapy for tics in children: acute and long-term effects on psychiatric and psychosocial functioning. J Child Neurol 2011;26(7):858–65.

[48] Espil FM, Woods DW, Specht MW, et al. Long-term outcomes of behavior therapy for youth with tourette disorder. J Am Acad Child Adolesc Psychiatry 2022;61(6):764–71.

[49] Wilhelm S, Peterson A, Piacentini J, et al. Randomized trial of behavior therapy for adults with tourette syndrome. Arch Gen Psychiatry 2012;69:795–803.

[50] Dreison KC, Lagges AM. Effectiveness of the Comprehensive Behavioral Intervention for Tics (CBIT) in a pediatric psychiatry clinic: a retrospective chart review. Clinical Practice in Pediatric Psychology 2017;5:180–5.

[51] Ricketts EJ, Gilbert DL, Zinner SH, et al. Pilot testing behavior therapy for chronic tic disorders in neurology and developmental pediatrics clinics. J Child Neurol 2015;31(4):444–50.

[52] Hoogduin K, Verdellen C, Cath D. Exposure and Response Prevention in the Treatment of Gilles de la Tourette's Syndrome: Four Case Studies. Clin Psychol Psychother 1997;4(2):125–35.

[53] Verdellen CW, Keijsers GP, Cath DC, et al. Exposure with response prevention versus habit reversal in Tourettes's syndrome: a controlled study. Behav Res Ther 2004; 42(5):501–11.

[54] Nissen JB, Kaergaard M, Laursen L, et al. Combined habit reversal training and exposure response prevention in a group setting compared to individual training: a randomized controlled clinical trial. Eur Child Adolesc Psychiatry 2019;28(1):57–68.

[55] Rizzo R, Pellico A, Silvestri PR, et al. A randomized controlled trial comparing behavioral, educational, and pharmacological treatments in youths with chronic tic disorder or tourette syndrome. Front Psychiatr 2018;9. https://doi.org/10.3389/fpsyt.2018.00100.

[56] Andrén P, Wachtmeister V, Franzé J, et al. Effectiveness of behaviour therapy for children and adolescents with tourette syndrome and chronic tic disorder in a naturalistic setting. Child Psychiatry Hum Dev 2021;52(4): 739–50.

[57] Sukhodolsky DG, Woods DW, Piacentini J, et al. Moderators and predictors of response to behavior therapy for tics in Tourette syndrome. Neurology 2017;88(11): 1029–36.

[58] Nissen JB, Parner ET, Thomsen PH. Predictors of therapeutic treatment outcome in adolescent chronic tic disorders. BJPsych Open 2019;5(5):e74.

[59] McGuire JF, Piacentini J, Brennan EA, et al. A meta-analysis of behavior therapy for Tourette Syndrome. J Psychiatr Res 2014;50:106–12.

[60] Woods DW, Conelea CA, Himle MB. Behavior therapy for Tourette's disorder: utilization in a community sample and an emerging area of practice for psychologists. Prof Psychol Res Pract 2010;41(6):518–25.

[61] Ricketts EJ, Goetz AR, Capriotti MR, et al. A randomized waitlist-controlled pilot trial of voice over Internet protocol-delivered behavior therapy for youth with chronic tic disorders. J Telemed Telecare 2016;22(3): 153–62.

[62] Himle MB, Freitag M, Walther M, et al. A randomized pilot trial comparing videoconference versus face-to-face delivery of behavior therapy for childhood tic disorders. Behav Res Ther 2012;50(9):565–70.

[63] Blount TH, Raj JJ, Peterson AL. Intensive outpatient comprehensive behavioral intervention for tics: a clinical replication series. Cognit Behav Pract 2018;25(1): 156–67.

[64] Rachamim L, Zimmerman-Brenner S, Rachamim O, et al. Internet-based guided self-help comprehensive behavioral intervention for tics (ICBIT) for youth with tic disorders: a feasibility and effectiveness study with 6 month-follow-up. Eur Child Adolesc Psychiatry 2022; 31(2):275–87.

[65] Hollis C, Hall CL, Jones R, et al. Therapist-supported online remote behavioural intervention for tics in children and adolescents in England (ORBIT): a multicentre, parallel group, single-blind, randomised controlled trial. Lancet Psychiatr 2021;8(10):871–82.

[66] McGuire JF, Piacentini J, Storch EA, et al. Defining tic severity and tic impairment in Tourette Disorder. J Psychiatr Res 2021;133:93–100.

[67] Conelea CA, Woods DW, Zinner SH, et al. Exploring the chronic tic disorders on youth: results from the Tourette Syndrome Impact Survey. Child Psychiatry Hum Dev 2011;42(2):219–42.

[68] Reese HE, Vallejo Z, Rasmussen J, et al. Mindfulness-based stress reduction for Tourette syndrome and chronic tic disorder: a pilot study. J Psychosom Res 2015;78(3):293–8.

[69] Döpfner M, Rothenberger A. Behavior therapy in tic-disorders with co-existing ADHD. Eur Child Adolesc Psychiatry 2007;16(1):89–99.

[70] Greenberg E, Albright C, Hall M, et al. Modified comprehensive behavioral intervention for tics: treating children with tic disorders, Co-Occurring ADHD, and Psychosocial Impairment. Behav Ther 2022. https://doi.org/10.1016/j.beth.2022.07.007.

Advances in Psychiatry and Behavioral Health 3 (2023) 33–41

ADVANCES IN PSYCHIATRY AND BEHAVIORAL HEALTH

Treatment of Misophonia

M. Zachary Rosenthal, PhD[a,b,*], Yanyan Shan, MA[a,b], Jacqueline Trumbull, MA[a,b]

[a]Department of Psychiatry & Behavioral Sciences, Duke University, DUMC, 6400 Pratt Street, North Pavilion, 6th Floor, Room 6043, Durham, NC 27705, USA; [b]Department of Psychology & Neuroscience, Duke University, Durham, NC, USA

KEYWORDS
- Misophonia • Treatment • Psychotherapy • Unified protocol • Process-based therapy
- Multi-disciplinary treatment

KEY POINTS
- Introduces misophonia and reviews published psychotherapy treatment studies.
- Outlines a multi-disciplinary strategy for treatment.
- Describes the application of two transdiagnostic psychotherapies with emerging evidence in misophonia (Unified Protocol and Process-Based Therapy).
- Suggests an agenda for future research and treatment development.

Misophonia was recently defined as a disorder characterized by intolerance of specific auditory stimuli and associated cues causing significant psychological distress and interference in social, occupational, or academic functioning [1]. Aversive stimuli in this context may be labeled as "triggers" that are commonly repetitive sounds produced by others. Primary triggering stimuli in misophonia most often (but not always) originate from facial (eg, nose noises, throat-clearing) or oral (eg, lip-smacking, chewing, drinking) sources. However, there are individual differences in the types of cues and contexts (eg, the same sound may have different effects when produced by specific people) associated with misophonia symptoms [2,3].

Individuals with impairing levels of misophonia symptoms may have strong multi-modal emotional responses to contexts in which triggering cues are anticipated or encountered. For example, common responses include central (eg, insula) [4] and peripheral nervous system activation (eg, increased heart rate and skin conductance) [5], negative affect (eg, irritation, anger, anxiety, disgust) [6,7], and behavioral patterns that can be conceptualized as consistent with freeze (eg, hypervigilance), flight (eg, escape or avoidance behavior), and fight behaviors (eg, interpersonally aggressive verbal behavior) [8]. These responses are highly distressing and different than how most others might react [1].

Jastreboff and Jastreboff are credited for coining the term misophonia over 20 years ago [9]. The term translates to hatred or dislike (miso) of sound (phonia). However, this literal translation is misleading, as the condition is neither uniquely associated with the affective experience of hate or dislike, nor are auditory cues the only stimuli that can function as triggers. The first pilot studies directly examining misophonia were published only 9 years ago [5,10]. Since then, over 60 published empirical studies have investigated misophonia, with roughly 25% of these published over the last year in the first special section in a peer-reviewed scientific journal dedicated to misophonia (*Frontiers in Neuroscience*).

Recent reviews suggest that misophonia may be associated with a wide variety of mental health problems [1–3]. The majority of studies have used self-report

---

Corresponding author, E-mail address: mark.rosenthal@duke.edu

https://doi.org/10.1016/j.ypsc.2023.03.009
2667-3827/23/ © 2023 Elsevier Inc. All rights reserved.

methodologies and have found that misophonia symptom severity is positively correlated transdiagnostically with, for example, neuroticism, anxiety symptoms, depressive symptoms, difficulties with emotion regulation, affective instability, anxiety sensitivity, some obsessive-compulsive disorder (OCD) symptoms, perfectionism, and somatic pain [11–19]. Additionally, adults with misophonia may be significantly more likely than those without misophonia to self-report a lifetime history of attention-deficit/hyperactivity disorder (ADHD), OCD, bipolar disorder, substance use disorder, post-traumatic stress disorder, and conversion disorder [17,20].

Two recent studies have used structured psychiatric diagnostic interviews as a more rigorous approach to the assessment of misophonia and associated mental health problems. In one study, 575 adults presenting for treatment at a clinic in Amsterdam were interviewed using the Mini International Neuropsychiatric Interview [21], a structured interview assessing 15 current psychiatric problems (Jager and colleagues, 2020a) [14]. Results indicated that most (72%) participants did not meet the full criteria for a current psychiatric disorder. The most common current disorders were mood disorders (10.1%), anxiety disorders (9%), ADHD (5.4%), and personality disorders (5%).

Rosenthal and colleagues [8] conducted the first study to characterize diagnsotic and statistical manual of mental disorders (DSM-5) disorders using structured diagnostic interviews in a nationally recruited community sample of 207 adults with high misophonia symptoms. Results indicated that anxiety disorders were the most common type of current mental health problem (56.9%). Additionally, high rates of lifetime history of psychiatric disorders were observed, including diagnoses of any anxiety (73%), mood (61%), obsessive-compulsive (27%), substance use (26%), trauma-related (24%), eating (18%), or personality disorders (13%).

The findings from Jager and colleagues [14] suggest that most adults seeking outpatient treatment of misophonia in Amsterdam may not have a current psychiatric disorder. In contrast, Rosenthal and colleagues [8] indicate that adults across the United States with high misophonia symptoms may be most likely to meet the full criteria for a current anxiety disorder or lifetime history of any anxiety or mood disorders. A consistent interpretation of findings across all studies is that higher misophonia symptoms do not appear to be uniquely related to any specific psychiatric disorder. Accordingly, it is premature to conclude that any specific treatment protocol for any specific psychiatric disorder is best for the treatment of misophonia.

TREATMENT OF MISOPHONIA
Multi-Disciplinary Model: Audiology

There is no gold standard evidence-based treatment of misophonia, and it is not a disorder within the purview of any specific clinical discipline. Because it appears to be a problem at the intersection of various clinical fields, a multi-disciplinary treatment model may be valuable. For example, audiologists may be important in the assessment and treatment of misophonia as it is defined as a sound intolerance condition. Because misophonia may need to be differentiated from hyperacusis, audiologists may be helpful in assessment and treatment planning. For example, audiologists use evaluative measures to assess sensitivity thresholds and can discern if one is hypersensitive to auditory stimuli.

With regard to treatment, audiologists can work with patients to determine the pros and cons of using sound-based therapies. These approaches use patient-controlled devices unobtrusively placed in the ear canal to diminish (eg, noise cancellation), mask (eg, static brown or white noise), and change responses to auditory input. Although these interventions have not been tested empirically using randomized trials for the treatment of misophonia, promising support has come from clinical observations reported by Jastreboff and Jastreboff, who pioneered the adaptation of Tinnitus Retraining Therapy for patients with misophonia and report high rates of success in uncontrolled trials [22]. This approach uses sound therapy and behavioral training to change response patterns to triggering contexts and cues, and was reported by the developers to be highly effective in a clinical setting.

Multi-Disciplinary Model: Occupational Therapy

Because misophonia may occur in the context of multisensory over-responsivity, it may be valuable to include occupational therapists in a multi-disciplinary assessment and treatment approach. Occupational therapists emphasize improvement of functioning across key domains of life. Because occupational therapists are the experts in sensory processing within health care, they may offer helpful coping strategies to manage misophonia effectively. Occupational therapy includes treatments designed to help improve central sensory processing through interventions designed to enhance sensory integration functioning. Treatments may identify and intervene upon environmental barriers to adaptive sensory processing or train new adaptive reactions to emotionally evocative sensory cues. Like approaches used by audiologists, there are no randomized controlled trials evaluating the efficacy of occupational therapy interventions with misophonia. However, these interventions have a long history of being used to improve sensory processing, and, as such, may be worth considering for those with misophonia.

Multi-Disciplinary Model: Mental Health

Some early clinical observations [22] and the large study by Jager and colleagues [14] indicate that adults with misophonia may present for treatment without co-occurring psychiatric disorders. On the other hand, there is a growing body of research and clinical observations pointing to misophonia occurring in the context of varied and debilitating psychiatric disorders [8] and an associated need for mental health professionals to be involved in the treatment of this disorder. Accordingly, evaluation and treatment recommendations from mental health providers are indicated in a multi-disciplinary model of care for misophonia.

Treatment Studies

Most publications describing possible psychotherapies for misophonia have been small case studies (Table 1) [23–35]. These treatments were mostly conducted using branded (eg, acceptance and commitment therapy; ACT) and non-branded interventions from the family of cognitive behavioral therapies (CBTs), and the authors reported descriptions of successful treatment in one or several individuals.

Examples of non-branded interventions include cognitive restructuring [23,24,26,30–32,35], relaxation exercises [26,28,32,35], counter-conditioning [27,28], acceptance and distress tolerance strategies [25,26,29,30,33,35], exposure and response prevention [23–26,30–32,34], interpersonal communication skills [24,32,33], attentional control skills [24,30,34], and parent management training [26,32]. Case studies are useful beginning points for treatment development and provide a direction for clinicians in the absence of a clear gold standard of care. However, these case studies do not provide compelling evidence of efficacy for any particular intervention.

OPEN TRIALS

Three open trials have been conducted to treat misophonia [36–38]. Schröder and colleagues [38] conducted an uncontrolled trial involving 90 adults with misophonia, showing promise for a cognitive behavioral approach using brief group therapy. In this trial, 48% of participants improved on a clinician rating of outcome, and 30% reported a significant reduction in symptoms on a self-report measure of misophonia. The treatment included four main components: (1) attentional shifting away from trigger stimuli, (2) counter-conditioning to disrupt classically conditioned associations between neutral/positive stimuli that have become paired with negative emotional experiences, (3) stimulus manipulation exercises (allowing the participant to manipulate trigger sounds), and (4) relaxation exercises. Because this intervention occurs in a group, validation and support from other sufferers may also be an important component of this treatment.

Frank and McKay reported that 18 participants received 12 sessions of exposure therapy before or after stress management training [36]. The exposure procedure used an inhibitory learning model, emphasizing altered expectations for the target sounds along with the deliberate practice of hearing sounds on an individual hierarchy. Rather than targeting habituation of psychological distress when exposed to triggers, the inhibitory learning approach to exposure enhances patient motivation to approach triggering cues and contexts by changing the features of these cues or their responses to them in an effort to change expectations, increase psychological flexibility, enhance valued actions, and increase the perception of control over reactions to misophonic cues. This study demonstrates that without habituation to certain sounds, inhibitory learning-based exposure procedures may be a promising way to enhance perceived control over emotional reactions to misophonia triggers.

Finally, Jager and colleagues [37] used an open trial to evaluate the efficacy of eye movement desensitization and reprocessing (EMDR) therapy in treating misophonia in eight participants. Misophonia-related emotionally disturbing memories were addressed with EMDR in an average of 2.6 sessions lasting 60 to 90 minutes. Participants reported a statistically significant 20% average reduction (with a large effect size estimate of $d = 1.14$) in symptoms of misophonia on a self-report measure of misophonia. No statistically significant changes were observed in psychological distress or impairment in functioning on secondary outcome measures. Due to the uncontrolled experimental design of these open trials, no definitive conclusions can be drawn from these studies about treatment efficacy, though these are valuable studies pointing to possible treatments to further evaluate.

RANDOMIZED CLINICAL TRIAL

Jager and colleagues [39] conducted the only randomized controlled trial for misophonia (Table 2). Using

TABLE 1
Case Studies of Misophonia Treatment

Studies	Treatment	Cognitive Restructuring	Relaxation Exercises	Counter-Conditioning	Acceptance and Distress Tolerance	ERP	Interpersonal Skills	Attention Control	Parenting Training	Age	Gender	Comorbidity	# of sessions	Baseline	Post	Symptom Reduce
Bernstein [24], 2013	CBT	✓				✓	✓	✓		19	Female	None	6	NA	NA	NA
Dozier [27], 2015(a)	NRT			✓						48	Female	NA	14	MAQ41	MAQ9	MAQ78%
Dozier [28], 2015(b)	NRT		✓	✓						21	Female	None	4	MAQ49	MAQ13	MAQ73%
McGuire [31], 2015	CBT	✓				✓				17	Female	None	10	MQ55 MSS12	MQ37 MSS7	MQ33% MSS42%
										11	Female	None	18	MQ31 MSS5	MQ25 MSS4	MQ19% MSS20%
Reid [34], 2016	CBT	✓				✓		✓		14	Female	OCD, MDD, phobia, ADHD	14	AMISOS17	AMISOS7	AMISOS59%
Kamody [29], 2017	DBT		✓		✓					16	Female	social anxiety	7I+35G	AMISO22 MAQ51	AMISO10 MAQ16	AMISO 55% MAQ 71%
Schneider [35], 2017	DBT and ACT		✓		✓					17	Male	None	10	AMISOS14	AMISOS8	AMISOS57%
Altınöz 2018	CBT	✓				✓				18	Female	NA	6	MAS6 MPRS6 AMISOS11	MAS2 MPRS2 AMISOS4	MAS67% MPRS67% AMISOS64%
Muller [32], 2018	CBT		✓			✓	✓		✓	14	Female	None	24	NA	NA	NA
Dover [26], 2021	CBT	✓	✓		✓	✓	✓		✓	10	Female	OCSD	30	AMISOS10 MQ27	AMISOS3 MQ6	AMISOS70% MQ78%
Lewin [30], 2021	UP	✓			✓	✓		✓		4 cases, NA			10	MAQ25 AMISOS13 / MAQ18 AMISOS15 / MAQ12 AMISOS9 / MAQ54 AMISOS17	MAQ13 AMISOS9 / MAQ25 AMISOS12 / MAQ3 AMISOS6 / MAQ13 AMISOS10	MAQ48% AMISOS31% / MAQ+39% AMISOS20% / MAQ75% AMISOS33% / MAQ76% AMISOS42%
Cowan [25], 2022	EASE [1]	✓			✓	✓				14	Female	NA	6	NA	NA	NA
Petersen [33], 2022	ACT				✓		✓			12	Female	NA	16	AMISOS10	AMISOS5	AMISOS50%

Abbreviations: ACT, acceptance and commitment therapy; ADHD, attention deficit hyperactivity disorder; AMISO, Amsterdam Misophonia Scale; CBT, cognitive behavioral therapy; DBT, dialectic behavioral therapy; EASE, experiential acceptance and stimulus engagement; ERP, exposure and reaction prevention; MAQ, misophonia assessment questionnaire; MAS, misophonia activation scale; MPRS, misophonia psychological response scale; MQ, misophonia questionnaire; MSS, misophonia severity scale; NA, not applicable; NRT, neural repatterning technique; OCD, obsessive-compulsive disorder; OCSD, obsessive-compulsive spectrum disorder; 7I+35G, 7 individual sessions and 35 group sessions.

TABLE 2
Open Trials and Randomized Clinical Trial of Misophonia Treatment

Studies	Treatment	Cognitive Restructuring	Relaxation Exercises	Counter-Conditioning	Attention Control	ERP	Stimulus manipulation	Others	Participants	Age	Comorbidity	# of Sessions	Symptom Reduce
Open Trials													
Schröder [38], 2017	Group-CBT		✓	✓	✓		✓		90	36	NA	8	AMISOS-R 33%
Frank [36], 2019	Inhibitory Learning	✓				✓			18	35	56%	12	NA
Jager [37], 2021	EMDR							Desensitization and reprocessing	10	35	50% Axis I, 60% Axis II	2.6	AMISOS-R 20%
Randomized Clinical Trial													
Jager [39], 2020	Group-CBT	✓	✓	✓	✓		✓	Psychoeducation for family and friends	27	31	NA	12	AMISOS-R 32%

Abbreviations: AMISOS-R, Amsterdam misophonia scale—revised; CBT, cognitive behavioral therapy; EMDR, eye movement desensitization and reprocessing; NA, not applicable.

a cross-over design, adults with misophonia ($N = 54$) were randomly assigned to 3 months of weekly CBT in a group therapy format or to a waitlist. Participants were assessed at baseline, 3 months (following CBT or waitlist), 6 months (after cross-over), and between months 15 and 18 (1-year follow-up). CBT groups included task concentration, arousal reduction, positive affect labeling, and stimulus manipulation. Across all participants, symptoms of misophonia reduced by 32% after 3 months of CBT (a large effect size estimate of $d = 1.97$). Clinical improvement was observed in 37% of the CBT group compared to 0% in the waiting list group. Those who responded to CBT at post-treatment demonstrated no significant changes in symptoms of misophonia 1 year later, suggesting the effects of CBT maintained over time.

This randomized trial is the clearest evidence supporting the use of any specific treatment of misophonia. However, it should be noted that the comparison condition was an unblinded wait list control without any active intervention components. Additional studies are needed comparing this protocol to credible control conditions featuring non-specific factors such as psychoeducation, therapist time and attention, validation, and/or support. Nonetheless, the findings of this trial and, collectively, the combined findings across the preliminary case studies and open trials largely indicate that components from CBTs (eg, cognitive restructuring, exposure and counter-conditioning, relaxation exercises, interpersonal communication, and acceptance-based skills) may be reasonable for clinicians to consider and in need of future study as treatments of misophonia in both youth and adults.

TRANSDIAGNOSTIC APPROACHES TO PSYCHOTHERAPY

Unified Protocol

As outlined, early studies suggest misophonia (a) is not best accounted for by any psychiatric disorder, (b) is associated with various transdiagnostic psychological problems, and (c) pilot studies developing promising treatments have used various interventions from the family of CBTs. Accordingly, when considering which treatment approaches to scientifically evaluate, it is unclear whether it is appropriate to use a specific branded psychotherapy protocol designed for a specific diagnosis. Although untested, transdiagnostic psychotherapies may be a flexible and pragmatic alternative. The Unified Protocol (UP) is a reasonable candidate for transdiagnostic psychotherapy to consider, as it has been developed

and evaluated for use with a wide range of "emotional disorders," including anxiety and mood disorders [40].

The UP is a 16-week skills-based treatment that consists of five core modules: mindful emotional awareness, cognitive flexibility, identifying and changing emotional avoidance, increasing tolerance of emotion-related physical sensations, and emotional exposures [41]. Patients with misophonia may be characterized by problems with emotional reactivity, limited access to emotion regulation strategies, and intolerance of elevated physical sensations when exposed to trigger sounds [13,42]. The core modules in the UP target these processes. The transdiagnostic approach of the UP has demonstrated efficacy against single-disorder treatments in multiple studies [41,43]. This success may be due to the high rates of co-occurrence between emotional disorders, with anxiety and depressive disorders having lifetime rates of co-occurrence as high as 75% [43]. As examples of efficacy, the UP has demonstrated improvements in anxiety [41], OCDs [44], and dysregulated anger across a range of clinical presentations [45]. Patients with misophonia may have high rates of co-occurring mental health problems [8,14], suggesting that the UP may be a helpful approach to consider.

Although a recent case study examined UP as a possible treatment of adolescents with misophonia [46], controlled clinical trials are needed before conclusions can be made about the efficacy of UP for misophonia. Our own research team is currently conducting preliminary open trials and developing a manual using the UP to treat adults with misophonia. Of eight participants treated with the UP, none dropped out of the treatment, and all reported that they found the treatment helpful. Patients also reported that learning about their own unhelpful coping mechanisms was important, as was enhanced skill use for emotional responses to trigger sounds [47].

Process-Based Therapy (PBT)

Although manualized models of psychotherapy such as the UP may be helpful, another candidate approach that is transdiagnostic and highly flexible is the PBT framework [48]. In PBT, therapists leverage evidence-based therapeutic processes that are common across therapies (eg, strong therapeutic alliance, empathy, support, motivational enhancement) and specific procedures used across protocols for various diagnoses and problems (eg, the list of interventions in Table 1). PBT assessment features functional analyses to identify maladaptive and adaptive patterns and measurement-based care using both qualitative and psychometrically validated quantitative measures of functioning and change processes. Additionally, targets for treatment are collaboratively selected in a sequence that is acceptable to patients and intended to impact other targets in a network of related change processes. This enables an emphasis on patient strengths and empowerment, with assumptions of non-linear change leading to iterative and flexible changes in targets and therapeutic procedures throughout treatment.

When using PBT for misophonia, a therapist and patient determine through functional analyses that there are problematic patterns before, during, or after being triggered across attentional (eg, hypervigilance), cognitive (eg, internal, stable, and global attributions), physiological (eg, sympathetic arousal), social (eg, verbal confrontations), or other behavioral (eg, avoidance or escape behavior) levels of functioning. After discerning specific personally-relevant patterns, problematic patterns are collaboratively prioritized for targeted change. Next, therapeutic procedures known empirically to impact targeted patterns are offered by the therapist, and the patient chooses the one they are most willing and able to do (eg, to reduce physiological arousal when triggered, the patient could choose any protocol known to reduce sympathetic arousal). The intervention is administered, the patient applies the intervention in their daily life, and measures are taken to determine the effects of the intervention. When progress is made on a prioritized target, the patient selects the next most prioritized target to address, and the process repeats itself until patients are satisfied that they have met treatment goals. PBT is an approach that our group is currently testing for misophonia, with a manual under development iteratively based on patient feedback. As such, it is unknown if this approach is efficacious for misophonia.

RESEARCH AGENDA FOR TREATMENT DEVELOPMENT
Mechanistic Translational Studies
Studies identifying underlying neurobehavioral mechanisms of misophonia are needed to develop optimal interventions that target precise biological, social, or behavioral change processes. Candidate targets include difficulties with attention (eg, hypervigilance toward possible misophonic cues), cognition (eg, attributional styles, hopelessness), behavior (eg, avoidance, escape), social (eg, indirect aggression), and emotional (eg, sensitivity, reactivity) processes. As researchers seek to discover underlying biopsychosocial change processes in misophonia, it will be important to do so using multi-method studies with objective laboratory-based measures. Processes that are unique to misophonia and those shared with other sound intolerance or mental health conditions need to be elucidated empirically using thoughtful experimental and statistical approaches.

Global Research with Diverse Participants
To date, most studies investigating misophonia have included disproportionately White, educated women as participants. It may be that these demographic factors align with access to knowledge about misophonia or motivation to participate in research. However, some studies using sampling methodologies with more representative approaches have not reported gender differences in misophonia symptoms [49]. Similarly, no studies have explored ethnicity, race, or multicultural considerations related to misophonia. To understand the nature and features of misophonia for all people, it is essential for researchers to use sampling methods that include diverse participants.

Multi-Disciplinary Treatment Models
Although a multi-disciplinary model of evaluations and treatment is recommended as a general strategy, there are no studies empirically testing this approach. To determine for whom, how, and why this model may be helpful, multi-disciplinary research is needed. This could include direct testing of such an approach compared to usual treatment or discipline-specific interventions. This also could include using adaptive designs that begin with fewer resources and, for those who are non-responsive, randomizing participants to higher resource treatment approaches.

Psychoeducation and Support
It is uncommon for clinical providers or the lay public to have extensive knowledge about misophonia. This overall lack of public awareness about misophonia frequently translates into patients and loved ones needing foundational psychoeducation and support in how to make sense of and manage misophonia. Particularly for caregivers and those with somewhat less impairing misophonia presentations, it may be that psychoeducation and support can serve as an important, low-cost, and scalable component of an overall treatment approach. Studies are needed to examine whether, for whom, and how such approaches can be helpful.

Digital Health
Another recommended approach for treatment development is the use of digital health-based models of care. This could include, for example, interventions using mobile phones with misophonia support apps to screen,

educate, support, and provide specific real-time interventions targeting underlying mechanistic change processes (eg, attentional hypervigilance, emotional reactivity, indirect interpersonal aggression, approach or avoidance behavior, cognitive reframing, or defusion). In addition, digital health approaches that train novel coping skills in virtual environments or with augmented reality could directly target underlying mechanistic targets of change and, in some instances, provide real-time feedback and tailored interventions based on user input and machine learning. These platforms can provide immersive and engaging experiences that may be more desirable for some than conventional treatment approaches such as psychotropic medication or psychotherapy.

CLINICS CARE POINTS

- Misophonia symptoms can occur with or without psychiatric disorders or other health problems. Start treatment with a multi-disciplinary strategy of evaluations and treatment recommendations across audiology, occupational therapy, and mental health providers.

- There are no cures, evidence-based medications, or proven treatments for misophonia. Aim to enhance functioning using interventions known to impact primary processes underlying problematic patterns (physiological arousal, attention, cognition, behavior, communication).

- Given the absence of a proven mental health treatment of misophonia, transdiagnostic evidence-based therapies (eg, UP) and flexible patient-centered frameworks leveraging evidence-based change process may be useful to tailor interventions to the individual (eg, PBT), although require further evaluation.

- Habituation-based exposure therapy is not indicated, but inhibitory learning models of exposure therapy may be helpful as part of a broader treatment approach.

FUNDING

Funding for this work was provided by anonymous supporters of the Duke Center for Misophonia and Emotion Regulation.

DISCLOSURE

The authors have nothing to disclose.

REFERENCES

[1] Swedo SE, Baguley DM, Denys D, et al. Consensus definition of misophonia: a delphi study. Front Neurosci 2022;16:841816.

[2] Brout JJ, Edelstein M, Erfanian M, et al. Investigating misophonia: a review of the empirical literature, clinical implications, and a research agenda. Front Neurosci 2018; 12:36.

[3] Potgieter I, MacDonald C, Partridge L, et al. Misophonia: a scoping review of research. J Clin Psychol 2019;75(7): 1203–18.

[4] Kumar S, Tansley-Hancock O, Sedley W, et al. The brain basis for misophonia. Curr Biol 2017;27(4):527–33.

[5] Edelstein M, Brang D, Rouw R, et al. Misophonia: physiological investigations and case descriptions. Front Hum Neurosci 2013;7:296.

[6] Remmert N, Schmidt KMB, Mussel P, et al. The Berlin Misophonia Questionnaire (BMQ): development and validation of a symptom-oriented diagnostical instrument for the measurement of misophonia. PsyArXiv 2021. https://doi.org/10.31234/osf.io/mujya.

[7] Rosenthal MZ, Anand D, Cassiello-Robbins C, et al. Development and initial validation of the duke misophonia questionnaire. Front Psychol 2021;12:709928.

[8] Rosenthal MZ, McMahon K, Greenleaf AS, et al. Phenotyping misophonia: psychiatric disorders and medical health correlates. Front Psychol 2022;13:941898.

[9] Jastreboff MM, Jastreboff PJ. Components of decreased sound tolerance: hyperacusis, misophonia, phonophobia. ITHS News Letter 2001;2(5–7):1–5.

[10] Schröder A, Vulink N, Denys D. Misophonia: diagnostic criteria for a new psychiatric disorder. PLoS One 2013; 8(1):e54706.

[11] Cassiello-Robbins C, Anand D, McMahon K, et al. A Preliminary investigation of the association between misophonia and symptoms of psychopathology and personality disorders. Front Psychol 2021;11:519681.

[12] Cusack SE, Cash TV, Vrana SR. An examination of the relationship between misophonia, anxiety sensitivity, and obsessive-compulsive symptoms. J Obsessive Compuls Relat Disord 2018;18:41–8.

[13] Guetta RE, Cassiello-Robbins C, Trumbull J, et al. Examining emotional functioning in misophonia: the role of affective instability and difficulties with emotion regulation. PLoS One 2022;17(2):e0263230.

[14] Jager I, de Koning P, Bost T, et al. Misophonia: phenomenology, comorbidity and demographics in a large sample. PLoS One 2020;15(4):e0231390.

[15] McKay D, Kim SK, Mancusi L, et al. Profile Analysis of psychological symptoms associated with misophonia: a community sample. Behav Ther 2018;49(2):286–94.

[16] Quek TC, Ho CS, Choo CC, et al. Misophonia in singaporean psychiatric patients: a cross-sectional study. Int J Environ Res Public Health 2018;15(7):1410.

[17] Rouw R, Erfanian M. A large-scale study of misophonia. J Clin Psychol 2018;74(3):453–79.

[18] Siepsiak M, Sobczak AM, Bohaterewicz B, et al. Prevalence of misophonia and correlates of its symptoms among inpatients with depression. Int J Environ Res Public Health 2020;17(15):5464.

[19] Wu MS, Lewin AB, Murphy TK, et al. Misophonia: incidence, phenomenology, and clinical correlates in an undergraduate student sample. J Clin Psychol 2014;70(10):994–1007.

[20] Kılıç C, Öz G, Avanoğlu KB, et al. The prevalence and characteristics of misophonia in Ankara, Turkey: population-based study. BJPsych Open 2021;7(5):e144.

[21] Sheehan DV, Lecrubier Y, Sheehan KH, et al. The mini-international neuropsychiatric interview (M.I.N.I): the development and validation of a structured diagnostic psychiatric interview for DSM-IV and ICD-10. J Clin Psychiatry 1998;59(Suppl 20):22–33.

[22] Jastreboff PJ, Jastreboff MM. Treatments for decreased sound tolerance (hyperacusis and misophonia). Semin Hear 2014;35(2):105–20.

[23] Altınöz AE, Ünal NE, Altınöz ŞT. The effectiveness of cognitive behavioral psychotherapy in misophonia: a case report. Turk J Clin Psychiatry 2018;21(4):414–7.

[24] Bernstein RE, Angell KL, Dehle CM. A brief course of cognitive behavioural therapy for the treatment of misophonia: A case example. Cogn Behav Ther 2013;6:e10.

[25] Cowan EN, Marks DR, Pinto A. Misophonia: a psychological model and proposed treatment. J Obsessive Compuls Relat Disord 2022;32:100691.

[26] Dover N, McGuire JF. Family-based cognitive behavioral therapy for youth with Misophonia: a case report. Cogn Behav Pract 2021. https://doi.org/10.1016/j.cbpra.2021.05.005.

[27] Dozier TH. Counterconditioning treatment for Misophonia. Clin Case Stud 2015;14(5):374–87.

[28] Dozier TH. Treating the initial physical reflex of misophonia with the neural repatterning technique: a counterconditioning procedure. Psychol Thought 2015;8(2):189–210.

[29] Kamody RC, Del Conte GC. Using dialectical behavior therapy to treat misophonia in adolescence. Prim Care Companion CNS Disord 2017;19(5). https://doi.org/10.4088/PCC.17l02105.

[30] Lewin AB, Dickinson S, Kudryk K, et al. Transdiagnostic cognitive behavioral therapy for misophonia in youth: methods for a clinical trial and four pilot cases. J Affect Disord 2021;291:400–8.

[31] McGuire JF, Wu MS, Storch EA. Cognitive-behavioral therapy for 2 youths with misophonia. J Clin Psychiatry 2015;76(5):573–4.

[32] Muller D, Khemlani-Patel S, Neziroglu F. Cognitive-behavioral therapy for an adolescent female presenting with misophonia: a case example. Clin Case Stud 2018;17(4):249–58.

[33] Petersen JM, Twohig MP. Acceptance and commitment therapy for a child with misophonia: a case study. Clin Case Stud 2022. https://doi.org/10.1177/153465012211 261 15346501221126136.

[34] Reid AM, Guzick AG, Gernand A, et al. Intensive cognitive-behavioral therapy for comorbid misophonic and obsessive-compulsive symptoms: a systematic case study. J Obsessive Compuls Relat Disord 2016;10:1–9.

[35] Schneider RL, Arch JJ. Case study: a novel application of mindfulness-and acceptance-based components to treat misophonia. J Contextual Behav Sci 2017;6(2):221–5.

[36] Frank B, McKay D. The suitability of an inhibitory learning approach in exposure when habituation fails: a clinical application to misophonia. Cogn Behav Pract 2019;26(1):130–42.

[37] Jager I, Vulink N, de Roos C, et al. EMDR therapy for misophonia: a pilot study of case series. Eur J Psychotraumatol 2021;12(1):1968613.

[38] Schröder AE, Vulink NC, van Loon AJ, et al. Cognitive behavioral therapy is effective in misophonia: an open trial. J Affect Disord 2017;217:289–94.

[39] Jager IJ, Vulink NC, Bergfeld IO, et al. Cognitive behavioral therapy for misophonia: a randomized clinical trial. Depress Anxiety 2020;38(7):708–18.

[40] Barlow DH, Sauer-Zavala S, Carl JR, et al. The nature, diagnosis, and treatment of neuroticism back to the future. Clin Psychol Sci 2014;2(3):344–65.

[41] Barlow DH, Farchione TJ, Bullis JR, et al. The unified protocol for transdiagnostic treatment of emotional disorders compared with diagnosis-specific protocols for anxiety disorders: a randomized clinical trial. JAMA Psychiatr 2017;74(9):875–84.

[42] Dozier TH, Morrison KL. Phenomenology of misophonia: initial physical and emotional responses. Am J Psychol 2017;130(4):431–8.

[43] Steele SJ, Farchione TJ, Cassiello-Robbins C, et al. Efficacy of the Unified Protocol for transdiagnostic treatment of comorbid psychopathology accompanying emotional disorders compared to treatments targeting single disorders. J Psychiatr Res 2018;104:211–6.

[44] Sakiris N, Berle D. A systematic review and meta-analysis of the Unified Protocol as a transdiagnostic emotion regulation based intervention. Clin Psychol Rev 2019;72:101751.

[45] Cassiello-Robbins C, Sauer-Zavala S, Brody LR, et al. Exploring the effects of the mindfulness and countering emotional behaviors modules from the Unified Protocol on dysregulated anger in the context of emotional disorders. Behav Ther 2020;51(6):933–45.

[46] Tonarely-Busto NA, Phillips DA, Saez-Clarke E, et al. Applying the unified protocol for transdiagnostic treatment of emotional disorders in children and adolescents to misophonia: a case example. Evid Based Pract Child Adolesc Ment Health 2022;1–15. https://doi.org/10.10 80/23794925.2022.2025631.

[47] McMahon K, Cassiello-Robbins C, Rosenthal MZ. Exploring the Acceptability and Efficacy of a Transdiagnostic Treatment for Misophonia. Misophonia Research Fund Annual Report 2021;1–3.

[48] S.C. Hayes, S.G. Hofmann (Eds.), Process-based CBT: the science and core clinical competencies of cognitive behavioral therapy, New Harbinger Publications, Inc, Oakland, CA, 2018.

[49] Jakubovski E, Müller A, Kley H, et al. Prevalence and clinical correlates of misophonia symptoms in the general population of Germany. Front Psychiatry 2022;13:012424.

Sports Psychiatry

Advances in Psychiatry and Behavioral Health 3 (2023) 43–55

ADVANCES IN PSYCHIATRY AND BEHAVIORAL HEALTH

Obsessive–Compulsive Disorder in Sports–Beyond Superstitions

Check for updates

Carla D. Edwards, MSc, MD, FRCPC[a,*], Cindy Miller Aron, LCSW, CGP, FAGPA[b,c]

[a]Department of Psychiatry and Behavioural Neurosciences, McMaster University, St. Joseph's Healthcare Hamilton, West 5th Campus, Administration B3, Hamilton, ON, L8N 3K7, Canada; [b]Department of Psychiatry, University of Wisconsin School of Medicine and Public Health, Madison, WI, USA; [c]Ascend Consultation in Healthcare/Illinois Sports Performance Center, 737 North Michigan Avenue Suite 1925, Chicago IL 60611, USA

KEYWORDS
- Obsessive-compulsive disorder • Athlete • Sport • Mental health • Obsessions • Compulsions

KEY POINTS
- While superstitions, routines, and peculiar behaviors in sports have been well characterized, they are distinguishable from the features of obsessive-compulsive disorder (OCD).
- OCD is a distinct mental health disorder with potentially debilitating consequences for those afflicted.
- Symptoms of OCD may begin in childhood and follow a waxing and waning course throughout an individual's lifetime.
- Comorbidities are common and may impact response to treatment.
- Interference by OCD symptoms in the function of an athlete can result in physical danger to the athlete, significant disruption in the training environment, and negative performance outcomes.

BACKGROUND

The concepts of superstitions, routines, and peculiar behaviors in sports have been well characterized and sometimes associated with "obsessions" and "compulsions." Numerous high-profile athletes have demonstrated intentional, repeated actions in specific sport scenarios, including Boston Red Sox short stop Nomar Garciaparra's extensive toe-tapping and glove routine before stepping into the batter's box, tennis great Rafael Nadal's ordering of his beverage bottles at his bench, and National Hockey League Hall of Fame goaltender Patrick Roy's post-tapping upon taking his position in front of the net. On a more subtle level, millions of athletes put on their equipment in the same order or wear the same articles of clothing to "increase their team's likelihood of winning" or somehow translate to their own best performance. These are distinctive from preperformance routines, which are learned cognitive and behavioral strategies intentionally used to optimize and enhance sport performance [1]. Preparticipation routines such as breathing and relaxation techniques, use of imagery, focus, and coping strategies are often linked with behavioral approaches and developed by an expert after a team or individual has been assessed. Superstitious and ritualistic behaviors can be seen in fans as well, with routines and actions geared to help their team rally or win. Although these actions are often performed with the belief that they influence the outcome of the competition, there is no actual relationship to the outcome.

While there have been numerous studies characterizing the nature and frequency of superstitions, repetitive behavior, and obsessive and compulsive features

---

*Corresponding author. Department of Psychiatry and Behavioural Neurosciences, McMaster University, 10b Victoria Street South, Kitchener, ON N2G 1C5. E-mail address: edwardcd@mcmaster.ca
Twitter: @Edwards10Carla

https://doi.org/10.1016/j.ypsc.2023.03.002
2667-3827/23/

in athletes, few studies report on the impact of obsessive-compulsive disorder (OCD) in sport [2,3].

To demonstrate the key differences between concepts that will be discussed in this article, it is important to understand their definitions.

A. Superstitions: actions that are deliberate, repetitive, formal, executed sequentially, and distinct from technical performance aspects of the sport, which the athletes believe to have influence over outcomes [4,5].

B. Rituals: a series of actions that are always performed in the same way [6].

C. Obsessions: intrusive thoughts, images, or urges that are recurrent and persistent, which cause the individual to experience distress and to try to suppress or neutralize them with another thought or action [7].

D. Compulsions: repetitive behaviors that the individual feels driven to perform according to rigid rules in response to an obsession, with the intent of reducing distress or preventing a feared outcome [7].

E. OCD: The presence of obsessions, compulsions, or both (as defined in C and D above) which causes clinically significant distress, functional impairment, are time-consuming (eg, consume more than 1 hour per day), and are not attributable to substances or another medical condition [7].

F. Obsessive-compulsive features: the presence of obsessive and compulsive symptoms without meeting full criteria for the disorder.

This review will describe how OCD presents in athletes and its impact on the experience of the athlete and the sport environment. Comorbidities and management approaches will also be explored.

CLINICAL FEATURES OF OCD

Epidemiology and Course

Little data regarding the epidemiology of OCD in athletes have been reported as of the submission date of this article. Several studies have reported the prevalence of obsessive-compulsive symptoms, including one that identified that a majority of its target population of professional tennis players had superstitious rituals and magical thinking, and the athletes scored more highly on the Yale-Brown Obsessive Compulsive Scale than controls (although the scores remained in the subclinical range) [3]. Another study, which screened 270 collegiate athletes from a division 1 university for OCD using the Florida Obsessive Compulsive Inventory, reported that 16.7% of the participants screened positive for OCD, and 5.2% fulfilled OCD criteria for diagnosis

[2]. The 12-month international prevalence of OCD in the general population has been reported to be between 1.1% and 1.8% [7], and the lifetime prevalence of OCD has been reported as 2.3% [8]. Although the mean age of onset in the United States is 19.5 years, 25% of cases are reported to start by 14 years of age, and 25% of affected males have onset before the age of 10 years. The course of OCD is often chronic, with a waxing and waning pattern, and the content of the obsessions and compulsions can change to reflect content appropriate to developmental stage of the individual [7]. The course and trajectory are often complicated by comorbidities. Untreated OCD can result in chronic, waxing and waning symptoms that can follow an episodic or deteriorating course. Early-onset OCD can lead to a lifetime of symptoms although 40% of affected children and adolescents can achieve remission by early adulthood. Remission rates of untreated adults are low [7].

Genetics and Heritability of OCD

There is an elevated prevalence of OCD in family members of individuals with OCD. Substantial heritability of OCD and related disorders has been confirmed through twin and family aggregate studies [9,10], as well as population-based studies [11]. Concordance rates in monozygotic versus dizygotic twins indicate an OCD heritability estimate of 48% [9]. A large multigenerational family clustering study of nearly 25,000 individuals with OCD, who were identified through the Swedish national registers, reported that the risk of OCD was increased in individuals who were more closely related to an affected individual (ie, proband) [11]. This study also found that shared environmental factors did not contribute additional risk to the development of OCD and estimated the genetic contribution of OCD to be 50% [11]. A significant portion of the specific genetic contribution to OCD is unknown [12].

Obsessions

The most common obsessions involve contamination, violent or sexual imagery, aggression, doubting, symmetry, and order [13]. Broader themes include forbidden or taboo thoughts (including religious, sexual, or violent content) and fears of harming oneself or others [7]. Obsessions are egodystonic and unwanted, and affected individuals are often horrified and distressed by their content, which may lead to a delay in identification and treatment [14]. Obsessions are not a reflection of the individual's true thoughts, nor are they an indication of the person's character. Individuals with OCD are often loath to endorse symptoms because of shame and fear of repercussions [15,16]. Obsessions are frequently unrealistic or irrational, and not merely excessive worries about real-life problems [17]. Individuals with OCD generally retain insight (to variable degrees) regarding the irrationality and excessive nature of their obsessive-compulsive behaviors [18].

Compulsions

The most common physical compulsions include washing, ordering, checking, and hoarding, while mental compulsions include counting, praying, repeating words, reassurance seeking, and mental undoing [13,19]. Compulsions are more easily identified in children because they are observable [7]; however, individuals with OCD become adept at hiding their compulsions in public settings or avoiding people and settings that may trigger their symptoms [20,21].

Functional Consequences and Impairment

Impairment is associated with symptom severity and may span numerous life domains, including time spent engaging with symptoms, avoidance of triggering situations, and interference with relationships [7]. Consequences may include academic or work-related delays or incompletions because the product never feels "just right," compromised health due to avoidance of medical appointments and investigations, dermatological problems related to excessive washing, or difficulty maintaining relationships because of harm or sexual obsessions.

For athletes, obsessions and compulsions can include those commonly experienced by the general population and may also extend into specific context relevant to their sport. Consider the cyclist who, while replacing their wheel, must install and remove their wheel seven times to "counteract" their obsessive thought that not doing it 7 times would result in a relative dying. Or the soccer player who must repeat a drill until his execution of a skill felt "just right" (which could require several hours). Although affected individuals exert tremendous effort to control and contain their obsessions and compulsions for purposes of concealment or to maintain function, higher levels of illness severity may result in symptoms spilling into the sport environment. The interference by OCD symptoms in the function of a training or competing athlete can result in physical danger to the athlete, significant disruption in the training environment, and negative performance outcomes. Potential dangers include the use of toxic cleaning products (eg, bleach) either topically or through ingestion to combat contamination obsessions or engaging in risk-taking behaviors to prevent an obsession-related feared outcome (eg, racing downhill on a bike at high speed or holding their breath under water for an excessive period of time to "undo" a distressing thought or image).

Suicide Risk

Suicidality is a relevant phenomenon in patients with OCD. There is a greater risk of suicidality with OCD patients than in the general population [22]. It has been reported that up to 25% of patients with OCD have attempted suicide [23,24]. A systematic review reported the mean prevalence rate of suicide attempts in affected individuals as 14.2%, and lifetime prevalence rates of suicidal ideation at 26.3% to 73.5% (mean 44.1%) [25]. Factors associated with increased suicide risk with OCD include severity of symptoms, unacceptable thoughts, presence and severity of comorbid mood, anxiety and substance use disorders, a history of suicidal behavior, and emotional-cognitive symptoms such as hopelessness and alexithymia [25]. Early detection and treatment with combined psychotherapy and pharmacotherapy are essential for the prevention of suicidal behavior.

NEUROANATOMY AND NEUROBIOLOGY OF OCD

Converging evidence from numerous studies suggest that OCD is a complex disorder whose etiology arises from dysfunction within several brain regions [26]. One model that illustrates the interconnection of the cortico-striato-thalamo-cortical circuit has provided the framework for subsequent imaging studies [27]. Functional brain imaging studies in OCD have largely generated consistent results, showing increased activation in regions of the orbitofrontal cortex, anterior cingulate cortex, and portions of the basal ganglia (particularly the caudate nucleus) when symptoms are active [28,29]. These areas of increased activation demonstrate normalization with successful treatment upon further testing [28,30,31]. These treatments, including medications and exposure and response prevention (ERP), are described in the "Clinical management of OCD" section.

Some cases of OCD have been traced to neuroanatomical etiologies [9]. Evidence for the role of the basal ganglia, particularly the globus pallidus and caudate, in the pathophysiology of OCD has been described in case reports of neurological conditions such as Sydenham chorea [32] and ischemic events [33,34]. A syndrome of childhood-onset OCD has been proposed to be associated with an autoimmune response to infection with group A *Streptococcus*. Pediatric autoimmune neurological disorder associated with *Streptococcus* (PANDAS) and pediatric autoimmune neurological syndrome have an abrupt, dramatic onset of obsessive-compulsive behaviors and associated neurological symptoms such as deterioration in handwriting [35,36]. Antibodies from serum of children with PANDAS has been found to bind specifically to striatal cholinergic interneurons (CINs), and immunoglobulin G has been shown to bind to CINs in the striatum of mice, but not in other brain regions [37]. This evidence suggests that striatal CINs may be the cellular targets for rapid-onset OCD in children.

Drug response data demonstrating reduction in clinical symptoms in response to treatment with serotonergic agents led to the hypothesis that dysfunction in brain serotonergic systems may underlie the pathophysiology of OCD [38]. Emerging data from studies based on imaging, genomics, and cerebrospinal fluid biology are providing momentum for the potential role of the glutamatergic system in the neurobiology of OCD [39–42].

CASE ILLUSTRATION #1

Maya (name and details fictionalized) was a 21-year-old elite diver who was diagnosed with OCD during hospitalization following a recent episode of severe behavioral disturbance in the training environment. On the day of the disturbance, Maya had gone to her coach's office to discuss the recent death of a friend. She became overwhelmed with self-directed disgust about hating her own life while her friend had not lived to the age of 21 years. The resultant panic attack caused her to behave in an impulsive, irrational manner that led to an involuntary hospitalization.

Maya recalled symptoms of OCD since the age of 6 years but kept them hidden because of embarrassment about her ritualistic behaviors. Her obsessions and compulsions changed based on what she was learning about or exposed to. She had chronic symptoms of harm OCD (fear of doing something to harm herself or others). She feared accidently harming young children when they were in her presence and bent her fingers or caused herself to bleed to prevent that from happening.

She experienced graphic images and urges that caused significant distress. While cycling downhill, she had thoughts of hitting the brakes and flying over her handlebars. She did things in sets of 3 (eg, 3, 6, 9, 3 cubed), including removing and reinstalling the wheels of her bicycle in sets of three to help herself feel in control.

Maya had many scars on the back of her hands from a combination of excessive handwashing, punching things when she felt out of control, and damaging her hands when she had harm obsessions. Her coach sometimes commented on the state of her hands (Fig. 1) and interpreted it as intentional self-harm.

Additional obsessions included

- Food that was not prepared by her was contaminated
- Orange objects, food or medications, were contaminated with the toxic herbicide agent orange
- Medications were contaminated or altered, or she had already taken them, which resulted in the need for an extensive, elaborate, and time-consuming inspection and counting routine before taking her medications
- All surfaces were contaminated
- She had a sexually transmitted infection after any intimacy
- Speaking about her thoughts would spread them to other people

Other functional impacts included difficulty living with roommates and having romantic partners because of her symptoms. She was prohibited from training if her hands were bleeding or appeared unhealthy. Interruption of compulsions resulted in having to start from the beginning. She preferred isolation to anyone else knowing about her OCD.

Case Discussion

Maya's case illustrates significant daily functional impairment resultant from severe OCD symptomatology that first appeared in childhood. Symptoms were continuous, and the constant efforts required to neutralize and contain them were exhausting. Obsessions and compulsions were present inside and outside

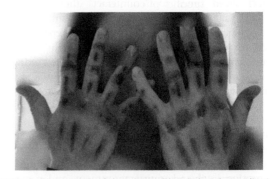

FIG. 1 Photograph of damage to Maya's hands resultant from behaviors related to obsessive-compulsive disorder. The background has been blurred to remove potentially identifying features.

of the sport environment, and despite her efforts to keep her symptoms secret, teammates, the training environment, and team staff were affected by the expression of her symptoms. The use of caustic cleansers on her hands caused significant damage to her skin, and compulsive risk-taking behavior undertaken to counteract obsessions created several dangerous situations.

SPORT-SPECIFIC OCD-RELATED DISRUPTIONS

OCD manifestations that may create disturbance in sport include

- Rigidity about nutrition could result in challenges navigating eating and drinking during travel and competition
- Contamination concerns could cause difficulties and distress in high-traffic areas such as airports and in enclosed spaces such as on airplanes or elevators
- Distracting intrusive thoughts during an intense effort, workout, or competition could place the athlete at risk of injury
- Rigid and elaborate self-care and bedtime routines could create challenges during team travel
- Physical compulsions witnessed by teammates and coaches could cause them to feel uncomfortable being around the affected individual and lead to prohibition from training and competitions

COMORBIDITIES AND OTHER ASSOCIATED CONDITIONS

Comorbid conditions have been reported in up to 90% of individuals with OCD [8,43]. Illnesses that commonly co-occur with OCD include anxiety disorders (eg, panic disorder, generalized anxiety disorder, social anxiety disorder, and specific phobia), mood disorders, and obsessive-compulsive personality disorder [7]. Disorders experienced more frequently by individuals with OCD than by those without include obsessive-compulsive-related disorders such as body dysmorphic disorder (BDD), trichotillomania (pathological hair-pulling), and excoriation disorder (skin picking) [7].

OCD and Eating Disorders

The entanglement between eating disorders (EDs) and OCD has been an enduring point of inquiry and diagnostic confusion both in and out of the sport context. The Diagnostic and Statistical Manual of Mental Disorders, fifth edition, (DSM-5) notes that OCD should not be diagnosed if OCD-like symptoms consist solely of ritualized eating behaviors that are better explained by an ED

[6]. In 1 global study, 18% of the general population with anorexia nervosa and 15% with bulimia nervosa had a concurrent diagnosis of OCD [44]. The prevalence and risk of OCD and ED is highest in cases of anorexia nervosa, binge/purge type [45]. Curiosity and persistence in the exploration of the individuals' history can reveal underlying issues that need to be addressed, while simultaneously clarifying the diagnostic picture. These disorders can also be experienced in a nonconcurrent manner, as 10% of individuals with OCD are diagnosed with an ED at some point in their lifetimes, and acquiring both conditions increases the likelihood of more severe pathology [46]. Additionally, OCD- and ED-afflicted individuals frequently have symptoms of posttraumatic stress disorder, depression, and social anxiety [46]. The variation in prevalence of EDs can be sport-specific, with sports that are aesthetically judged, have weight classes or are gravitational in nature, or have an emphasis on lean muscle mass placing athletes at higher risk of EDs [47]. The prevalence of disordered eating or EDs in athletes has been estimated at up to 19% in male athletes and 6% to 45% in female athletes [48].

OCD and Orthorexia Nervosa

Although orthorexia nervosa (ON) is not formally recognized in the DSM-5, it has been increasingly recognized since the term was introduced in the late 1990s. Orthorexia presents as a pathological obsession with healthy eating and control over food intake. This can lead to the ritualistic establishment of a restricted diet, including preparation, checking ingredients, and strict avoidance of certain foods. Afflicted athletes place an exaggerated importance on the value of healthy foods. ON involves a dramatic shift from the act of nourishment to elimination of most foods because of fear of impurities. This rigid belief can cause the athlete to avoid social situations that involve food, creating disruption in their psychosocial environment, and leading to significant anxiety related to eating. As foods are restricted, weight is lost, nutritional deficiencies occur, and performance declines [49]. The rigid, restrictive behaviors can resemble anorexia nervosa as well as OCD. There is conflicting evidence and controversy regarding whether orthorexia is on the ED spectrum or the OCD spectrum although it is generally more closely associated with EDs [50]. Elite athletes are at higher risk of developing ON given the cultural focus on appropriate food intake to enhance performance [51].

OCD and Body Dysmorphic Disorder

BDD has been examined through the lens of obsessive-compulsive spectrum disorder for more than a century [52]. In the DSM-5, it is grouped with "OCD and other related disorders" [7] and is characterized by preoccupation with an imagined or slight defect in appearance. This preoccupation causes significant distress in the individual, creating impairment socially, occupationally, or in other areas of the affected individual's life [52].

Similarities between BDD-related preoccupations and OCD-related obsessions include intrusiveness, persistence, repetitiveness, and the fact that they are unwanted thoughts that are recognized as one's own. Most individuals with BDD have at least 1 compulsion, such as checking oneself in the mirror, seeking reassurance, skin picking, excessive grooming, or comparing themselves with others [7].

Muscle dysphoria is a subset of BDD in the DSM-5 in which the afflicted individual is preoccupied with their body and/or build being too small or lacking in musculature. This has garnered increasing attention during the last 2 decades. Its distinguishing feature primarily focuses upon increased muscle size. Body builders, many of whom are athletes, can become preoccupied with concerns that their body is not muscular and/or lean enough, creating ongoing distress [53].

OCD and Perfectionism

Perfectionism is well researched in sport and manifests in psychological, emotional, and behavioral tendencies [54]. Adaptive perfectionistic strivings are expressed by athletes who derive satisfaction from intensive training and competition and have the ability to tolerate their own imperfections without excessive self-criticism [55]. Perfectionism can be a powerful driver and motivator for achievement, even if there is an unrealistic establishment of personal standards [54]. Perfectionism can become maladaptive when athletes find themselves troubled by thoughts that are intrusive, persistent, negative, and self-deprecating and that are not amenable to typical mental skills work. Rumination focused on an excessive concern for mistakes can be a manifestation of OCD. Athletes with high degrees of perfectionism may be more susceptible to the negative consequences of traumatic life events. Maladaptive perfectionism in combination with a high-perceived-stress response put an athlete at greater risk of performance breakdowns [55].

CASE ILLUSTRATION #2

Mark (name and details fictionalized) was a 29-year-old male professional endurance athlete who presented at an outpatient mental health clinic for evaluation of mood. He described fluctuation in mood, depressive symptoms,

irritability, and anxiety. While he was highly successful between the ages of 18 and 24 years, drug and alcohol misuse between ages 24 and 29 caused him to drop out of elite sport. Several months before the assessment, he entered sobriety, embraced lifestyle changes, and viewed therapy as an integral component of his support. Return to sport was part of his "hero's journey." Mark focused on what he ate, his mileage, heart rate, and weight and maintained a meticulous focus on training and performance times. He viewed himself as a perfectionist and did not believe that his approach to sport was problematic or substantially different from his peers. A previous medication (selective serotonin reuptake inhibitor [SSRI]) had no impact on symptoms. Given his persistent agitation, anxiety, and obsessive thinking, psychiatric assessment was recommended.

Despite being highly functioning at work, he was disappointed in his professional achievements. He expressed deep feelings of self-loathing, harbored regret about failures in his athletic career, and had a burning desire to "'prove himself as a winner." He envisioned becoming well known for his use of sobriety as the pathway to athletic success. During assessment, he endorsed mild depression as well as occasional agitation and anxiety when he was alone at home. Anxiety at work primarily surrounded his need to be desired by the younger women in that setting. He spent increasingly longer periods of time tracking his interactions with different women and ruminating about whether they found him attractive. Mark described a significant childhood worry about his parents dying. Upon arriving home from school 1 day at the age of 12 years, he walked in on his parents having sex. He described the experience as "terrifying" and viewed the experience as traumatic. The experience amplified his fears of harm coming to his parents, and he eventually lived with his mother when his parents divorced.

Approximately 1 year into treatment, Mark abruptly shifted to a plant-based diet and hyperfocused on his running. He engaged in significant nutritional rigidity, which included counting every piece of food consumed, counting calories, and measuring exact portions. He increased his mileage against coaching recommendations, neglected rest periods, and described his long runs as an almost spiritual experience. He unintentionally lost weight and failed to meet competition goals. This led to a cycle of increased volume and intensity of training, which left him increasingly depleted and depressed. He developed chronic overuse injuries. His obsession with young women at work increased, as did his sexual activity with them. As he felt unable to control his thoughts and behaviors, food restrictions increased because of his frustration with his perceived "failures." Once muscle wasting became observable, his fatigue became debilitating, and he had increasing difficulty getting out of bed for training. His mood plummeted and sense of despair soared. In an episode of emotional dysregulation, he broke down and sobbed on the floor, feeling hopeless and unable to move. He was evaluated for suicidal ideation in the emergency department and was released the following morning to his outpatient supports.

After this experience, Mark was open to considering the concerns raised by his health care providers. He took a leave of absence from sport to recover from a mental health and general physical health standpoint and attended to his disordered eating and comorbidities of hypothyroidism and low testosterone. He adhered to treatment recommendations and recovered over the course of 6 to 12 months. In this process, he shifted sports and explored geographical relocation to support his new professional and athletic interests.

Case Discussion

Mark's case presented a challenging diagnostic picture with his presenting symptoms of mild depression, moderate agitation and anxiety, a history of substance misuse, and a positive family history of mood disorder. Additional salient features included irrational childhood fears about his parents, difficulty with emotional attunement, fears and obsessions about sexuality, and excessive rigidity related to food, work, and exercise. He later developed orthorexia, overexercising/exercise dependence, and severe depression, which impaired performance. Mark was diagnosed with major depressive disorder with atypical features and prescribed bupropion (once it was assured that nutritional intake was adequate and that there was no purging) in addition to escitalopram. He was referred to an endocrinologist to address hypothyroidism and low testosterone and then to a nutritionist to increase his caloric and nutritional intake. Psychotherapeutic approaches involved a combination of insight-oriented work integrated with cognitive behavior therapy (CBT) techniques for managing anxiety, mood, and compulsions. This combination of biopsychosocial interventions fostered a considerable integration of self and capacity for interpersonal and professional success.

SCREENING AND DIAGNOSTIC CONSIDERATIONS

Although the timing between OCD symptom onset, assessment, and treatment can be delayed, patients are often aware of their symptoms long before they are on anyone else's radar [56]. Signs and symptoms that should raise suspicion and lead to diagnostic screening include

- Excessive resistance to change
- Excessive time spent on routine tasks
- Rigidity in thinking or behavior
- Refusal to touch surfaces with bare hands
- Excessive handwashing or checking
- Routines that must be carried out to completion in the same way every time
- Interruption in compulsions results in significant distress

Although there are several diagnostic interviews for OCD, the most common assessment instruments are the Yale-Brown Obsessive Compulsive Scale [57–59], the Yale-Brown Obsessive Compulsive Scale adapted for children [59,60], and the Obsessive-Compulsive Inventory-Revised [61]. These instruments assess for historic and current obsessions and compulsions, degree of symptom severity, time consumed by symptoms, and magnitude of distress experienced.

CLINICAL MANAGEMENT OF OCD

As no data regarding the management of OCD in athletes had been reported at the time of submission of this article, we present an overview of management approaches for OCD in the general population within the context of general principles of mental health management in athletes. Numerous factors influence the initial choice of treatment approach and setting. General principles of treatment planning should involve consideration of the following elements [62].

- Nature of OCD symptoms
- Symptom severity
- Comorbid conditions (including treatment)
- Treatment history
- Current treatment
- Side effect profiles
- Availability of psychotherapy
- Patient preference
- Engagement in treatment
- Role of supports in illness accommodation and treatment (eg, are they able to support efforts—however painful—at ERP in their loved ones?)

Treatment should be provided in the least restrictive setting to provide safe and effective care [22,63]. Hospital-based treatment may be required if there are concerns about safety, self-care, or significant functional impairment [62]. Residential treatment may be required for individuals needing intensive multidisciplinary treatment and monitoring [64], and partial hospitalization programs may be indicated for individuals who need daily psychotherapy, medication monitoring, and other psychosocial treatments [65]. Patients who are unable to leave their homes because of symptoms such as hoarding and contamination concerns may require home-based care. Initial treatment can typically be started in the outpatient setting, and early focus on education and establishing a therapeutic alliance is important [62].

Psychological Treatment

While athletes represent a highly motivated group who regularly engage in goal setting and practice, they may be reluctant to engage in psychotherapy because of stigma, minimization of symptoms, and less positive attitudes toward mental health services than the general population [66].

Cognitive and behavioral therapy approaches—in particular, CBT featuring ERP—have been demonstrated to be effective in the treatment of OCD [67–69]. ERP is the first-line psychotherapy for OCD and has been associated with large treatment effects [70,71]. ERP targets the negative reinforcement of compulsions and avoidance and involves gradual and systematic exposure to distress-evoking stimuli while refraining from distress-reducing behaviors [18]. Response to CBT is equivalent or superior to pharmacotherapy [72–74]. Other therapeutic techniques that have demonstrated benefits in managing OCD include acceptance and commitment therapy and mindfulness training [75,76]. Severe anxiety or depression can interfere with the individual's ability to engage in the cognitive and behavioral homework that is typically required in CBT [62].

Pharmacological Treatment

When considering pharmacological agents for use in athletes, it is recommended that the clinician remain mindful of adverse effects that may impact athletic performance (such as sedation and weight gain).

SSRIs and clomipramine are the mainstay of pharmacological treatment for OCD. Numerous randomized control trials (RCTs) confirmed that clomipramine and SSRIs were superior to placebo for treating OCD [77–81]. RCTs and meta-analyses demonstrated significant benefits from the SSRIs fluoxetine (20–60 mg), sertraline (150–200 mg), fluvoxamine (100–300 mg; max 200 mg in children younger than 11 years), paroxetine (20–60 mg, pediatric starting dose 10 mg), and escitalopram (5–20 mg) with no difference separating agents when pooled response rates are considered. Dose ranges reflect US Food and Drug

Administration (FDA) indications; however, escitalopram does not have an FDA indication for OCD. Both citalopram and escitalopram have been shown to be safe and effective in treating OCD in large, double-blind European trials [82,83]. Response rates to SSRIs have been reported at twice those of placebo (40%–60% vs <20%) [73,74,84–86]. Second-line agents include clomipramine (150–250 mg, pediatric dosing 100–200 mg), mirtazapine (no FDA indication, adult dosing only, 15–45 mg), and venlafaxine XR (no FDA indication, adult dosing only, 75–225 mg) [72,84,87,88]. While clomipramine performed similarly to the SSRIs in terms of efficacy, SSRIs are generally preferred because of their better-tolerated side effect profile, especially in athletes. Common adverse effects reported with clomipramine include dry mouth, constipation, blurred vision, urinary retention, orthostatic hypotension, weight gain, and sedation [22,84,89,90], while serious side effects may include cardiac arrhythmias, seizures, drug interactions, and toxicity during overdose [22,90]. Effective pharmacological treatment for OCD typically requires moderate to high doses and the need to wait several weeks (up to 12 weeks) for the patient to demonstrate clinical response (which is defined as a reduction in baseline symptoms by 25% to 35%) [25,62,91,92].

Augmentation with certain atypical antipsychotic medications (such as risperidone) can be used for treatment-resistant cases [63,93–95]. Antidepressants that do not bind with high affinity to the serotonin transporter are not generally effective for OCD [39]. Childhood onset, longer duration of illness, and diminished insight are associated with a poorer response to SSRIs [96].

Glutamate modulators have been studied as potential augmenting agents for treatment-resistant OCD. N-acetylcysteine (NAC, 600 mg-3000 mg/d, delivered in divided doses) showed greater efficacy in reducing OCD symptoms when combined with an SSRI in 3 of 5 RCTs [97,98]. NAC is not currently regulated by the FDA. Trials of lamotrigine (up to 100 mg/d), topiramate (up to 400 mg/d), riluzole (up to 100 mg/d), memantine (up to 20 mg/d), and intravenous ketamine (single dose of 0.5 mg/kg) have yielded preliminary evidence of efficacy when the drugs are added to SSRIs in patients with treatment-resistant OCD [98–100]. One case report described the effect of intranasal ketamine on OCD symptoms [101,102].

Combined Treatment

The combination of psychological and pharmacological treatments outperformed pharmacological approaches alone, but not CBT alone [61,103]. Combined treatment may enhance treatment response and improve relapse prevention [88].

Additional Treatments

Beyond the described psychological and pharmacological treatments, there are few evidence-based alternatives. A form of repetitive transcranial magnetic stimulation has been approved by the FDA for treatment of OCD [104]. The most severe and refractory cases may require consideration of neurosurgical interventions such as stereotactic ablation [105,106] or deep brain stimulation [107,108].

Treatment Caveats

Before choosing pharmacological agents for the treatment of any condition involving athletes competing in high-performance or international settings, care should be taken to refer to worldwide databases of prohibited substances, as some agents may be prohibited during competitions or at all times (depending on the agent and the sport). Resources such as the Global Drug Reference Online provide athletes and support personnel with information about the prohibited status of specific medications based on the current World Anti-Doping Agency (WADA) Prohibited list [109]. If a medication is prohibited in competition, a Therapeutic Use Exemption would be required to enable the athlete to maintain treatment without incurring an adverse analytic finding and an antidoping rule violation resulting in sanction.

SUMMARY

OCD is distinctly different from superstitions, sport rituals, and preperformance routines in their definitions and functional impact. It is a chronic disorder that can significantly impact function and quality of life beginning in childhood. Although most of the obsessions and compulsions are experienced privately, more severe forms can spill into professional and sport settings. When this happens, the athlete, training environment, team staff, and facility staff may be impacted by the symptoms. Specific sport-focused manifestations of the most common obsessions and compulsions can be anticipated, and the presence of symptoms should trigger assessment. Comorbidities are common and influence the course of treatment and outcomes. Untreated OCD can have a chronic and debilitating course. Safe and successful treatments are available for OCD and its comorbid conditions, and early identification of these symptoms may lead to earlier treatment

and mitigate the development of more severe pathology. Established first-line treatment modalities for OCD are limited to CBT with ERP and SSRIs; however, 25% to 40% of patients fail to respond to either of these approaches [18]. Treatment typically requires higher dosages of medications and long periods of time before a response is identified. Partial hospitalization programs, residential treatment, and neuromodulation treatments may be required for refractory cases. Further understanding of the neurobiology of OCD may help to develop new treatments and interventions.

Future research is needed to explore epidemiology and treatment outcomes of OCD in the athlete population.

CLINICS CARE POINTS

- Screen for obsessive-compulsive disorder (OCD) if indicators of common obsessions and compulsions are identified, including excessive rigidity in thoughts and behavior, excessive time spent on tasks, and excessive checking and cleaning behaviors.
- Screen for OCD if features of common comorbidities are present, such as peculiar eating behavior, perfectionism, or excessive concern about physical appearance.
- Recommend psychotherapy with a provider experienced in cognitive behavioral therapy with exposure and response prevention for treatment of OCD.
- Consider pharmacotherapy with a selective serotonin reuptake inhibitor early in the clinical management course to improve outcomes, being mindful of adverse effects that may impact athletic performance (such as sedation and weight gain).
- Pharmacotherapy may require higher doses and longer periods of time before treatment response emerges.

DISCLOSURE

The authors have nothing to disclose.

REFERENCES

[1] Cohn PI. Preperformance routines in sport: Theoretical support and practical applications. Sport Psychol 1990; 4:301–12.

[2] Cromer L, Kaier E, Davis J, et al. OCD in college athletes. Aust J Pharm 2017;174:595–7.

[3] Marazziti D, Parra E, Amadori, et al. Obsessive-compulsive and depressive symptoms in professional tennis players. Clinical Neuropsychiatry 2021;18(6):304–11.

[4] Bleak JL, Frederick CM. Superstitious behavior in sport: levels of effectiveness and determinants of use in three collegiate sports. J Sport Behav 1998;21:1–15.

[5] Womack M. Why Athletes Need Ritual: A study of magic among professional athletes. In: Hoffman S, editor. Sport and religion. Champaign. IL: Human Kinetics; 1992. p. 191–202.

[6] Available at: https://www.oxfordlearnersdictionaries.com/us/definition/english/ritual_1?q=rituals. Accessed November 19, 2022.

[7] American Psychiatric Association. Diagnostic and statistical manual of mental disorders (DSM-5). Washington, DC: American Psychiatric Publishing; 2013. p. 237–42.

[8] Ruscio AM, Stein DJ, Chiu WT, et al. The epidemiology of obsessive-compulsive disorder in the National Comorbidity Survey Replication. Mol Psychiatry 2010;15(1):53–63.

[9] Fernandez TV, Leckman JF, Pittenger C. Genetic susceptibility in obsessive-compulsive disorder. Handb Clin Neurol 2018;148:767–81.

[10] Monzani B, Rijsdijk F, Harris J, et al. The structure of genetic and environmental risk factors for dimensional representations of DSM-5 obsessive-compulsive spectrum disorders. JAMA Psychiatr 2014;71:182–9.

[11] Mataix-Cole D, Boman M, Monzani B, et al. Population-based multigeneral family clustering study of obsessive-compulsive disorder. JAMA Psychiatr 2013;70:709–17.

[12] Grice DE. Don't worry, the genetics of obsessive-compulsive disorder is finally catching up. Biol Psychiatry 2020;87:1017–8.

[13] Hollander E, Kim S, Khanna S, et al. Obsessive-Compulsive Disorder and Obsessive-Compulsive Spectrum Disorders: Diagnostic and Dimensional Issues. CNS Spectr 2007;12(S3):5–13.

[14] Hollander E. Obsessive-compulsive disorder: the hidden epidemic. J Clin Psychiatry 1997;58(suppl 12):3–6.

[15] Torres AR, Prince MJ. The Importance of Epidemiological studies on obsessive-compulsive disorder (Editorial). Rev Bras Psiquiatr 2004;26(3):141–2.

[16] Simonds LM, Elliot SA. OCD patients and non-patients groups reporting obsessions and compulsions: phenomenology, help-seeking, and access to treatment. Br J Med Psychol 2001;74:431–49.

[17] AACAP facts for families #60: obsessive compulsive disorder in children and adolescents. Available at: https://www.aacap.org/AACAP/Families_and_Youth/Facts_for_Families/FFF-Guide/Obsessive-Compulsive-Disorder-In-Children-And-Adolescents-060.aspx Updated October 2018. Accessed November 20, 2022.

[18] Goodman WK, Storch EA, Sheth SA. Harmonizing the neurobiology and treatment of obsessive-compulsive disorder. Am J Psychiatr 2021;178(1):17–29.

[19] Williams MT, Farris SG, Turkheimer E, et al. Myth of the pure obsessional type in obsessive–compulsive disorder. Depress Anxiety 2011;28(6):495–500.

[20] Fennel D. The World of obsessive-compulsive disorder: the experiences of living with OCD7. NY: NYU Press; 2022. p. 92.

[21] Geller DA, March J. Practice parameter for the assessment and treatment of children and adolescents with obsessive-compulsive disorder. J Am Acad Child Adolesc Psychiatry 2012;51(1):98–113.

[22] American Psychiatric Association. Practice guideline for the treatment of patients with obsessive-compulsive disorder. Arlington, VA: American Psychiatric Association; 2007. Available at: http//www.psych.org/psych_pract/treatg/pg/prac_guide.cfm. Accessed December 13, 2012.

[23] Torres AR, Prince MJ, Bebbington PE, et al. Obsessive-compulsive disorder: prevalence, comorbidity, impact, and help-seeking in the British National Psychiatric Morbidity Survey of 2000. Am J Psychiatr 2006;163:1978–85.

[24] Torres AR, Ramos-Cerqueira AT, Ferrao YA, et al. Suicidality in obsessive-compulsive disorder: prevalence and relation to symptom dimensions and comorbid conditions. J Clin Psychiatry 2011;72:17–26 [quiz 119-120].

[25] Albert U, De Ronchi D, Maina G, et al. Suicide Risk in Obsessive-Compulsive Disorder and Exploration of Risk Factors: A Systematic Review. Curr Neuropharmacol 2019;17(8):681–96.

[26] Yuste R. From the neuron doctrine to neural networks. Nat Rev Neurosci 2015;16:487–97.

[27] Milad MR, Rauch SL. Obsessive-compulsive disorder: beyond segregated cortico-striatal pathways. Trends Cogn Sci 2012;16:43–51.

[28] Saxena S, Rauch SL. Functional neuroimaging and the neuroanatomy of obsessive-compulsive disorder. Psychiatr Clin North Am 2000;23:563–86.

[29] Breiter HC, Rauch SL, Kwong KK, et al. Functional Magnetic resonance imaging of symptom provocation in obsessive-compulsive disorder. Arch Gen Psychiatry 1996;53:595–606.

[30] Schwartz JM, Stoessel PW, Baxter LR Jr, et al. Systematic changes in cerebral glucose metabolic rate after successful behavior modification treatment of obsessive-compulsive disorder. Arch Gen Psychiatry 1996;53:109–13.

[31] Benkelfat C, Nordahl TE, Semple WE, et al. Local cerebral glucose metabolic rates in obsessive-compulsive disorder. Patients treated with clomipramine. Arch Gen Psychiatry 1990;47:840–8.

[32] Asbahr FR, Garvey MA, Snider LA, et al. Obsessive-compulsive symptoms among patients with Sydenham chorea. Biol Psychiatry 2005;57:1073–6.

[33] Thobois S, Jouanneau E, Bouvard M, et al. Obsessive-compulsive disorder after unilateral caudate nucleus bleeding. Acta Neurochir 2004;146:1027–31 [discussion 1031].

[34] Grados MA. Obsessive-compulsive disorder after traumatic brain injury. Int Rev Psychiatry 2003;15:350–8.

[35] Swedo SE, Leonard HL, Garvey M, et al. Pediatric autoimmune neuropsychiatric disorders associated with streptococcal infections: clinical description of the first 80 cases. Am J Psychiatr 1998;155:264–71.

[36] Murphy TK, Patel PD, McGuire JF, et al. Characterization of the pediatric acute-onset neuropsychiatric syndrome phenotype. J Child Adolesc Psychopharmacol 2015;25:14–25.

[37] Xu J, Liu RJ, Fahey S, et al. Antibodies from children with PANDAS bind specifically to striatal cholinergic interneurons and alter their activity. Am J Psychiatr 2021;178:48–64.

[38] Goodman WK, McDougle CJ, Price LH, et al. Beyond the serotonin hypothesis: a role for dopamine in some forms of obsessive-compulsive disorder? J Clin Psychiatry 1990;51(Suppl):36–43 [discussion: 55-58].

[39] Brennan BP, Rauch SL, Jensen JE, et al. A critical review of magnetic resonance spectroscopy studies of obsessive-compulsive disorder. Biol Psychiatry 2013;73:24–31.

[40] Stewart SE, Mayerfield C, Arnold PD, et al. Meta-analysis of association between obsessive-compulsive disorder and the 3c region of neuronal glutamate transporter gene SLC1A1. Am J Med Genet B Neuropsychiatr Genet 2013;162B:367–79.

[41] Bhattacharyya S, Khanna S, Chakrabarty K, et al. Anti-brain autoantibodies and altered excitatory neurotransmitters in obsessive-compulsive disorder. Neuropsychopharmacology 2009;34:2489–96.

[42] Chakrabarty K, Bhattacharyya S, Christopher R, et al. Glutamatergic dysfunction in OCD. Neuropsychopharmacology 2005;30:1735–40.

[43] Katzman MA, Bleau P, Blier P, et al. Canadian clinical practice guidelines for the management of anxiety, post-traumatic stress and obsessive-compulsive disorders. BMC Psychiatr 2014;14(Suppl 1):S1.

[44] Mandelli L, Draghetti S, Albert U, et al. Rates of comorbid obsessive-compulsive disorder in eating disorders: A meta-analysis of the literature. J Affect Disord 2020 Dec 1;277:927–39.

[45] Drakes DH, Fawcett EJ, Rose JP, et al. Comorbid obsessive-compulsive disorder in individuals with eating disorders: An epidemiological meta-analysis. J Psychiatr Res 2021;141:176–91.

[46] Danner UN, Sternheim LC, van Oppen P, et al. The relationship between eating disorders and OCD symptom dimensions: An explorative study in a large sample of patients with OCD. Journal of Obsessive Compulsive and Related Disorders 2002;35.

[47] Wells KR, Jeacocke NA, Appaneal R, et al. The Australian Institute of Sport (AIS) and National Eating Disorders Collaboration (NEDC) position statement on disordered eating in high performance sport. Br J Sports Med 2020;54(21):1247–58.

[48] Bratland-Sanda S, Sundgot-Borgen J. Eating disorders in athletes: overview of prevalence, risk factors and recommendations for prevention and treatment. Eur J Sport Sci 2013;13(5):499–508.

[49] Bennett K. Treating athletes with eating disorders: bridging the gap between sport and clinical worlds. New York, NY: Routledge; 2021.

[50] Zagaria A, Vacca M, Cerolini S, et al. Associations between orthorexia, disordered eating, and obsessive-compulsive symptoms: A systematic review and meta-analysis. Int J Eat Disord 2022;55(3):295–312.

[51] Uriegas NA, Winkelmann ZK, Pritchett K, et al. Examining Eating Attitudes and Behaviors in Collegiate Athletes, the Association Between Orthorexia Nervosa and Eating Disorders. Front Nutr 2021;8:763838. https://doi.org/10.3389/fnut.2021.763838.

[52] Phillips KA, Pinto A, Menard W, et al. Obsessive–compulsive disorder versus body dysmorphic disorder: a comparison study of two possibly related disorders. Depress Anxiety 2017;24(6):399–409.

[53] Esco MR, Olson MS, Williford HN. Muscle dysmorphia: An emerging body image concern in men. Strength Condit J 2005;27(6):76.

[54] Aron CM, LeFay SM. Post-traumatic Stress Disorder and Other Trauma-Related Disorders. In: Reardon CL, editor. Mental health care for elite athletes. Switzerland: Springer; 2022. p. 69–78.

[55] Aron CM, Harvey S, Hainline B, et al. Post-traumatic stress disorder (PTSD) and other trauma-related mental disorders in elite athletes: a narrative review. Br J Sports Med 2019;53(12):779–84.

[56] Hollander E, Kwon JH, Stein DJ, et al. Obsessive-compulsive and spectrum disorders: overview and quality of life issues. J Clin Psychiatry 1996;57(suppl 8):3–6.

[57] Yale-Brown Obsessive Compulsive Scale. https://pandasnetwork.org/wp-content/uploads/2018/11/y-bocs-w-checklist.pdf Retrieved November 23, 2022.

[58] Storch EA. Measuring obsessive-compulsive symptoms: common tools and techniques. International OCD Foundation. Summer 2005. Available at: https://iocdf.org/expert-opinions/expert-opinion-measuring-oc-symptoms/. Accessed November 23, 2022.

[59] YBOCS-SR. Available at: https://static1.squarespace.com/static/58cab82ff5e231f0df8d9cad/t/60945b3af4680c68037f8188/1620335418443/YBOCS-II-SR.pdf. Accessed November 23, 2022.

[60] Scahill L, Riddle MA, McSwiggin-Hardin M, et al. Children's Yale-Brown Obsessive Compulsive Scale: reliability and validity. J Am Acad Child Adolesc Psychiatry 1997;36:844–52.

[61] Foa EB, Huppert JD, Leiberg S, et al. The Obsessive-Compulsive Inventory: Development and validation of a short version. Psychological Assessment 2002;14(4):485–96.

[62] Koran L. Obsessive-Compulsive Disorder : An Update for the Clinician. Focus 2007;5(3):281–388. Available at: https://focus.psychiatryonline.org/doi/epdf/10.1176/foc.5.3.foc299. Accessed December 13, 2022.

[63] Koran L, Simpson HB. Guideline Watch (March 2013): Practice guideline for the treatment of patients with obsessive-compulsive disorder. Available at: https://psychiatryonline.org/pb/assets/raw/sitewide/practice_guidelines/guidelines/ocd-watch.pdf. Accessed December 13, 2022.

[64] Stewart SE, Stack DE, Farrell C, et al. Effectiveness of intensive residential treatment (IRT) for severe, refractory obsessive-compulsive disorder. J Psychiatr Res 2005;39:603–9.

[65] Bystritsky A, Saxena S, Maidment K, et al. Quality-of-life changes among patients with obsessive-compulsive disorder in a partial hospitalization program. Psychiatr Serv 1999;50:412–4.

[66] Stillman MA, Glick I, McDuff D, et al. Psychotherapy for mental health symptoms and disorders in elite athletes: a narrative review. Br J Sports Med 2019;53(12): 767–71.

[67] Rosa-Alcazar AI, Sanchez-Meca J, Gomez-Conesa A, et al. Psychological treatment of obsessive-compulsive disorder: a meta-analysis. Clin Psychol Rev 2008;28: 1310–25.

[68] Hoffmann SG, Smits JA. Cognitive-behavioral therapy for adult anxiety disorders: a meta-analysis of randomized placebo-controlled trials. J Clin Psychiatry 2008; 69:621–32.

[69] Abramowitz JS. Effectiveness of psychological and pharmacological treatments for obsessive-compulsive disorder: a quantitative review. J Consult Clin Psychol 1997; 65:44–52.

[70] Ost LG, Havnen A, Hansen B, et al. Cognitive behavioral treatments of obsessive-compulsive disorder. A systematic review and meta-analysis of studies published 1993-2014. Clin Psychol Rev 2015;40:156–69.

[71] McGuire JF, Piacentini J, Lewin AB, et al. A meta-analysis of cognitive behavior therapy and medication for child obsessive-compulsive disorder: moderators of treatment efficacy, response and remission. Depress Anxiety 2015;32:580–93.

[72] Foa E, Liebowitz M, Kozak M, et al. Randomized, placebo-controlled trial of exposure and ritual prevention, clomipramine, and their combination in the treatment of obsessive-compulsive disorder. Am J Psychiatr 2005;162:151–61.

[73] Sousa MB, Isolan LR, Oliveira RR, et al. A randomized clinical trial of cognitive-behavioral group therapy and sertraline in the treatment of obsessive-compulsive disorder. J Clin Psychiatry 2006;67:1133–9.

[74] Belotto-Silva C, Diniz JB, Malavazzi DM, et al. Group cognitive-behavioral therapy versus selective serotonin reuptake inhibitors for obsessivecompulsive disorder: a practical clinical trial. J Anxiety Disord 2012;26: 25–31.

[75] Twohig MP, Hayes SC, Plumb JC, et al. A randomized clinical trial of acceptance and commitment therapy versus progressive relaxation training for obsessive-compulsive disorder. J Consult Clin Psychol 2010;78: 705–16.

[76] Hanstede M, Gidron Y, Nyklicek I. The effects of a mindfulness intervention on obsessive-compulsive symptoms in a non-clinical student population. J Nerv Ment Dis 2008;196:776–9.

[77] Goodman WK, Price LH, Delgado PL, et al. Specificity of serotonin reuptake inhibitorsin the treatment of obsessive-compulsive disorder. Comparison of fluvoxamine and desipramine. Arch Gen Psychiatry 1990;47: 577–85.

[78] Pittenger C, Bloch MH. Pharmacological treatment of obsessive-compulsive disorder. Psychiatr Clin North Am 2014;37:375–91.

[79] Katz RJ, DeVeaugh-Geiss J, Landau P. Clomipramine in obsessive-compulsive disorder. Biol Psychiatry 1990;28: 401–14.

[80] Goodman WK, Price LH, Rasmussen SA, et al. Efficacy of fluvoxamine in obsessive-compulsive disorder. A double-blind comparison with placebo. Arch Gen Psychiatry 1989;46:36–44.

[81] Perse TL, Greist JH, Jefferson JW, et al. Fluvoxamine treatment of obsessive-compulsive disorder. Am J Psychiatr 1987;144:1543–8.

[82] Montgomery SA, Kasper S, Stein DJ, et al. Citalopram 20 mg, 40 mg and 60 mg are all effective and well tolerated compared with placebo in obsessive-compulsive disorder. Int Clin Psychopharmacol 2001;16:75–86.

[83] Stein DJ, Tonnoir B, Andersen EW. Escitalopram in the treatment of OCD [abstract NR717 plus poster]. Toronto, Ont., Canada: Presented at The 159th annual meeting of the American Psychiatric Association; 2006.

[84] Piccinelli M, Pini S, Bellantuono C, et al. Efficacy of drug treatment in obsessive-compulsive disorder. A meta-analytic review. Br J Psychiatry 1995;166:424–43.

[85] Stein DJ, Andersen EW, Tonnoir B, et al. Escitalopram in obsessive compulsive disorder: a randomized, placebo-controlled, paroxetine referenced, fixed-dose, 24-week study. Curr Med Res Opin 2007;23:701–11.

[86] Soomro GM, Altman D, Rajagopal S, et al. Selective serotonin re-uptake inhibitors (SSRIs) versus placebo for obsessive compulsive disorder (OCD). Cochrane Database Syst Rev 2008;CD001765.

[87] Denys D, van Megen HJ, van der Wee N, et al. A double-blind switch study of paroxetine and venlafaxine in obsessive-compulsive disorder. J Clin Psychiatry 2004; 65:37–43.

[88] Kordon A, Kahl KG, Broocks A, et al. Clinical outcome in patients with obsessive-compulsive disorder after discontinuation of SRI treatment: results from a two-year follow-up. Eur Arch Psychiatry Clin Neurosci 2005;255:48–50.

[89] Lopez-Ibor JJ Jr, Saiz J, Cottraux J, et al. Double-blind comparison of fluoxetine versus clomipramine in the treatment of obsessive compulsive disorder. Eur Neuropsychopharmacol 1996;6:111–8.

[90] Decloedt EH, Stein DJ. Current trends in drug treatment of obsessive compulsive disorder. Neuropsychiatr Dis Treat 2010;6:233–42.

[91] Bloch MH, McGuire J, Landeros-Weisenberger A, et al. Meta-analysis of the dose-response relationship of SSRI in obsessive-compulsive disorder. Mol. Psychiatry 2010;15(8):850–5.

[92] Albert U, Marazziti D, Di Salvo G, et al. A systematic review of evidence-based treatment strategies for obsessive-compulsive disorder resistant to first-line pharmacotherapy. Curr Med Chem 2017. https://doi.org/10.2174/0929867325666171222163645.

[93] Albert U, Carmassi C, Cosci F, et al. Role and clinical implications of atypical antipsychotics in anxiety disorders, obsessive-compulsive disorder, trauma-related, and somatic symptom disorders: a systematized review. Int Clin Psychopharmacol 2016;31(5):249–58.

[94] Albert U, Salvo GD, Solia F, et al. Combining drug and psychological treatments for Obsessive-Compulsive Disorder: what is the evidence, when and for whom. Curr Med Chem 2018;25(41):5632–46.

[95] Dold M, Aigner M, Lanzenberger R. etc al. Antipsychotic augmentation of serotonin reuptake inhibitors in treatment-resitant obsessive-compulsive disorder: a meta-analysis of double-blind, randomized, placebo-controlled trials. Int J Neuropsychopharmacol 2013; 16:557–74.

[96] Denys D, Burger H, van Megen H, et al. A score for predicting response to pharmacotherapy in obsessive-compulsive disorder. Int Clin Psychopharmacol 2003; 18:315–22.

[97] Kayser RR. Pharmacotherapy for treatment-resistant obsessive-comulsive disorder. J Clin Psychiatry 2021; 81(5). https://doi.org/10.4088/JCP.19ac13182.

[98] Stein DJ, Costa DLC, Lochner C, et al. Obsessive–compulsive disorder. Nat Rev Dis Prim 2019;5(1):52.

[99] Pittinger C, Bloch MH. Pharmacological Treatment of obsessive-compulsive disorder. Psychiatr Clin North Am 2014 Sep;37(3):375–91.

[100] Sheshachala K, Narayanaswamy JC. Glutamatergic augmentation strategies in obsessive-compulsive disorder. Indian J Psychiatry 2019;61(Suppl 1):S58–65.

[101] Adams TG, Bloch MH, Pittenger C. Intranasal ketamine and cognitive-behavioral therapy for treatment-refractory obsessive-compulsive disorder. J Clin Psychopharmacol 2017;37(2):269–71.

[102] Rodriguez CI, Lapidus KAB, Zwerling J, et al. Challenges in testing intranasal ketamine in obsessive-compulsive disorder. J Clin Psychiatry 2017;78(4):466–7.

[103] Simpson HB, Foa EB, Liebowitz MR, et al. A randomized, controlled trial of cognitive-behavioral therapy for augmenting pharmacotherapy in obsessive-compulsive disorder. Am J Psychiatr 2008; 165:621–30.

[104] Carmi L, Tendler A, Bystrytsky A, et al. Efficacy and safety of deep transcranial magnetic stimulation for obsessive-compulsive disorder: a prospective multi-center randomized double-blind placebo controlled trial. Am J Psychiatr 2019;176:931–8.

[105] Dougherty DD, Baer L, Cosgrove GR, et al. Prospective long-term follow up of 44 patients who received cingulotomy for treatment refractory obsessive-compulsive disorder. Am J Psychiatr 2002;159:269–75.

[106] Sheth SA, Neal J, Tangherlini F, et al. Limbic system surgery for treatment-refractory obsessive-compulsive disorder: a prospective long-term follow up of 64 patients. J Neurosurg 2013;118:491–7.

[107] Greenberg BD, Gabriels LA, Malone DA Jr, et al. Deep brain stimulation of the ventral internal capsule/ventral striatum for obsessive-compulsive disorder: worldwide experience. Mol Psychiatry 2010;15:64–9.

[108] Bourne SK, Eckhardt CA, Sheth SA, et al. Mechanisms of deep brain stimulation for obsessive-compulsive disorder: effects upon cells and circuits. Front Integr Neurosci 2012;6:29.

[109] Global Drug Reference Online. Available at: www.globaldro.com. Accessed December 13, 2022.

Advances in Psychiatry and Behavioral Health 3 (2023) 57–68

ADVANCES IN PSYCHIATRY AND BEHAVIORAL HEALTH

Eating Disorders and Disordered Eating in Athletes During Times of Transition

A Narrative Systematic Review of the Literature

Claudia L. Reardon, MD[a],*, Ryan Benoy, MD[a], Mary Hitchcock, MA, MS[b]

[a]Department of Psychiatry, University of Wisconsin School of Medicine and Public Health, 6001 Research Park Boulevard, Madison, WI 53719, USA; [b]University of Wisconsin-Madison, Ebling Library for the Health Sciences, 2339 Health Sciences Learning Center, 750 Highland Avenue, Madison, WI 53705, USA

KEYWORDS
• Eating disorders • Athletes • Sport • Transition • Retirement • Injury • Pandemic • Pregnancy

KEY POINTS
- Times of transition in sports are high-risk periods for development of disordered eating and eating disorders.
- Disordered eating and eating disorders that develop in athletes during times of transition in sports may go undiagnosed
- Psychoeducational and other prevention programming on and screening for disordered eating and eating disorders during times of transition should be implemented for athletes.

INTRODUCTION/BACKGROUND

Increasing attention is being paid to athletes' mental health [1,2]. In recent years, it has become more appreciated that many mental health symptoms and disorders occur at rates at least as high as and sometimes higher than those in the general population [1]. Eating disorders stand out as an example of mental health disorders that affect athletes at rates even higher than those of the general population [3].

Moreover, times of transition, such as injury and retirement, are established as times of increased risk of mental health symptoms and disorders in athletes [4,5]. However, much research describing mental health symptoms during those times focuses on depression, anxiety, sleep disturbance, general psychological distress, and substance use problems [6,7]. Less is written about eating disorders in athletes during times of transition out of sport. These times of transition may

be temporary (eg, a few days for a minor injury or illness, a few months for the off-season, or a year or more for pregnancy and postpartum) or permanent (eg, retirement due to any number of factors). Recently, the COVID-19 pandemic has contributed to temporary and sometimes permanent transitions out of sports. The pandemic has thus afforded researchers and clinicians the rare opportunity to look at large-scale transition out of competitive sport for almost all athletes around the world at a single juncture.

Knowing that athletes at any time point are at significant risk of eating disorders, this narrative review examines eating disorders during what are usually particularly stressful times—those of transition—in their careers. Although some research has described eating disorders during a single type of transition, such as retirement, we are unaware of any reviews that have holistically and comprehensively considered the spectrum of types

---

*Corresponding author, E-mail address: clreardon@wisc.edu

of transition out of sports. This narrative systematic review aims to summarize the literature on this topic.

METHODS

An experienced academic librarian (M.H.) developed a search strategy using PubMed (Medline), CINAHL, PsycINFO, and SportDiscus databases from inception until November 2022. Search terms included words related to transition (transition, retirement, retiring, former, injury, pandemic, COVID), population of interest (sport, athlete, college athlete, professional athlete, elite athlete, Olympic athlete, high school athlete, junior high school athlete, middle school athlete, amateur athlete, child athlete, LGBTQ+ athlete, older athlete, baseball, basketball, badminton, bobsledder, bodybuilder, bowler, bullfighter, canoeist, cricket player, croquet player, cyclist, endurance athlete, extreme sports, fencer, football, gladiator, golf, gymnastics, handball, hockey, jai alai, judo, lacrosse, lawn bowling, martial arts, mountaineer, netball, rower, rugby, runner, skater, skier, squash, skydiver, snowboarder, soccer, surfer, swimmer, table tennis, team handball, tennis, track and field, triathlete, volleyball, water polo, weightlifter, windsurfer, wrestler), and symptoms and disorders in question (feeding and eating disorder, eating disorder, feeding disorder, body image, anorexia, anorexia nervosa, binge eating, binge eating disorder, bulimia, bulimia nervosa, hyperphagia, orthorexia, pica, purging, rumination, emotional eating) in various combinations and with various suffixes and conjugations of each word. Additional articles were reviewed for possible inclusion based on reference lists of the original articles found. Studies were selected if they included information on disordered eating, eating disorders, or body image in athletes during times of transition and excluded if they were not published in English.

RESULTS

Articles were retrieved and reviewed from all databases searched (Table 1). A total of 84 articles were ultimately deemed relevant for inclusion in this article. Where there was disagreement among the authors about salience of articles for inclusion, discussion was held until agreement was reached.

General Information

Athletes across most sports engage in significant physical activity. With that comes high energy needs. Athletes must develop a lifestyle in which they ingest sufficient calories to support their very active lifestyles.

TABLE 1
Number of Articles Reviewed and Retrieved from Various Databases

Database	Number of Articles Reviewed
PubMed (Medline)	877
CINAHL	311
PsycINFO	20
SPORTDiscus	354
Total	1562
Duplicates	620
Final unique items	942

With anything that suddenly and markedly decreases their level of physical activity, their caloric needs—and perception of their needs—might change. Ideally, athletes would be able to seamlessly continue to meet their caloric needs in a balanced manner, adjusting intake based on hunger cues and a healthy "food as fuel" attitude in keeping with the model of intuitive eating [8]. However, this is not often something in which they receive any support or guidance [9]. Left to figure it out themselves, food and eating can become major sources of concern during times of transition, as athletes have often dedicated many years of close attention to their physical bodies [10].

Athletes may "overcompensate" for the decreased physical activity by markedly and inappropriately decreasing their caloric intake or increasing physical activity in whatever forms remain available to them [8,11–21]. They may feel they do not deserve to eat and may feel guilty when they do so, now that they are not exercising as much [22]. This can be a setup for disordered eating. A common pattern that can develop may be significant caloric restriction or excessive exercise with subsequent binge eating in response to inevitable extreme hunger cues and/or innate biological drives for nourishment [21]. Full-blown eating disorders that may develop during these times, as defined in the Diagnostic and Statistical Manual of Mental Disorders, fifth edition (DSM-5), include anorexia nervosa, bulimia nervosa, and binge eating disorder, among others [23].

Specific Types of Transition
Retirement
Regardless of the impetus for retirement, it inevitably usually involves long-term changes in behaviors related to nutrition, body, and exercise [24]. The reality is that

this often results in loss of lean muscle mass and fitness, altered body composition, and changes in dietary practice when optimal nutrition becomes less immediately salient for one's success in their occupation [25].

Retirement has been shown to be associated with disordered eating, although comparisons with the general population have been scant. For example, Oltmans and colleagues [26] surveyed 297 Dutch former athletes across multiple sports, with a mean age of 50 years and mean duration since retirement of 17 years, and reported that 28% endorsed disordered eating in the previous four weeks. This was a greater risk for those athletes who reported career dissatisfaction (3–4 times higher risk) or adverse life events (eg, death of a spouse, significant change in financial status) and for female athletes (31%) compared to male athletes (24%). In another study that looked at only male athletes in a single sport (ice hockey), disordered eating was reported by 8% of 123 players with an average age of 35 years and average duration of retirement of 7 years [27]. In a third study, Gouttebarge and colleagues [13] surveyed 282 former elite Dutch athletes across multiple sports, with an average age of 51 years and average duration of retirement of 20 years; they reported a 4-week prevalence of eating disorders (as defined by the Eating Disorder Screen for Primary Care) of 27%. In a fourth study, Gouttebarge and colleagues [15] surveyed retired professional rugby players (N = 295) and found that 62% reported "adverse nutrition behavior," which was defined as endorsement of all of the following: consuming healthy meals less than 5 days per week, eating regularly throughout the day less than 3 days per week, having breakfast before 10:30 AM less than three days per week, and having a final meal before 20:30 less than 3 days per week. Authors have pointed out obvious differences in demographics and sport culture across these types of studies that likely impacted results [26].

There are important aspects of retirement to consider. Retirement can be voluntary (eg, planned in advance after reaching a certain milestone in sport) or involuntary (eg, after a significant injury, loss of sponsorship, or failure to ascend to the next competitive level). Voluntary retirement is associated with overall better psychological adjustment [28], which may include better food and body-related adjustments.

The degree of athletic identity is also an important predictor of ease of retirement; higher degrees of athletic identity predict a harder time adjusting [29], and this can include greater body-image-related difficulties [30]. That is, athletes who continue to identify as athletes will tend to maintain expectations about certain body types and fitness levels, even when no longer participating in competitive sports at the same level [30,31]. If retiring athletes maintain a presence in their athletic environments (eg, by serving as team managers, coaches, or other sport staff or by participating in social media related to their sport), they are more likely to continue to identify as athletes, to experience continued body objectification, to be identified as athletes by others around them, and to not develop new aspects to their identity [20]. Any efforts to stray from athletic identities can be challenging given that the world of sports is where athletes' occupational skills may lie [24]. Furthermore, media can critically portray images of retired athletes as if the expectation is that they maintain the same bodies as they did when competing [32,33]. Retired athletes who have been in the public eye may worry about public perception and describe feeling fearful of "letting themselves go" [34]. Efforts to maintain their same body types as when actively competing may lead to exercise addiction (Box 1) [35], muscle dysmorphia (preoccupation with the idea that one's body is not sufficiently lean and muscular) [36], or orthorexia nervosa (obsessive attention to healthy eating with excessive control over quality of food eaten) [37]. These are not official diagnoses in the DSM-5, but nonetheless have received research attention [23]. Proposed features of exercise addiction parallel those of other addictive disorders [1,35].

Conversely, having paid attention to and remained open to other (nonsport) life areas and identities when they were active competitors and developing a new life focus following transition out of sport are associated with higher body satisfaction after retirement [38].

The timing after retirement is an important factor as well. Early months after retirement appear to be the most difficult regarding eating and body image concerns [24]. This is when significant body composition changes may be noticed by retiring athletes and when they are most likely to be closely holding on to prior body ideals and athlete identities [18,19]. They may go through "body grief" during this time [17–21,32,39–41], wherein they are mourning the loss of the physical body that represented years of dedication and hard work and what society may have regarded as ideal. Moreover, in the bigger picture, it is known that times of bodily change (such as puberty) can be high-risk periods for disordered eating [42]. Relatively early phases of retirement from sports are exactly that for many athletes: a time of bodily change.

There are nuanced findings regarding the specific time during the early phases of retirement when

---

BOX 1
Proposed Features of Exercise Addiction

- Tolerance: the need to increase the exercise duration, frequency, and/or intensity to perceive the desired benefit and to satisfy "cravings" for it
- Withdrawal: depressive or anxious symptoms or irritability when the individual suddenly reduces or stops exercise, with possible difficulty performing professional or social activities as a result of these symptoms
- Continued exercise despite knowing that it is causing physical, psychological, and/or social problems
- Inability to reduce or manage exercise despite the desire to do so
- Time: a great deal of time is spent preparing for, engaging in, and recovering from exercise
- Elimination of other life activities (eg, previously desired social, occupational, or recreational activities) to accommodate increasingly time-consuming exercise regimens

---

(Data from Reardon CL, Hainline B, Aron CM, et al. Mental health in elite athletes: International Olympic Committee consensus statement (2019). Br J Sports Med 2019;53(11):667–699; and Lichtenstein MB, Hinze CJ, Emborg B, et al. Compulsive exercise: Links, risks and challenges faced. Psychol Res Behav Manag 2017;10:85–95).

individuals are more susceptible to developing disordered eating or related concerns. Body image in retiring Olympic athletes (N = 16) across several sports has been shown to be worse 5 months after retirement (when body changes may be even more apparent) compared to 1.5 months after retirement (when body image scores did not yet separate from those in actively competing elite athletes) [18]. However, at some point, it appears that this trend might reverse. For example, athletes 5 years out from retirement report better body image than athletes who had been retired for less time [18–20,43]. By 15 years after retirement, athletes in 1 study reported better body image than their peers who were not athletes [40], although disordered eating per se may still be common and may not improve with time even that far out from retirement [26].

Some specific groups of athletes are at even greater risk of disordered eating in retirement. Athletes who are retiring from sports with high caloric needs may be at higher risk [21] and may engage in compulsive exercise, in a pattern matching that of exercise addiction, to try to match the energy requirements of their former sport [20]. Second, athletes who report having drastically controlled their food intake during their sport career report greater struggles with disordered eating and body image after retirement [20,21,30]. Third, a relevant consideration is whether a given athlete's "body sport ideal" overlapped with the "body social ideal" [32]. If they are similar, for example, in female distance runners for whom a thin body type is regarded as ideal by both standards, then retirement might be particularly difficult [32]. That is because retirement might simultaneously lead to a change from both the body sport ideal and body social ideal. On the other hand, male distance runners may have a

body sport ideal of thin, which conflicts with the body social ideal of muscular; for them, retirement brings an increased influence of body social ideals, which may or may not have an ultimate positive effect on body image [24]. Finally, athletes (such as gymnasts) whose retirement coincides with a time when adolescents are already typically undergoing profound physical changes may be at higher risk of distress associated with the additional physical changes that retirement brings [30].

Of note, it does not appear to be the case that retiring athletes are more likely to suffer from disordered eating and body dissatisfaction because they gain more weight than their nonathlete peers who are similarly aging. For example, 55% of retired gymnasts and swimmers report body dissatisfaction, 60% are trying to lose weight in retirement [17], and 73% report disordered eating behaviors [44], even though 74% are in the "healthy weight range" as defined by a body mass index of 18-25 kg/m^2 [17].

On the positive side, for some athletes who persisted through their sporting careers with an eating disorder, their symptoms may improve or even abate upon retirement, with cessation of the sport-related forces that drove them to disordered eating in the first place [19,40].

In summary, Box 2 lists characteristics of athletes that appear to place them at higher risk of disordered eating or worse body image during retirement.

Injury

Injury may bring with it all the above behaviors and fears when it comes to food and body that are seen in retirement or other types of transition out of sports. Importantly, sometimes athletes who are suffering

> **BOX 2**
> **Factors that May Place Athletes at Higher Risk of Disordered Eating/Eating Disorders or Worse Body Image During Retirement**
>
> - Involuntary retirement
> - Higher athletic identity during active sport participation
> - Continued self-identity as an athlete after retirement
> - Maintaining a presence in athletic environments after retirement
> - Early phases of retirement (especially around 5 months)
> - Retirement from sport that had high caloric needs
> - Drastic control of food intake while actively participating in the sport
> - Congruent "body sport ideal" and "body social ideal" (both thin or both muscular)
> - Retirement that coincides with periods of rapid growth/puberty in adolescents

from injury will engage in continued exercise despite recommendations not to exercise or will overexercise to compensate for those aspects of sport in which they currently are unable to participate so as to avoid weight gain or other bodily changes. This may be part of exercise addiction [45]. A relevant concept is that of "primary" versus "secondary" exercise addiction. The former has been described as occurring separate from an eating disorder, whereas the latter accompanies an eating disorder, with exercise used as a mechanism for weight control [45].

There is research that indeed demonstrates an association between injuries and disordered eating. Sundgot-Borgen (1994) surveyed all the elite female athletes in Norway (N = 603), ages 12-35 years, across multiple sport types [46]. Via administration of a structured clinical interview to those identified as at risk of eating disorders, traumatic events including injury were found to be associated with the subsequent onset of eating disorders [46]. Conversely, eating disorders—with consequent compromised bone mineral density such as that described in Relative Energy Deficiency in Sport—are associated with higher risk of injuries [47]. This could be a part of a vicious cycle of an athlete with an injury developing an eating disorder, with subsequent perpetuation or worsening of the injury because of inadequate nutrition and difficulty stopping exercise. For example, Gusfa and colleagues (2022) surveyed 308 adolescent athletes (ages 12-19 years) and found that disordered eating was significantly associated with female sport injury (although not with male sport injury) [48]. The authors' interpretation was that disordered eating led to injury because of compromised nutritional status [48], but the timing of development of disordered eating (whether before or after injury) in this study is unclear.

COVID-19 pandemic–related transitions

Buckley and colleagues [49] (2021), drawing upon their prior seminal work on disordered eating in athletes during retirement, appreciated that the COVID-19 pandemic represented a rare opportunity to study and learn about disordered eating and body image in athletes during times of transition. It has been established that in general populations, rates of eating disorders increased, and eating pathology in those previously diagnosed further worsened, during the pandemic [50–53]. Even among nonathletes, there was a fear of gaining the "quarantine 15 (pounds)" [54]. Buckley's results, then, were not surprising. They surveyed 93 current and 111 former athletes, representing 41 sports at various competitive levels, between the ages of 18 and 63 years, across genders, in the April-May 2020 time frame; this was during the time that most organized sports were suspended [49]. They reported that 34.8% reported worsened body image, and 32.8% reported a worsened food relationship directly as a result of COVID-19. Disordered eating occurred most commonly in the forms of body preoccupation, dietary restriction, fear of body composition changes, and binge eating. There were no differences between individual versus team sports, type of sport (eg, endurance, esthetic), or level of competition (eg, club versus national or international). Athletes who were retired and female athletes were at the highest risk. Interestingly, it was fear of bodily changes—regardless of whether there actually were bodily changes—that was significantly associated with worsened body image, and this comports with other research studies [55]. Firoozjah and colleagues [56] (2022) reported some similar concerns in their study of 124 Iranian male adolescent athletes across six sports during the COVID pandemic. Similar to Buckley, they reported disordered eating and body image concerns in their sample. Unlike Buckley, they did find a difference between individual and team sport athletes: individual sport athletes suffered more than team sport athletes from disordered eating and worse body image. They reflected that individual sports tend to emphasize "leanness" as a means to improving performance, and pandemic-related stressors may have exacerbated this pressure. A 2022 systematic scoping review suggested that athletes have been among the most at-risk groups—along with young women in general and individuals highly fearful of COVID—for pandemic-associated disordered eating [50].

There are many factors that may have contributed to disordered eating and worsened body image in athletes during the pandemic. During the early days of the pandemic, athletes had sudden, unanticipated loss of access to training facilities, team/group practices, and competitions, which likely fueled their fear of bodily changes and their accompanying disordered eating practices to cope and compensate for less-organized sporting activities [49]. Food insecurity, unemployment, and other financial stressors (including for professional athletes, whose seasons and competitions—and associated paychecks—were cancelled) on the one hand and an increase in food access at home (where most people were spending much of their time) and boredom eating on the other hand may have contributed [49]. Athletes may have had sudden changes in their living situations, for example, with collegiate or professional athletes moving "back home" to types and amounts of foods to which they were unaccustomed—a change complicated by periods of panic buying and fluctuating food access. All the while they were increasingly having to look at themselves on Zoom [49] or other virtual platforms—akin to having to look in a mirror constantly. They were also spending more time on social media—with attendant social comparisons—and newly using virtual platforms that allowed obsessive comparison of training metrics with others more readily [49].

On the positive, some athletes who had dealt with other types of transitions before the pandemic may have been better equipped to cope with the major transition that the pandemic wrought [49]. They had prior experience sitting with uncertainty and loss of control and could use any skills previously learned.

Higher rates of eating pathology in athletes during the pandemic were coupled with, in many cases, less access to health care resources due to lockdowns and overall increased psychopathology leading to increased demand for all mental health services [57]. This led athletes with emerging eating disorder pathology to be less able than they usually would have been to connect with services.

Pregnancy

Pregnancy is a unique transition that necessarily represents a departure from usual sport participation for almost all athletes in almost all sports who experience it and that brings significant bodily change. Some athletes may need to alter their training and body composition to become pregnant [58]. Pregnancy can be a high-risk time for exacerbation of disordered eating in general populations [59], but its impact on body image and disordered eating has been studied little within sporting populations.

There may be fear of bodily changes that then "have to be reversed" quickly by athletes–in their perception–after childbirth. Some athletes have likened pregnancy to being injured regarding the loss of bodily control [60]. There may be an attendant desire to err on the side of minimizing weight gain and to return to one's prepregnancy body as quickly as possible—even if unhealthy to do so. In fact, eating disorders in pregnancy appear to be associated with an increased risk of adverse pregnancy and neonatal outcomes, such as antepartum hemorrhage, preterm birth, small size for gestational age, and microcephaly [61], although these findings are not specific to athletes. Beyond pregnancy, breastfeeding may perpetuate feelings of continued loss of control over one's body [61,62].

On the other hand, some pregnant athletes may welcome the changes or experience a mixture of positive and negative reactions [63]. They may feel relieved to "take a break" from the pressure to maintain perfect fitness and to feel less responsible for what happens to their bodies [63]. In 1 small (N = 20) study of elite Spanish sportswomen, most participants described some negative reactions to the bodily changes, and all reported a desire to recover their previous bodies as soon as possible [60]. In a small (N = 34) study of elite Norwegian sportswomen, participants experienced higher body dissatisfaction but lower rates of clinical eating disorders postpartum than before and during pregnancy, while control subjects had constant rates of eating disorders across all time points [64].

Off-season

As the previous paragraphs describe several examples of short- or long-term transitions out of sport that have been associated with worse body image and eating behaviors in athletes, it may follow that athletes would fear bodily changes such as weight gain during the off-season, when working out significantly less, and that eating pathology may follow. However, this is minimally mentioned in the literature. In 1 study on collegiate female athletes, weight gain during the off-season was reported as a common reason for nutrition consultations, but any association with disordered eating or disturbed body image was not described [65]. On the other hand, some athletes may view the off-season as an opportunity to be more relaxed about their eating habits, not in a manner that is problematic, but rather one that is appropriately flexible and less disordered than during the regular season. They may welcome a break from what may be experienced during the active sports season as "routine and ceaseless monitoring" of their bodies [66].

Assessment

We found no comprehensive, validated athlete-specific eating disorder or disordered eating screening tools for times of transition. However, recently, a work group of the International Olympic Committee published its Sports Mental Health Assessment Tool 1 (SMHAT-1), which includes several screening tools packaged together for use in athletes [67]. It is recommended to use the SMHAT-1 at various time points during an athlete's career, including times of transition such as major injury/illness, surgery, at the end of a competitive cycle, and retirement [67]. The Brief Eating Disorder in Athletes Questionnaire (BEDA-Q) is the disordered eating screening tool included in the SMHAT-1 and appears an acceptable choice for athletes during times of transition [67]. Thus, clinicians may incorporate the entire SMHAT-1, or only the BEDA-Q if primarily concerned about disordered eating, at high-risk times of transition such as any of the aforementioned circumstances.

If the related concept of exercise addiction/overexercise is a concern, the assessment of this can be challenging because athletes are required to train at high intensities [1]. However, the Athletes' Relationships with Training scale is a self-report measure of unhealthy training behaviors associated with eating disorders that has demonstrated strong psychometric properties and clinical utility [43]. Additionally, the Compulsive Exercise Test athlete version has been described as potentially more sensitive than eating disorder screening tools designed for the general population in detecting eating disorders in athletes, as athletes significantly underreport eating psychopathology on standard self-report questionnaires [68]. For

this reason, clinical interviews as compared to the use of screening tools may yield more sensitive results [69].

Prevention

Psychoeducational and other prevention programs targeting difficulties associated with sport transitions—with the literature especially having focused on the transition of retirement—have been recommended in numerous articles [12,13,28,30,38,70–72]. Some mention that this should include an explicit focus on eating and body image concerns in transitioning athletes [28,70]. Esopenko and colleagues (2020) recommended that athletes should have an exit examination with a nutritionist or team doctor regarding changing nutritional needs and anticipated bodily changes—and psychological challenges associated with these bodily changes—after retirement [28]. Shander and Petrie [38] (2021) suggest that before retirement, sport professionals should help athletes begin career planning, identify coping strategies, nurture identities outside of sport, and develop support networks outside of sport, and their findings suggest that ultimately this will help with all aspects of transition, including those related to food and body. Papathomas and colleagues [73] described 10 tips from Olympians for dealing with body-related concerns during retirement based on their extensive interviews with this population (Box 3).

However, the evidence base supporting particular programs to ease eating/body concerns during transitions is minimal. The Bodies in Motion (BIM) program has received some attention. It is facilitated by female professionals (eg, licensed mental health professionals, registered dieticians, athletic trainers) in athletics departments, and athletes from women's sports teams are introduced to psychological strategies, tools, and perspectives to help them respond to ubiquitous pressures in heathier and more functional ways and ultimately to develop a more positive and compassionate perspective toward themselves and their bodies [74]. Barrett and colleagues (2022) studied the impact during sport retirement (retirement duration of two to six years) of having participated in BIM during active collegiate sport participation [75]. While the sample size was small (N = 12) and disordered eating per se was not studied, results suggested positive impacts of having participated in BIM on body image in retirement. The impact during other types of transition is unknown. We did not find any published results on the impact of other eating disorder or disordered eating prevention programs—

BOX 3
Ten Tips From Olympians for Dealing with Body-Related Concerns During Anticipated Transitions Such as Retirement

- Seek professional support early, ideally before the transition.
- Prepare a structured detraining plan to follow.
- Seek new sport and exercise experiences.
- Have a goal/focus—but not necessarily a sporting one.
- Speak to those who have done it; learn from your sporting peers.
- Work to accept the body will change and that it is a normal process.
- Practice self-compassion by allowing your body the break it needs.
- Practice body appreciation; be thankful for what it did and what it still can do.
- Focus on health above performance.
- Be patient—it will take time to adjust to the transition regardless of preparation.

(Data from Papathomas A, Petrie T, Moesch K. Body image experiences in retired Olympians: knowledge, awareness, and prevention. Final report for the IOC Olympic Studies Centre Advanced Olympic Research Grant Programme. September 2021).

including the well-known Female Athlete Body project [76]—specifically on transitioning athletes [77,78].

DISCUSSION

Athletes will inevitably experience transitions during their sporting careers. Some may weather these changes without apparent significant hardship. Although this is an underrepresented area of the sport mental health literature, it is clear that body image and eating challenges are common during these times. Some clinicians who are able to continue working with athletes during and after transitions out of sport anecdotally have long appreciated that this is a high-risk time for disordered eating. However, for many athletes, their treatment teams change, or their access to mental health and other medical services completely dissolves, after their sport participation ceases—right when they may be most in need. Thus, these difficulties may often go unnoticed, and there appear to be insufficient clinicians and researchers "in the know"—involved in this whole spectrum of care—to draw attention to this issue in clinical and research realms. It is therefore no surprise that the literature on these topics is sparse.

This raises the larger issue of what arguably is a duty to care for athletes not only during their sporting careers but beyond [26,79,80]. Sport needs a better system of continuity of care for athletes, recognizing that athletes are worthy of health care not only when they are capable of actively producing results on the playing field but also well beyond that. Perhaps that especially

should be the obligation when health care issues that arise after transition—such as eating disorders and disordered eating—appear to be a direct result of their years of active sport participation.

Knowledge of and attention to the reported risk factors for eating disorders, disordered eating, and other body image concerns in transitioning athletes can help clinicians to have heightened awareness of the possibility of these problems. For example, if an athlete is retiring (especially if unplanned), experiencing an acute injury or an illness lasting more than a very brief period of time (including prolonged removal from the sport due to COVID-19 factors), or is pregnant/postpartum, the clinician should be particularly certain to screen for disordered eating and arrange for treatment if needed. If anything, health care providers should be even more available than usual during these transitions and should be educated in the challenges that come with bodily changes (or fear of bodily changes) and compensatory behaviors that commonly occur and might lead to full-blown eating disorders during this time. An early intervention can then be used, which may help prevent progression from symptoms to outright and persistent eating disorders.

Even better than an early treatment intervention, relevant psychoeducational and other prevention programs should be undertaken by athletes before they ever experience transitions. This may relate to how to healthily, intuitively, and flexibly adjust to new nutrition and exercise habits during transition and may target body image concerns. Athletes do not appreciate, because they are not taught, that extreme dietary and exercise habits during times of transition are not sustainable and are harmful. Prevention services on these topics depend on health care systems and sports organizations ensuring services are designed and delivered in a manner that is longitudinally accessible.

An understanding of the culture of sports by clinicians providing care for transitioning athletes is important [81]. Athletes may not respond well to clinicians who are naive to the world of sport and who, for example, do not understand why they cannot simply "just eat and exercise like a normal person" now that they have exited from sport. If the clinician does not evince truly "getting it," the athlete or former athlete is unlikely to bring up these concerns.

Several important future research and clinical directives emerge from this review.

- More research is needed on the longitudinal course of disordered eating and eating disorders that develop within times of transition. Retirement has been relatively more studied in this regard, but we know little about differences across sports and about persistence of symptoms that develop during the full complement of types of transitions. Generally, we know that eating disorders tend to be long-term conditions that often persist for many years [82]. However, we do not know if that is the case in all circumstances involving sport transition. For example, it is possible that once an athlete returns to their sport from injury, pregnancy, or the off-season, symptoms abate relatively quickly. On the other hand, it is possible that once such symptoms have gotten a foothold, they persist. Arguing for the latter is the fact that when female athletes in particular develop eating disorders within active phases of sport participation, their symptoms often persist at least six years or more into retirement [25], especially when compared to male athletes in a similar context [83]. Social reinforcement of thin body ideals may perpetuate eating disorders in certain populations such as women even after the inciting context has become less salient.
- Validated screening tools relevant to disordered eating and eating disorders for use with athletes during times of transition should be developed, validated, and employed.
- Impacts of disordered eating and eating disorders during transitions on different demographic groups, across genders, LGBTQ+ status, and racial and ethnic groups should be studied.
- Prevalence studies that use larger sample sizes and control groups matched from the general population should be undertaken.

- Studies that use clinical diagnosis (eg, of eating disorders) from medical professionals, as opposed to self-report questionnaires, should be used.
- Studies of specific programs and supports targeting disordered eating and eating disorders during times of transition should be carried out toward the end of determining short- and long-term effectiveness.

SUMMARY

Times of transition in sports are an underappreciated high-risk period for development of eating disorders and disordered eating in athletes. We need to work toward supporting athletes through these transitions with evidence-based interventions and to support research that furthers our understanding of these risks and how to mitigate them. It is the moral duty of those working in sports to work toward these goals.

CLINICS CARE POINTS

- Athletes who are experiencing transitions out of sport—whether temporary or permanent—should be screened for mental health symptoms and disorders, including disordered eating.
- Clinicians and institutions should take steps to ensure continued access to health care for athletes during times of transition out of sport.
- Clinicians and institutions should take steps to help athletes plan for transitions out of sport well in advance of any actual transitions.

DISCLOSURE

The authors have nothing to disclose.

REFERENCES

[1] Reardon CL, Hainline B, Aron CM, et al. Mental health in elite athletes: International Olympic Committee consensus statement (2019). Br J Sports Med 2019; 53(11):667–99.

[2] Chang C, Putukian M, Aerni G, et al. Mental health issues and psychological factors in athletes: detection, management, effect on performance and prevention: American Medical Society for Sports Medicine Position Statement. Clin J Sport Med 2020;30(2):e61–87.

[3] Sundgot-Borgen J, Torstveit MK. Prevalence of eating disorders in elite athletes is higher than in the general population. Clin J Sport Med 2004;14:25–32.

[4] Arnold R, Fletcher D. A research synthesis and taxonomic classification of the organizational stressors encountered

by sport performers. J Sport Exerc Psychol 2012;34: 397–429.

[5] Wylleman P, Reints A. A lifespan perspective on the career of talented and elite athletes: perspectives on high-intensity sports. Scand J Med Sci Sports 2010; 20(Suppl 2):88–94.

[6] van Ramele S, Aoki H, Kerkhoffs GMMJ, et al. Mental health in retired professional football players: 12-month incidence, adverse life events and support. Psychol Sport Exerc 2017;28:85–90.

[7] Simon JE, Docherty CL. Current health-related quality of life is lower in former Division I collegiate athletes than in non-collegiate athletes. Am J Sports Med 2014;42(2): 423–9.

[8] Plateau CR, Petri TA, Papathomas A. Learning to eat again: intuitive eating practices among retired female collegiate athletes. Eat Disord 2017;25(1):92–8.

[9] Silva AM, Nunes CL, Matias CN, et al. Champ4life Study Protocol: a one-year randomized controlled trial of a lifestyle intervention for inactive former elite athletes with overweight/obesity. Nutrients 2020;12(2): 286.

[10] Jones L, Avner Z, Denison J. After the dust settles": Foucauldian narratives of retired athletes' "re-orientation" to exercise. Front Sports Act Living 2022;4:901308.

[11] Cosh S, Crabb S, Lecouteur A. Elite athletes and retirement: identity, choice, and agency. Aust J Psychol 2013;65:89–97.

[12] Gouttebarge V, Aoki H, Kerkhoffs GM. Prevalence and determinants of symptoms related to mental disorders in retired male professional footballers. J Sports Med Phys Fitness 2016;56:648–54.

[13] Gouttebarge V, Jonkers R, Moen M, et al. The prevalence and risk indicators of symptoms of common mental disorders among current and former Dutch elite athletes. J Sports Sci 2017;35:2148–56.

[14] Gouttebarge V, Frings-Dresen MHW, Sluiter JK. Mental and psychosocial health among current and former professional footballers. Occup. Med. Oxf 2015;65: 190–6.

[15] Gouttebarge V, Kerkhoffs G, Lambert M. Prevalence and determinants of symptoms of common mental disorders in retired professional Rugby Union players. Eur J Sport Sci 2016;16:595–602.

[16] Kerr ZY, DeFreese JD, Marshall SW. Current physical and mental health of former collegiate athletes. Orthop J Sports Med 2014;2:2325967114544107.

[17] Papathomas A, Petrie TA, Plateau CR. Changes in body image perceptions upon leaving elite sport: The retired female athlete paradox. Sport Exerc Perform Psychol 2018;7:30–45.

[18] Stephan Y, Bilard J. Repercussions of transition out of elite sport on body image. Percept Mot Skills 2003;96:95–104.

[19] Kerr G, Dacyshyn A. The retirement experiences of elite, female gymnasts. J Appl Sport Psychol 2000;12:115–33.

[20] Stirling AE, Cruz LC, Kerr GA. Influence of retirement on body satisfaction and weight control behaviors:

perceptions of elite rhythmic gymnasts. J Appl Sport Psychol 2012;24:129–43.

[21] Cooper H, Winter S. Exploring the conceptualization and persistence of disordered eating in retired swimmers. J Clin Sport Psychol 2017;11:222–39.

[22] Putukian M. Mind, Body and Sport: how being injured affects mental health. In: Mind, body, and sport: understanding and supporting student-athlete mental wellness. NCAA. 2014. Available at: https://www.ncaa.org/sports/2014/11/5/mind-body-and-sport-how-being-injured-affects-mental-health.aspx. Accessed November 18, 2022.

[23] American Psychiatric Association. Diagnostic and statistical manual of mental disorders (DSM-5). Washington, DC: American Psychiatric Publishing; 2013.

[24] Buckley GL, Hall LE, Lassemillante AM, et al. Retired athletes and the intersection of food and body: a systematic literature review exploring compensatory behaviours and body change. Nutrients 2019;11:1395.

[25] Thompson A, Petrie T, Tackett B, et al. Eating disorder diagnosis and the female athlete: a longitudinal analysis from college sport to retirement. J Sci Med Sport 2021;24(6): 531–5.

[26] Oltmans E, Confectioner K, Jonkers R, et al. A 12-month prospective cohort study on symptoms of mental health disorders among Dutch former elite athletes. Phys Sportsmed 2022;50(2):123–31.

[27] Gouttebarge V, Kerkhoffs GMMJ. A prospective cohort study on symptoms of common mental disorders among current and retired professional ice hockey players. Phys Sportsmed 2017;45(3):252–8.

[28] Esopenko C, Coury JR, Pieroth EM, et al. The psychological burden of retirement from sport. Curr Sports Med Rep 2020;19(10):430–7.

[29] Lavallee D. The effect of a life development intervention on sports career transition adjustment. Sport Psychol 2005;19:193–202.

[30] Warriner K, Lavallee D. The retirement experiences of elite female gymnasts: self identity and the physical self. J Appl Sport Psychol 2008;20(3):301–17.

[31] Martin LA, Fogarty GJ, Albion MJ. Changes in athletic identity and life satisfaction of elite athletes as a function of retirement status. J Appl Sport Psychol 2014;26: 96–110.

[32] Greenleaf C. Athletic body image: exploratory interviews with former competitive female athletes. Wom Sport Phys Act 2002;11(1):63–8.

[33] Cosh S, Crabb S, Kettler L, et al. The normalisation of body regulation and monitoring practices in elite sport: A discursive analysis of news delivery sequences during skinfold testing. Qual Res Sport Exerc Health 2015;7: 338–60.

[34] PA. Webinar: athlete body image-the impact of retirement. In: Loughborough University. Available at: https://www.lboro.ac.uk/schools/sport-exercise-health-sciences/events/2021/athlete-body-image-impact-of-retirement/. Accessed November 18, 2022.

[35] Lichtenstein MB, Hinze CJ, Emborg B, et al. Compulsive exercise: Links, risks and challenges faced. Psychol Res Behav Manag 2017;10:85–95.

[36] Murray SB, Rieger E, Touyz SW, et al. Muscle dysmorphia and the DSM-V conundrum: where does it belong? A review paper. Int J Eat Disord 2010;43:483–91.

[37] Dunn TM, Bratman S. On orthorexia nervosa: A review of the literature and proposed diagnostic criteria. Eat Behav 2016;21:11–7.

[38] Shander K, Petrie T. Transitioning from sport: life satisfaction, depressive symptomotology, and body satisfaction among retired female collegiate athletes. Psychol Sport Exerc 2021;57:102045.

[39] Marquet L, Brown M, Tafflet M, et al. No effect of weight cycling on the post-career BMI of weight class elite athletes. BMC Public Health 2013;13:510.

[40] O'Connor PJ, Lewis RD, Kirchner EM, et al. Eating disorder symptoms in former female college gymnasts: Relations with body composition. Am J Clin Nutr 1996;64:840–3.

[41] Stephan Y, Torregrosa M, Sanchez X. The body matters: psychophysical impact of retiring from elite sport. Psychol Sport Exerc 2007;8:73–83.

[42] Moore SR, McKone KMP, Mendle J. Recollections of puberty and disordered eating in young women. J Adolesc 2016;53:180–8.

[43] Chapa DA, Hagan KE, Forbush KT, et al. The Athletes' Relationships with Training scale (ART): a self-report measure of unhealthy training behaviors associatd with eating disorders. Int J Eat Disord 2018;51(9):1080–9.

[44] Kerr G, Berman E, De Souza MJ. Disordered eating in women's gymnastics: perspectives of athletes, coaches, parents, and judges. J Appl Sport Psychol 2006;18(1):28–43.

[45] Freimuth M, Moniz S, Kim SR. Clarifying exercise addiction: differential diagnosis, co-occurring disorders, and phases of addiction. Int J Environ Res Publ Health 2011;8:4069–81.

[46] Sundgot-Borgen J. Risk and trigger factors for the development of eating disorders in female elite athletes. Med Sci Sports Exerc 1994;26:414–9.

[47] Rauh MJ, Barrack M, Nichols JF. Associations between the female athlete triad and injury among high school runners. Int J Sports Phys Ther 2014;9(7):948–58.

[48] Gusfa D, Mancine R, Kennedy S, et al. The relationship between disordered eating behaviors and injury rates in adolescent athletes. Int J Eat Disord 2022;55(1):131–4.

[49] Buckley GL, Hall LE, Lassemillante AM, et al. Disordered eating & body image of current and former athletes in a pandemic; a convergent mixed methods study-What can we learn from COVID-19 to support athletes through transitions? J Eat Disord 2021;9:73.

[50] Linardon J, Messer M, Rodgers RF, et al. A systematic scoping review of research on COVID-19 impacts on eating disorders: a critical appraisal of the evidence and recommendations for the field. Int J Eat Disord 2022; 55(1):3–38.

[51] Vuillier L, May L, Greville-Harris M, et al. The impact of the COVID-19 pandemic on individuals with eating disorders: the role of emotion regulation and exploration of online treatment experiences. J Eat Disord 2021;9(1):18.

[52] Robertson M, Duffy F, Newman E, et al. Exploring changes in body image, eating and exercise during the COVID-19 lockdown: a UK survey. Appetite 2021;159:6.

[53] Monteleone AM, Cascino G, Marciello F, et al. Risk and resilience factors for specific and general psychopathology worsening in people with eating disorders during COVID-19 pandemic: a retrospective Italian multicentre study. Eat Weight Disord Stud Anorexia Bulimia Obes 2021;10:1–10.

[54] Castellini G, Cassioli E, Rossi E, et al. The impact of COVID −19 epidemic on eating disorders: a longitudinal observation of pre versus post psychopathological features in a sample of patients with eating disorders and a group of healthy controls. Int J Eat Disord 2020; 53(11):1855–62.

[55] Keel PK, Gomez MM, Harris L, et al. Gaining "the quarantine 15:" perceived versus observed weight changes in college students in the wake of COVID-19. Int J Eat Disord 2020;53(11):1801–8.

[56] Firoozjah MH, Shahrbanian S, Homayouni A, et al. Comparison of eating disorders symptoms and body image between individual and team sport adolescent athletes during the COVID-19 pandemic. J Eat Disord 2022;10(1):119.

[57] Shaw H, Robertson S, Ranceva N. What was the impact of a global pandemic (COVID-19) lockdown period on experiences within an eating disorder service? A service evaluation of the views of patients, parents/carers and staff. J Eat Disord 2021;9(1):11.

[58] Zanker CL. Regulation of reproductive function in athletic women: an investigation of the roles of energy availability and body composition. Br J Sports Med 2006; 40(6):489–90.

[59] Martinez-Olcina M, Rubio-Arias JA, Reche-Garcia C, et al. Eating disorders in pregnant and breastfeeding women: a systematic review. Medicina 2020;56(7):352.

[60] Martinez-Pascual B, Alvarez-Harris S, Fernandez-de-Las-Penas C, et al. Pregnancy in Spanish elite sportswomen: a qualitative study. Womens Health 2017;57(6):741–55.

[61] Mantel A, Hirschberg AL, Stephansson O. Association of maternal eating disorders with pregnancy and neonatal outcomes. J Am Med Assn 2020;77(3):285–93.

[62] Schmied V, Lupton D. Blurring the boundaries: breastfeeding and maternal subjectivity. Sociology Health Illn 2001;23(2):234–50.

[63] Warren S, Brewis J. Matter over Mind?: examining the experience of pregnancy. Sociol 2004;38(2):219–36.

[64] Sundgot-Borgen J, Sundgot-Borgen C, Myklebust G, et al. Elite athletes get pregnant, have healthy babies and return to sport early postpartum. BMJ Open Sport Exerc Med 2019;5:e000652.

[65] Quatromoni PA. Clinical observations from nutrition services in college athletics. J Am Diet Assoc 2008; 108(4):689–94.

[66] Manley A, Williams S. We're not run on numbers, we're people, we're emotional people': Exploring the experiences and lived consequences of emerging technologies, organizational surveillance and control among elite professionals. Organization 2022;29:1–22.

[67] Gouttebarge V, Bindra A, Blauwet C, et al. International Olympic Committee (IOC) Sport Mental Health Assessment Tool 1 (SMHAT-1) and Sport Mental Health Recognition Tool 1 (SMHRT-1): towards better support of athletes' mental health. Br J Sports Med 2021;55(1): 30–7.

[68] Plateau CR, Arcelus J, Meyer C. Detecting eating psychopathology in female athletes by asking about exercise: use of the compulsive exercise test. Eur Eat Disorders Rev 2017;25:618–24.

[69] Martinsen M, Bratland-Sanda S, Eriksson AK, et al. Dieting to win or to be thin? A study of dieting and disordered eating among adolescent elite athletes and non-athlete controls. Br J Sports Med 2010;44: 70–6.

[70] Rossell K. How retired professional cheerleaders adjust to retirement. Dissertation. John F. Kennedy University. May 2020Available at: https://www.proquest.com/openview/2b878e10ac909ab017506e097f1d6360/1?pq-origsite=gscholar&cbl=18750&diss=y. Accessed 12 November 2022.

[71] Coleman N, Roberts WO. Mental health aspects of voluntary and involuntary sport retirement. Curr Sports Med Rep 2021;20(12):651–4.

[72] Barker-Ruchti N, Achubring A. Moving into and out of high-performance sport: the cultural learning of an artistic gymnast. Phys Educ Sport Pedag 2016;21(1): 69–80.

[73] Papathomas A, Petrie T, Moesch K. Body image experiences in retired Olympians: knowledge, awareness, and prevention. Final report for the IOC Olympic Studies Centre Advanced Olympic Research Grant Programme. Switzerland: Lausanne; September 2021.

[74] Voelker DK, Petrie TA, Huang Q, et al. Bodies in motion: an empirical evaluation of a program to support positive body image in female collegiate athletes. Body Image 2019;28:149–58.

[75] Barrett S, Petrie T, Voelker D, et al. The body satisfaction and psychological well-being of retired women athletes: a long-term qualitative analysis of Bodies in Motion. Body Image 2022;43:143–53.

[76] Stewart TM, Pollard T, Hildebrandt T, et al. The female athlete body project study: 18-month outcomes in eating disorder symptoms and risk factors. Int J Eat Disord 2019;52:1291–300.

[77] Becker CB, McDaniel L, Bull S, et al. Can we reduce eating disorder risk factors in female college athletes? A randomized exploratory investigation of two peer-led interventions. Body Image 2012;9(1):31–42.

[78] Martinsen M, Bahr R, Borresen R, et al. Preventing eating disorders among young elite athletes: a randomized controlled trial. Med Sci Sports Exerc 2014;46(3): 435–47.

[79] Sinclair DA, Orlick T. Positive transitions from high-performance sport. Sport Psychol 1993;7(2):138–50.

[80] Stambulova N, Alfermann D, Statler T, et al. Position stand: career development and transitions of athletes. Int J Sport Exercise Psychol 2009;7(4):395–412.

[81] Reardon CL, Gorczynski P, Hainline B, et al. Anxiety disorders in athletes: a clinical review. Advanc Psychiatr Behav Health 2021;1:149–60.

[82] Eddy KT, Tabri N, Thomas JJ. Recovery from anorexia nervosa and bulimia nervosa at 22-year follow up. J Clin Psychiatry 2017;78(2):184–9.

[83] Glazer JL. Eating disorders among male athletes. Curr Sports Med Rep 2008;7(6):332–7.

Advances in Psychiatry and Behavioral Health 3 (2023) 69–79

ADVANCES IN PSYCHIATRY AND BEHAVIORAL HEALTH

Retirement from Elite Sport

Factors Associated with Adjustment and Holistic Health Outcomes

Daniel M. Zimet, PhD[a,*], David R. McDuff, MD[b], Virginia N. Iannone, PhD[c], Timothy P. Herzog, EdD[d,1], Richard P. Moser, PhD[e]

[a]Daniel M Zimet, LLC, Columbia, MD, USA; [b]University of Maryland School of Medicine, 110 South Paca Street 4th floor, Baltimore, MD 21201, USA; [c]Stevenson University, 10945 Boulevard Circle, Owings Mills, MD 21117, USA; [d]Reaching Ahead LLC, Annapolis, MD, USA; [e]Behavioral Research Program, National Cancer Institute, 9609 Medical Center Drive, Room 3E602, Rockville, MD 20850, USA

KEYWORDS

• Sports • Athlete transition • Retirement • Mental health • Well-being

KEY POINTS

• Sixty percent of athletes experienced significant mental health concerns during their adjustment to life after sport.
• Transition experiences of different athletes are highly variable, potentially adversely affecting the cognitive, mental, behavioral, and physical health and social well-being.
• A surprise/sudden retirement was most predictive of a difficult transition, accounting for 10.3% of the variance.
• Career satisfaction, athlete identity, positivity of team atmosphere, and gender accounted for an additional 12% of the variance.

INTRODUCTION

"I think it is just crazy how we spend most of our lives competing at such a high level, and then one day, it's just over. We are expected to just move on with our lives. You push your body and mind to its limit and then you don't. You exert yourself every day and then you don't. You have a strict diet and schedule every day and then you don't. You have coaches looking out for you every day and then you don't. You have goals and then you don't. You have a group of friends and teammates you see every day and then you don't. You have a purpose and then you don't. I wish there was something or somebody to help me understand what was going on in my mind and body when all this just stopped." Division 1 distance and individual medley swimmer and Athlete Transition Study participant.

More than 522,000 National Collegiate Athletic Association (NCAA) athletes competed in 2022 [1], each with a 5-year eligibility limit. Adding in non-NCAA athletes and people retiring from the professional, national, and Olympic ranks suggests that more than 100,000 elite-level US athletes transition out of competitive sports each year. This transition often occurs when an athlete is in their twenties, when coping strategies and support systems may not be fully developed. Prior studies suggest that 16% to 20% of athletes experience difficulties during their transition out of competitive sport, including financial hardship, identity crisis, emotional distress, loneliness, grief, depression,

---

[1] Present address: 2152 Renard Court, Annapolis, MD 21041, USA.

*Corresponding author. 10801 Hickory Ridge Road #220, Columbia, MD 21044. *E-mail address:* danielmzimet@gmail.com

anxiety, sleep disturbances, and substance misuse that may persist for 12 to 18 months or longer [2–5]. Leaving sports constitutes a major life transition, necessitating significant changes in priorities, identity, and lifestyle [6,7].

Elite sports environments and the individuals who compete within them are diverse, resulting in unique career experiences. Events associated with an athlete's retirement are similarly diverse. Subsequently, an adjustment period can range from easy, short, and simple to difficult, prolonged, and complex. Some research on factors explaining adjustment outcomes, including demographics (eg, gender), sport played, and level of competition, have had mixed or indeterminate results. Factors contributing to an easier transition into retirement may include educational attainment, financial stability, vocational and life skills training, career satisfaction, occupational opportunities, the voluntariness of leaving the competitive sport, pre-retirement planning, social support, and positive coach–athlete relationships [8–10]. Difficult transitions are associated with a lack of these factors, as well as intense athlete identity, poor life balance while competing, and experiencing a severe injury, chronic pain, or another poor health status [2,11]. For example, a difficult transition is common when retirement is a surprise/occurs suddenly, and is unplanned, such as with deselection, suspension, or a career-ending injury [2]. It is similarly challenging for athletes who experienced harassment, abuse, racial discrimination, trauma, chronic pain, or concussions with persistent symptoms [12,13]. According to Cooper and colleagues [14], 57% of retired British Olympians experienced a significant injury, 20% retired early because of an injury, and those injured are more likely to report chronic pain.

Adjustment quality often improves within the first 3 months of retirement [15] and for most within 12 to 18 months [6,16]. This steady improvement has been associated with increased financial stability, obtaining employment, using support systems, investing in new and meaningful interests (ie, identity diversification), and a holistic approach to healthy development by addressing multiple aspects of wellness [17].

In the past decade, transitioning athlete support programs have shifted from an athlete/sport focus to a dual-career developmental framework and whole-person emphasis, addressing sport and non-sport development [17]. The revised International Society of Sport Psychology Position Stand suggests that this framework encourages longitudinal attention and ongoing examination of sport, education, and occupational transitions to determine key struggles, lessons learned, and acquired coping skills [17]. Each athlete is viewed as having a holistic, multi-dimensional identity [18].

This article aims to describe the health impact of an elite athlete's retirement transition from a holistic, multi-dimensional health perspective. Additionally, this article seeks to add to the understanding of factors that prior research has associated with different adjustment experiences. Data for this article come from the Athlete Transition Study, whose broad aims are to clarify personal and career factors related to and contributing to an athlete's transition experience, holistic health during their retirement transition and at the time when they took the survey, and systems and individuals used for support during and after the transition period.

This article addresses the following.

1. Aspects of the athlete, their career, and conditions of their transition from sport, including demographics (ie, gender, age, ethnicity, retirement years), team atmosphere, pre-planning for retirement, career longevity and satisfaction, the strength of athlete identity, the suddenness of their retirement transition, and control over the decision to retire.

2. Evaluating the strength and significance of these perceptions and associations concerning how they impacted the athlete's health during the period of greatest adjustment difficulty while transitioning from competitive sport.

3. Assessing the utility and internal consistency of a 13-item Holistic Health Questionnaire (HHQ) as a tool for understanding the self-described period of greatest adjustment difficulty.

METHODS

Procedure: Participants were recruited using a convenience sampling approach from May 7, 2021, to August 9, 2022, and accessed through outreach efforts including 1) networking and social media (eg, Instagram, Facebook) and 2) direct emails to collegiate and professional sports organizations and support organizations for retired athletes. All elite athletes over 18 years old and retired for at least 3 months were eligible. Participants must have competed at the collegiate level or higher, or the equivalent for sports and nations that do not follow the US' developmental pathway. The anonymous survey was hosted on SurveyMonkey, accessed through the Website www.Athlete-TransitionStudy.com, and took approximately 23 minutes to complete. Participants were not compensated for their time. Stevenson University's Institutional Review Board approved this study (reference #20–017).

Predictor Variables: Participants were asked to rate on a four-point Likert scale ranging from Strongly Agree to Strongly Disagree their recollection of the following questions: I had been making plans for my retirement before it happened (*Plans*); My career was as long or longer than I anticipated (*Length*); I made the decision to retire—the decision was in my control (*Control*); Overall, I feel satisfied with my career in my sport (*Satisfied*); The last team/program/coach/gym I played for had a healthy/positive atmosphere (*Atmosphere*); My retirement came suddenly—it was a surprise (*Surprise*); Being an athlete defined by identity while I was transitioning out of playing my sport (*Identity*). The final predictor variable was *Gender* (ie, woman, man, and non-binary). The sample size was too small to study non-binary as a distinct group so they were excluded from the gender analysis.

Outcome Variable: A composite of 13 health questions was used to create the HHQ and included items related to cognitive, physical, behavioral, social, and mental health concerns or challenges. Nine of the thirteen items were created by the authors for this study, while two items each (4 total items) were taken from the Patient Health Questionnaire-2 (PHQ-2) and the Generalized Anxiety Disorder 2-Item (GAD-2). Participants were asked to consider the period of greatest difficulty during their transition out of sport and then indicate on a 4-point Likert scale (Never, Rarely, Sometimes, Often) their recollection of the following (1): I had problems with my thinking, memory, or attention (2); I exercised and kept to a healthy diet (reverse scored) (3); I experienced pain or other physical problems (eg, headaches) (4); I got easily frustrated, lost my temper, or felt like breaking things or fighting (5); I engaged in risky behaviors, such as gambling, partying, or overspending (6); I engaged in risky drug and alcohol use (7); I felt lonely and socially disconnected (8); I struggled to create structure in my life (9); I felt nervous, anxious or on edge (10); I was unable to stop or control worrying (11); I had little interest or pleasure in doing things (12); I felt down, depressed, or hopeless; and (13) I considered suicide. Total scores could range from 0 (no difficulty) to 39 (extreme difficulty).

Open-Ended Responses: The survey also contained an open-ended text box stating, "Please share anything else about your experience competing, retiring, or your life after elite sport that you'd like us to know, or that could be helpful to future athletes facing retirement." Answers to this question were used to emphasize important points in the introduction and discussion sections.

Statistical analysis: Descriptive analyses were first conducted to show the distribution of values among the predictor and outcome variables, including simple frequencies and measures of central tendency. Next, a multivariable linear regression model was conducted, regressing the HHQ scores on the eight predictor variables using a forward selection process. This method begins with an empty model and then adds in the variable that has the highest zero-order correction with the dependent variable, and subsequently adds additional variables (with an inclusion criterion of F to enter less than or equal to 0.05). The analysis stops when no remaining variables are significant, creating a final, parsimonious model that describes how much of the outcome variable (ie, HHQ) can be explained by each of the significant predictor variables. Total variance describes how much of the outcome can be explained by all the included variables combined, with scores ranging from 0.00 (no variance explained) to 1.00 (all variance explained).

RESULTS

Participants: The Athlete Transition Study collected self-reported information on 483 retired athletes (329 women [68.1%], 151 men [31.2%], and 3 non-binary [0.6%]). Participants competed in 36 different sports, the most common including swimming (n = 73; 15.1%), American football (n = 60; 12.4%), soccer (n = 58; 12.0%), and softball (n = 41; 8.4%). Nearly all played for a college/university (n = 481; 99.6%), and 61% of these collegiate athletes competed at the Division I level (N = 295). A subset of the total sample competed in a professional league (n = 122; 25.2%), on a national team (n = 99; 20.4%), or in the Olympics/Paralympics (n = 36; 7.4%). The self-described ethnicity of this sample was 77.4% White; 8.7% African American; 4.5% multi-racial; 4.3% Hispanic; 3.1% Asian; and 1.7% other/missing. Their ages ranged from 19 to 79 (mean = 34.3 years), and the number of years since their retirement ranged from 3 months to 57 years (mean = 10 years).

HHQ: The scores for the HHQ ranged from 0 to 39 with a mean of 16.11 (SD = 9.1), were positively skewed (0.037), and were relatively flat (kurtosis = 1.002). Internal consistency was assessed by calculating Cronbach's alpha for HHQ scores and was $\alpha = 0.90$. Item-total score correlations ranged from 0.33 to 0.81, and the overall Cronbach's alpha showed no significant change when dropping any item. All items contributed meaningfully to the overall score, and the scale would not be improved by dropping any item(s).

Perception of Various Aspects of their Career and Retirement: A minority of participants felt their retirement came suddenly (31.6%), and approximately half felt that their career was as long as they anticipated (50.4%). A majority agreed that being an athlete defined their identity while transitioning to retirement (84.4%), felt satisfied with their career (73.8%), had been making plans for retirement before it happened (54.3%), felt that the decision to retire was in their control (63.9%), and felt that the last team/program/coach they played for had a positive team atmosphere (69.8%).

Regression Model Results: Using a forward selection process and including all eight predictor variables, the final, parsimonious model included these variables entered in the following order: *Surprise; Satisfied; Identity Transition; Atmosphere; Gender.* The following variables were excluded as they did not meet the inclusion criteria: *Length, Control, and Plans* (Table 1). The following groups had significantly higher HHQ scores: women (compared with men); those who strongly agreed that being an athlete defined their identity (compared with those who strongly disagreed); and those who both strongly and somewhat agreed that their retirement came as a surprise (compared with those who strongly disagreed). The following groups had significantly lower HHQ scores: those who strongly agreed that they felt satisfied with their careers (compared with those who strongly disagreed); and those who both strongly and somewhat agreed that their team/program/coach/gym had a healthy/positive atmosphere (compared with those who strongly disagreed).

DISCUSSION

The main objective of the Athlete Transition Study is to provide a platform for elite athletes from every sport and competitive level to share their experience before, during, and after their transition out of sports. This article addresses two narrower aims within that broader objective. First, the authors aimed to develop and test the internal consistency of the HHQ, which asked participants to retrospectively share their perceptions of the period of greatest difficulty during their transition out of sports. The composite score of the HHQ provides a holistic view of the challenges that athletes transitioning out of sport face related to cognitive, physical, social, behavioral, and mental health outcomes. The HHQ composite scores and skewness suggest that most athletes had a reasonably good transition from their sport. Still, there was variability, which supports looking deeper into the specific domains addressed by the HHQ.

Second, the participants reflected on factors frequently cited in the athlete transition literature as significant predictors of adjustment outcomes. We endeavored to build a parsimonious list describing each variable's strength and distinct contribution (Table 2). Such an analysis can help identify athletes at risk of transition hardship and inform support systems on the most salient issues.

Predictors Associated with Transition Outcomes: A composite score of the HHQ was used to assess transition outcomes. Understanding what differentiates those athletes who easily adapted to life after competition from those who struggled has been a research focus for decades. In this study, we looked at eight commonly referenced retirement factors. We aspired to determine the strength and significance of each variable's unique contribution to our participants' period of adjustment difficulty (PAD) while controlling for the contribution made by the remaining variables in the model. Our analysis suggested that five of the original eight variables made significant and independent contributions as follows:

Retirement came as a surprise: Feeling that retirement was sudden and came as a surprise emerged as the variable with the strongest association with PAD outcome, explaining 10.3% of the variance. A sudden retirement might be brought about by a career-ending injury, getting cut or deselected from a roster, failing to qualify for a team (eg, Olympics), a significant organizational change, or an adverse life event (eg, the coach being fired, an altercation with the coach, legal difficulty, loss of financial support).

Athletes invest a great deal of time and effort at high personal costs to be at peak performance. Those suddenly thrust into retirement often experience an unanticipated and unwelcome end to pursuing a lifelong ambition. The jarring abruptness of that loss can come as a surprise, despite an athlete's intellectual knowledge that leaving sport eventually happens to everyone and having witnessed other athletes departing sport under the same conditions. Still, the suddenness can have massive and unexpected consequences with little time for emotional preparation. An analogy might be the sudden, unpredicted ending of a romantic relationship with the person you considered a soul-mate where, as they walk out the door, they break your knee in addition to your heart and tell you that a higher performing partner has replaced you.

TABLE 1
Results of the Final Parsimonious Multivariable, Linear, Regression Model

	Beta	Standard Error	R Square
Variable			
Surprise [1] [c]	−1.77[a]	.37	.105[a]
Strongly agree	5.09[a]	1.21	
Somewhat agree	4.21[a]	1.19	
Somewhat disagree	1.29	1.09	
Strongly disagree (Ref)	–	–	
Satisfied [2]	2.09[a]	.48	.058[a]
Strongly agree	−5.23[b]	1.80	
Somewhat agree	−1.89	1.72	
Somewhat disagree	−.58	1.82	
Strongly disagree (Ref)	–	–	
Identity [3]	−2.16[a]	.50	.043[a]
Strongly agree	5.33[a]	2.02	
Somewhat agree	2.63	2.02	
Somewhat disagree	1.22	2.25	
Strongly disagree (Ref)	–	–	
Atmosphere [4]	1.04[b]	.42	.016[a]
Strongly agree	−3.94[b]	1.38	
Somewhat agree	−2.76[b]	1.34	
Somewhat disagree	−2.88	1.47	
Strongly disagree (Ref)	–	–	
Gender [5]	−2.07[b]	.89	.010[b]
Woman	2.16[b]	.90	
Man (Ref)	–	–	
			Total R squared =.232

Holistic Health Questionnaire composite scores.
  Note.
  1)The following variables were excluded from the final model as they did not meet the inclusion criteria: *Length; Control; Plans.*
  2)R squared of final model =.23.
  [a] $P < .01$.
  [b] $P < .05$.
  [c] Indicates order in which variables were added to the model; first variable had the highest zero-order correlation with the outcome, second variable was the second highest that remains significant in the model, etc.

A sudden end to an athletic career may be impactful for at least three reasons. First, the event was not in the athlete's control, which contributes to feelings of help-lessness, and casts a shadow of injustice and unfairness on their career. Second, the athlete is left feeling like their athletic career lacked closure and that this vital part of their lives will forever be unfulfilled. Finally, the suddenness does not give the athlete time to mentally prepare or come to terms with the impending transition.

Career satisfaction: Feeling satisfied with one's career accomplishments was the second strongest contributing variable, describing an additional 5.8% of the variance. Reflecting positively on an athletic career can help with

TABLE 2
Simple Frequencies of Each Predictor Variable Showing Distribution of Responses

To What Extent do You Agree or Disagree with the Following Statements?	Participant Response Frequency			
	Strongly Agree	Somewhat Agree	Somewhat Disagree	Strongly Disagree
My retirement came suddenly—it was a surprise (*Surprise*)	15.7%	15.9%	19.2%	49.2%
My career was as long or longer than I anticipated (*Length*)	25.7%	23.9%	22.1%	28.3%
I made the decision to retire—the decision was in my control (*Control*)	37.0%	26.9%	17.8%	18.3%
Overall, I feel satisfied with my career in my sport (*Satisfied*)	32.2%	41.6%	18.9%	7.3%
The last team/program/coach/gym I played for had a healthy/positive Atmosphere (*Atmosphere*)	33.1%	36.7%	17.6%	12.7%
Being an athlete defined my identity while I was transitioning out of playing my sport (*Identity*)	42.2%	42.2%	11.2%	4.5%
I had been making plans for my retirement before it happened (*Plans*)	22.5%	31.8%	21.0%	24.7%
What is your gender?	Woman		Man	Other
	68.1%		31.3%	.6%

the transition because of corresponding feelings of self-worth, fulfillment, achievement, and having met one's goals. The achievements made the sacrifices and journey worthwhile. In contrast, feeling as though a career failed to meet their (or others') expectations or their perceived potential can leave an athlete feeling like they failed or underperformed. As career satisfaction is a matter of perception, it can be helpful for an athlete to focus on their accomplishments rather than their failures, as suggested by this swimmer: "Recognize all [of your] achievements, even if [your] ultimate goal was not realized. For example, I made it to Olympic trials but not to the Olympics. I've felt nothing but shame and embarrassment for years because of this, but as of recent I've learnt to be proud of my achievements."

Athletic identity at the time of transition: Perhaps the most frequently researched variable associated with the literature on athletic retirement is identity foreclosure, or the degree to which an athlete identifies themselves through their sport to the exclusion of other roles and interests. For this sample, identity foreclosure accounted for another 4.3% of the variance, suggesting that athletes transitioned better when they had a diverse identity that included but was not restricted to their role as an athlete. As said by this volleyballer, "I think one of the main things that led to life satisfaction after retirement was that my sport was never the SOLE purpose and focus of my life—I always had other activities, family and friends to help balance;" and this gymnast, "You lose your identity after graduating from a sport you've done your whole life. You don't know your interests and what else there is to life right after your sport ends because you never had the time to think about anything else, which is sad."

Team atmosphere: The next most important variable, accounting for 1.6% of the variance, was the athlete's perception that the atmosphere on their last team or program, or with their previous coach, was healthy and positive. Persistent feelings of anger, resentment, and bitterness can complicate the transition out of sports, a situation that is particularly significant when athletes experience bullying, abuse, or harassment. The reflections of this Division I softballer mirror several athletes who specifically identified abuse as causing psychological suffering long after retirement. "I have suffered extreme trauma from the emotional and mental abuse my collegiate coach inflicted. Most of my anxiety and depression stems from the trauma experienced in college." Another athlete wrote, "I left collegiate D1 sport due to an emotionally and verbally abusive coach, took a year off and then transitioned to collegiate club. It was the best decision for me but I felt like I missed out on a real D1 experience due to the trauma that I endured. Myself and my former teammates are still dealing with PTSD from these events."

Toxic sporting environments are often associated with coaching practices that are punitive, fear-based, demeaning, abusive, or otherwise hostile and dehumanizing. Athletes facing these conditions may suffer long-term adverse effects like chronic anxiety, depression, disordered eating, difficulty with trust, low self-esteem, substance misuse, dissociation, somatization, and symptoms of trauma-related disorders like post-traumatic stress disorder [13,19–22].

Gender: Female gender contributed 1% of the variance. Studies of mental health symptoms and disorders in current elite women athletes show higher rates of general psychological distress, anxiety, depression, disordered eating, and sleep disturbances than in current elite men athletes [23,24]. There are few studies on mental health symptoms in elite retired women athletes; however, in a study of retired women collegiate gymnasts (n = 473), Sweeney and colleagues [25] showed that those who specialized early, had surgery for sports injuries, and had a history of concussion were more likely to have accessed mental health services for anxiety disorders. In addition, those gymnasts with a history of disordered eating had higher current pain levels and lower physical functioning. Another study by Kerr and colleagues [26] of former collegiate athletes from different sports (n = 797; 52.8% women, 47.2% men) did not show gender differences in mental health and found that former athletes across genders had somewhat better psychological and physical health than the general population.

Although the mental health of the 204 retired elite gymnasts that Dr Larry Nassar sexually abused have not been systematically studied, their victim impact statements at his trial described a significant effect on their mental health, including depression, anxiety, loss of self-esteem, distorted body image, disordered eating, self-harm, and suicidal ideation [27]. Finally, in a study of former US women's Division I soccer athletes (n = 101), DeFreese and colleagues [11] found that many participants recommended physical activity/exercise, career guidance, mentorship programming, and mental health support to assist future retiring athletes.

Summary of Predictors Associated with Transition Outcomes: Together, these five variables explained 22.3% of the variance associated with an athlete's HHQ as measured during their PAD, or during their period of greatest adjustment difficulty following their decision to retire. Variables that dropped from the model included (1) the duration of my career was as long or longer than I anticipated; (2) the decision to retire was in my control; and (3) I made plans for retirement before it occurred. Although these elements often appear in research and treatment programs for transitioning athletes, data for participants in this study failed to show a sufficiently unique contribution from these variables to be retained in the model.

Components of the HHQ: Examining individual components of the HHQ provided additional insights into these challenges and are elucidated as follows:

Cognitive health: Forty-nine percent of this sample stated that they sometimes or often experienced problems with their thinking, memory, or attention during their PAD. Although we could not determine the origin of these concerns, many athletes indicated worries in line with this Lacrosse player, who stated, "I have real concerns about my concussion history and how it might impact me." Focusing and attention problems can also be symptoms of anxiety and depression or issues unrelated to their transition out of sports (eg, attention-deficit/hyperactivity disorder).

Exercise and diet: Twenty-six percent of participants indicated that they rarely or never engaged in exercise or kept to a healthy diet during their PAD. While training, elite athletes rigorously exercise for extended periods and are often required to ingest twice or more times the recommended calories for a non-athlete. Perhaps this professional soccer player summarized it best: "[The] biggest issues for me were nutrition and lack of structured exercise. I still ate like an elite athlete and didn't know how to make myself exercise without the sport performance as my end goal." A Division 1 volleyball player stated, "A major topic that nobody talks about is learning how to eat. The body can change drastically after playing, leading to body image issues and not being able to mentally accept those changes."

These challenges were reflected in the 53% of our sample who reported that they sometimes or often struggled to create structure in their life. Without the schedule, consequences, and control of a system that governs diet and exercise, many athletes struggle to build those habits autonomously. As stated by this elite rower, "I felt like I didn't know how to transition to a life that wasn't structured and where I wasn't training for something."

Many women participants identified negative body image as an issue during their PAD. One wrote, "A lot of my issues, beyond mental health, had to do with body image and learning a new way to exercise and take care of my body outside of training for competition." Another wrote, "As a female, the transition of uncontrollable body shape affects me a lot." Consider this poignant observation by a Division III sprint and relay swimmer: "Physical traits that were helpful in sports are often opposite of what is traditionally attractive, at least for women. It's a hard transition."

Pain: Fifty-six percent of our participants indicated that during their PAD, they sometimes or often experienced pain caused by their careers in sports. Chronic pain from injuries and strenuous bodily use over long periods is often associated with greater adjustment difficulty [28–30]. Consider these athlete's observations: "The physical pains I have now as an almost 50-year-old are crazy. My non-athlete sisters are in great shape, no pains, and I can barely walk some days;" and "I beat my body up badly. I needed knee replacement early to the point I couldn't do any activities." When asked to provide additional information to help us better understand this retired synchronized swimmer's adjustment, she simply wrote, "Lifelong debilitating body pain."

Mental health: The HHQ included two questions about anxiety from the GAD-2, two about depression from the PHQ-2, and one about suicidal ideation. Combining the GAD-2 and PHQ-2 items provided an estimate of the psychological or emotional distress experienced by our participants during their PAD. According to these data, 60.0% reported experiencing these symptoms in the sometimes and often range across all four items. Additionally, 11.7% said they sometimes or often thought about suicide during their PAD. These data indicate that an overwhelming number of athletes face significant mental health hardship during their transition out of sports. Consider this haunting observation by a semi-professional ice-hockey athlete, who stated, "It's Hell. People only pretend to care. My sport was everything to me. Meant more than anything and I'd give the rest of my life to go back and finish what I started. But I can't. Consequences linger. Pain is Physical, Mental, Emotional, etc. Nonstop pain."

Behavioral health: The Athlete Transition Study asked three questions on behavioral health. Participants sometimes or often endorsed the following items during their PAD: 35% had difficulty with frustration and anger; 33% engaged in gambling, partying, or overspending; and 28% stated that they engaged in risky drinking or drug use. One water polo athlete wrote, "Heavy drug use took over my life... My competitive nature from sports became a competitive life of drugs chasing a high. Hitting rock bottom and going to rehab helped me find myself and eventually my fiancé."

Social health: One of the most common laments of athletes, once they leave sports, is the loss of being a part of a team, as indicated by the 57% of participants who sometimes or often felt lonely and socially disconnected during their PAD. One athlete wrote, "Transitioning from sport also meant I lost my entire support system at once." A table tennis athlete who competed for a national team stated, "The most difficult thing I found by far was the lack of friends and social engagement outside of sport since I had spent so long within the sport building those relationships."

SUMMARY AND CONCLUSIONS

Although prior research indicates that 16% to 20% of elite athletes experience substantial adjustment problems during their transition out of sports [2], these data suggest a higher frequency across a range of health domains. Sixty percent of participants reported significant mental health concerns, and more than half had chronic pain and struggled to create structure in their lives. Considering the number of elite athletes who retire every year, these data indicate that retiring athletes are an at-risk population. A holistic questionnaire like the HHQ can help determine which athletes are struggling and in what specific holistic health domains. This information can be crucial when identifying at-risk athletes and making informed decisions about the need for support and treatment.

Prior research has identified a host of variables associated with adjustment outcomes. Our regression analysis suggested that, for the eight included variables, 22.3% percent of the variance associated with differential transition experiences came down to five variables. The most important of these, accounting for 10.5% of the total variance associated with post-career adjustment, was whether the moment they entered retirement was a surprise. Coaches, trainers, team doctors, and other staff will be aware when these situations arise. Before retirement, systems need to be initiated to improve the mental health literacy of these individuals, as well as an awareness of referral sources and building the expectation for following up on athlete welfare [31]. After retirement, the athlete, their family, and their social support system need to be aware of the difficulties associated with sudden retirement and encouraged to accept and offer increased support and treatment opportunities, including counseling, financial literacy, career assessment, and networking. Some have suggested expanding the exit health examination to include a mental health and well-being assessment such that a transition plan emphasizing holistic health can be created [32]. All these services can be included in a formal after-career program that focuses on (1): detraining (2); treatment of chronic injury and pain conditions (eg, osteoarthritis) (3); keeping a structured and healthy lifestyle (4); treatment of mental, cognitive, social, physical, and behavioral health problems and finding pathways toward wellness; and (5) education and employment [33].

Prior research has consistently reported on the impact of a toxic team environment. These data suggest that the legacy of that negativity can extend far beyond the point where the athlete leaves the team. Reports of abuse, harassment, racism, marginalization, and depersonalization of athletes need to be considered as examples of a broader problem within elite sports rather than rare exceptions to an otherwise healthy culture.

For many athletes, sport is more than just something they do—it is who they are. Recent models within the transition literature encourage a dual-career focus, where athletes see their competitive success as one prong and their development of a vocation or career within or outside of sport as a second prong. By developing interests, experiences, and education beyond sports, an athlete is better prepared to find work and, perhaps more importantly, invest their time in activities that have existential meaning and invigorate the pursuit of new goals [17].

Counseling with a mental health provider experienced with athletes can be a lifeline once competitive sport is no longer an individual's sole focus. For example, counseling can help athletes reassess how they perceive or value the time and costs associated with their careers. Whether or not an athlete played collegiate Division 1, made the roster of a professional team, advanced to the Olympic trials or made the Olympic team, or failed to medal or failed to gold medal, evaluating the success or failure of a career comes down to an appraisal of personal expectations. Once a career is over, all opportunities to meet unfulfilled ambitions end. Counseling an athlete on their identity is about who they want to become in the future.

Learning to reflect with pride and satisfaction on the past is similarly essential. Few athletes meet or exceed all their career ambitions; still, it is possible to remember their accomplishments positively.

This Division III gymnast expresses well how to think about transitioning into retirement: "A few things I wish I would have known as an athlete and transitioning out of my sport: There is so much more of a life out there beyond your sport. Don't forget that. You literally have the whole world open up to you and can do literally anything you want. Try new things, try new hobbies, and make new friends in more than one place in your life. (eg, work friends, gym friends, friends from a local group). Don't turn to negative coping mechanisms to cope with your retirement (not eating, over-exercising, drugs, alcohol, gambling, etc.) It is only going to make the transition harder and you will be miserable and miss out on so much of your life. Whatever happened to you throughout your sport, DOES NOT DEFINE YOU. Your sport in general does not define you. It can be a part of your life, but don't forget that you are so much more than being an athlete."

LIMITATIONS

There are several limitations of this study. First, the data collected about the participant's transition, PAD, and holistic health outcomes were retrospectively self-reported. In some cases, these events took place many years ago, leading to possible recall bias or inaccuracy. Second, this study used a convenience sample, so we cannot generalize to the larger population of retired athletes beyond these participants, nor can we calculate a response rate to assess for sampling bias. For example, this study may have recruited a disproportionate group of athletes more likely to have had retirement struggles and distress. Third, this sample is heavily represented by White (78%) and women (68%) athletes; therefore, the findings may not apply to men athletes or underrepresented ethnic athlete groups. Fourth, to keep the survey to a manageable length, many single-domain questions were explicitly created for the study, which limited the use of longer validated instruments (eg, alcohol misuse, emotional distress, chronic pain) that might have been more reliable. Fourth, there is no comparison group (eg, graduating college students) that would allow a comparison of athlete transition to collegiate educational/career transition difficulties. And finally, data were collected during the Coronavirus Disease 2019 (COVID-19) pandemic, which may have resulted in responses that were specifically impacted by that unique period.

DISCLOSURE

The authors have nothing to disclose.

REFERENCES

[1] Number of NCAA student athletes in the United States in 2022, by gender. 2022. Available at: https://www.statista.com/statistics/1098761/student-athletes-by-gender/. Accessed on 11 Apr 2023.

[2] Park S, Lavallee D, Tod D. Athletes' career transition out of sport: a systematic review. Int Rev Sport Exerc Psychol 2013;6(1):22–53.

[3] Stambulova N, Wylleman P. Athletes' career development and transitions. In: Papaioannou AG, Hackfort D, editors. Routledge companion to sport and exercise psychology: Global perspectives and fundamental concepts. Philadelphia, PA: Routledge/Taylor & Francis Group; 2014. p. 605–20.

[4] Lavallee D. Engagement in sport career transition planning enhances performance. J Loss Trauma 2019;24(1):1–8.

[5] Wylleman P. A developmental and holistic perspective on transitioning out of elite sport. In American Psychological Association Handbook of Sports and Exercise Psychology. Volume 1: Sport Psychology. Washington, DC: American Psychological Association; 2019. p. 201–16.

[6] Lally P. Identity and athletic retirement: A prospective study. Psychol Sport Exerc 2007;8:85–99.

[7] Alferman D, Stambulova N. Career transitions and career termination. In: Tenenbaum G, Eklund RC, editors. Handbook of sport psychology. 3rd edition. New York: Wiley; 2007. p. 712–36.

[8] Kuettel A, Boyle E, Schmid J. Factors contributing to the quality of the transition out of elite sports in Swiss, Danish, and Polish athletes. Psychol Sport Exerc 2016;29:27–39.

[9] Kiefer HR, Petrie TA, Walls R. The transition from collegiate sport: An analysis of the current retirement planning practices of NCAA institutions. J Study Sports Athletes Educ 2021;1–17.

[10] Harry M, Weight E. Post-collegiate athlete transitions and the influence of a coach. J Study Sports Athletes Educ 2021. https://doi.org/10.1080/19357397.2021.1916338.

[11] DeFreese J, Weight E, DeCicco J, et al. Examining a conceptual framework for transition experiences of former collegiate women's soccer athletes. J Intercoll Sport 2021;14(2):1–18.

[12] Greaves L, Hankivsky O, Kirby S. The dome of silence: Sexual harassment and abuse in sport. Winnipeg, Canada: Fernwood Publishing; 2000.

[13] Mountjoy M, Brackenridge C, Arrington M, et al. International Olympic Committee consensus statement: harassment and abuse (non-accidental violence) in sport. Br J Sports Med 2016;50(17):1019–29.

[14] Cooper DJ, Batt ME, O'Hanlon MS, et al. A Cross-Sectional Study of Retired Great British Olympians (Berlin 1936-Sochi 2014): Olympic Career Injuries, Joint Health in Later Life, and Reasons for Retirement from Olympic Sport. Sports Med Open 2021;7(1):54.

[15] Wippert P, Wippert J. Perceived Stress and Prevalence of Traumatic Stress Symptoms Following Athletic Career Termination. J Clin Sport Psychol 2008;2(1):1–16. Available at: https://journals.humankinetics.com/view/journals/jcsp/2/1/article-p1.xml.

[16] Douglas K, Carless D. Abandoning The Performance Narrative: Two Women's Stories of Transition from Professional Sport. J Appl Sport Psychol 2009;21(2):213–30.

[17] Stambulova N, Ryba T, Henriksen K. Career development and transition of athletes: The international society of sport psychology position stand revisited. Int J Sport Exerc Psychol 2021;19(4):524–50.

[18] Wylleman P. A developmental and holistic perspective on transitioning out of elite sport. In APA Handbook of Sports & Exercise Psychology Volume 1. Sports Psychology. Edited by Anshel MH, Petrie TA, Steinfeldt JA. Chapter 11, American Psychological Association, Washington DC, pp 201-216. Available at: https://doi.org/10.1037/0000123-011.

[19] Stirling AE. Definition and constituents of maltreatment in sport: establishing a conceptual framework for research practitioners. Br J Sports Med 2009;43(14):1091–9, Epub 2008 Nov 21. PMID: 19028734.

[20] Mountjoy M, Junge A, Magnusson C, et al. Beneath the Surface: Mental Health and Harassment and Abuse of Athletes Participating in the FINA (Aquatics) World Championships, 2019. Clin J Sport Med 2022;32(2):95–102, PMID: 34483238.

[21] Aron CM, Harvey S, Hainline B, et al. Post-traumatic stress disorder (PTSD) and other trauma-related mental disorders in elite athletes: a narrative review. Br J Sports Med 2019;53(12):779–84, Epub 2019 Apr 25. PMID: 31023859.

[22] Mountjoy M, Edwards C. Athlete Mental Health Impacts of Harassment and Abuse in Sport. In: Reardon CL, editor. Mental health care for elite athletes. Cham: Springer; 2022.

[23] Kilic Ö, Carmody S, Upmeijer J, et al. Prevalence of mental health symptoms among male and female Australian professional footballers. BMJ Open Sport Exerc Med 2021;7(3):e001043.

[24] Rice SM, Purcell R, De Silva S, et al. The Mental Health of Elite Athletes: A Narrative Systematic Review. Sports Med 2016;46(9):1333–53, PMID: 26896951; PMCID: PMC4996886.

[25] Sweeney E, Howell DR, Seehusen CN, et al. Health outcomes among former female collegiate gymnasts: the influence of sport specialization, concussion, and

disordered eating. Phys Sportsmed 2021;49(4):438–44, PMID: 33186080.

[26] Kerr ZY, DeFreese JD, Marshall SW. Current Physical and Mental Health of Former Collegiate Athletes. Orthop J Sports Med 2014;2(8):2325967114544107.

[27] Rahal S, Kozlowski K. 204 impact statements, 9 days, 2 counties, a life sentence for Larry Nassar. Detroit news; 2018. Available at: https://www.detroitnews.com/story/news/local/michigan/2018/02/08/204-impact-statements-9-days-2-counties-life-sentence-larry-nassar/1066335001/. Accessed 21 November 2022.

[28] Gouttebarge V, Jonkers R, Moen M, et al. The prevalence and risk indicators of symptoms of common mental disorders among current and former Dutch elite athletes. J Sports Sci 2017;35(21):2148–56.

[29] Brown JC, Kerkhoffs G, Lambert MI, et al. Forced Retirement from Professional Rugby Union is Associated with Symptoms of Distress. Int J Sports Med 2017;38(8):582–7.

[30] Mannes ZL, Waxenberg LB, Cottler LB, et al. Prevalence and Correlates of Psychological Distress among Retired Elite Athletes: A Systematic Review. Int Rev Sport Exerc Psychol 2019;12(1):265–94.

[31] Paul Gorczynski, Currie Alan, Gibson Kass, et al. Developing mental health literacy and cultural competence in elite sport. J Appl Sport Psychol 2021;33(4):387–401.

[32] Carmody S, Jones C, Malhotra A, et al. Put out to pasture: what is our duty of care to the retiring professional footballer? Promoting the concept of the 'exit health examination' (EHE)British. J Sports Med 2019; 53:788–9.

[33] Gouttebarge V, Goedhart E, Kerkhoffs G. Empowering the health of retired professional footballers: the systematic development of an After Career Consultation and its feasibility. BMJ Open Sport Exerc Med 2018;4(1): e000466.

Women's Mental Health

Advances in Psychiatry and Behavioral Health 3 (2023) 81–89

ADVANCES IN PSYCHIATRY AND BEHAVIORAL HEALTH

Perinatal Cannabis Use

A Clinical Review

Marissa L. Beal, DO[a],*, Julia R. Frew, MD[b,1]

[a]Department of Psychiatry & Behavioral Sciences, Johns Hopkins University School of Medicine, 550 Building, Suite 305, Baltimore, MD 21205, USA; [b]Department of Psychiatry, Geisel School of Medicine/Dartmouth Health, One Medical Center Drive, Lebanon, NH 03756, USA

KEYWORDS

• Cannabis • Marijuana • Pregnancy • Lactation • Perinatal

KEY POINTS

- The prevalence of cannabis use in women of childbearing age is increasing drastically in the United States.
- Cannabis use during pregnancy is likely associated with preterm birth, low birth weight, and long-term neuropsychiatric outcomes, though the current body of data has significant limitations.
- Providers should screen for cannabis use and cannabis use disorder among reproductive-age women and counsel them about the known and unknown risks of exposure in pregnancy and lactation.
- It is important to identify co-occurring mental health disorders and ensure adequate treatment during pregnancy and postpartum.
- There is a significant need for more research into outcomes, treatment, and public health initiatives related to cannabis use in pregnancy and postpartum.

INTRODUCTION/BACKGROUND

Cannabis use and cannabis use disorder (CUD) are increasing in prevalence during pregnancy and lactation and thus it is important for clinicians to acknowledge, screen, and discuss cannabis use with perinatal patients [1]. We present an evidence-based, clinically focused summary and guidelines for identifying and discussing cannabis use and CUD in pregnancy and lactation. Although we will discuss maternal-fetal outcome data related to perinatal cannabis use during pregnancy, this is not a systematic review, but a summary of the literature. We hope this review will help to guide discussions with patients related to the known and unknown risks of cannabis use during pregnancy.

Epidemiology

Cannabis use is common throughout the world and is one of the most used substances during pregnancy and lactation in the United States [1]. In 2020, 17.9% of people aged 12 or older reported using cannabis in the past year, up from 11% in 2002, with an increase in cannabis use for women in all age groups. Cannabis use in 2020 was the highest in the 18- to 25-year-old cohort of women, with 22.7% reporting use in the last month and 6.1% reporting daily or almost daily use, highlighting the increasing rate of cannabis use for women of childbearing age [1]. As the rate of use has increased in the general population and among women, this is also the case for pregnant women, with 8% reporting cannabis use in the past month in 2020 and

---

[1] Present address: One Medical Center Drive, Lebanon, NH 03756, USA.

*Corresponding author, *E-mail address:* mbeal4@jhmi.edu

https://doi.org/10.1016/j.ypsc.2023.03.013
2667-3827/23/ © 2023 Elsevier Inc. All rights reserved.

2.8% reporting daily use, up from 3.4% and 0.9%, respectively, in 2002 [1,2]. Pregnant women who use cannabis are also more likely to use other substances such as tobacco, alcohol, and illicit drugs [3].

The landscape for cannabis use is changing in the United States with a growing number of states legalizing or decriminalizing recreational cannabis use and legalizing medical use, although federally cannabis remains a schedule I drug. In the general population, perceived risk of cannabis use is much lower than for other illicit drugs, such as cocaine or opioids [1]. Perspectives regarding cannabis use during pregnancy are also changing. From 2005 to 2015, the perceived risk of cannabis use decreased among pregnant and nonpregnant women [4]. Pregnant women also perceived less risk during pregnancy if cannabis was legal in their state [5,6]. Following the legalization of cannabis in Colorado, more pregnant patients used cannabis, as evidenced by an increased rate of detection and concentration of tetrahydrocannabinol (THC) in meconium, indicating that legalization may further impact the prevalence of cannabis use in pregnant women [7,8].

Modes of Use
Cannabis can be consumed via smoking, vaping, or oral ingestion; the route of administration impacts the pharmacokinetics and timing of the onset of effect. Inhaled cannabis has a rapid onset of effect, entering the bloodstream and brain quickly after use [9]. When ingested orally, the time of onset is slower but effects last longer due to slowed absorption in the gastrointestinal tract [9]. Owing to its lipophilic nature, cannabis accumulates in the body and can be detected for 30 days or more after the last use, especially for chronic users [9]. Women tend to use cannabis via multiple routes of administration before conception [10]. There is also an added risk of contamination of cannabis with other toxins, pesticides, and substances such as opioids, which may increase the risk of use for pregnant patients, though systematic testing is limited [11].

Endocannabinoid System
The endocannabinoid system (ECS) consists of two receptors, CB1 and CB2. The most studied exogenous cannabinoids include THC and cannabidiol (CBD). THC is notably the more psychoactive compound causing symptoms of euphoria, anxiety, psychosis, cognitive effects, and psychomotor impairments [9]. THC is highly lipophilic and protein bound with a low molecular weight and thus readily crosses the blood-brain barrier, placenta, and into breastmilk. The ECS is implicated in pregnancy including gametogenesis, endometrial

proliferation, and placental development [12]. Alterations in the ECS may play a role in the development of reproductive pathology, such as miscarriage and preeclampsia, and some studies have shown an association with the use of cannabis and these outcomes though future research is needed to replicate these findings [12–15]. The ECS is also essential to brain development and neuronal differentiation and signaling and thus warrants consideration for the impacts of perinatal cannabis use on obstetric and fetal outcomes [16].

Cannabis Use Disorder
CUD is outlined in the Diagnostic and Statistical Manual of Mental Disorders, Fifth Edition (DSM-5) as a pattern of cannabis use leading to functional impairment or distress, with symptoms including taking cannabis in larger amounts or spending a great deal of time trying to obtain cannabis, cannabis use impacting social and physical functioning, and withdrawal and tolerance [17]. Severity of CUD is based on the number of symptoms present, ranging from mild to severe [17]. Data suggest that cannabis withdrawal syndrome is common [18], and is defined as symptoms of irritability, anger or aggression; anxiety; sleep difficulty; decreased appetite; restlessness; depressed mood; and physical symptoms such as abdominal pain, tremor, sweating, fever, chills or headache [17]. Similar to rates of cannabis use, CUD is increasing in women, with the highest rate in women ages 18 to 25 [1]. Alaska Native or American Indian and multiracial people are more likely to use cannabis than white, black, Hispanic, or Asian people [1]. It is estimated that 3 out of 10 people that use cannabis will develop a CUD [19]. There are a paucity of data on the management and treatment of CUD. The best evidence indicates that psychotherapeutic strategies, such as cognitive behavioral therapy (CBT) and motivational enhancement therapy (MET), may be helpful in reducing cannabis use [20,21]. There are no pharmacologic treatments approved for CUD currently and limited evidence for the use of other psychotropic medications for the treatment of CUD [22].

Outcomes
The data related to cannabis use and maternal-fetal outcomes are limited and there are significant gaps in the literature. It is important to recognize that many of the studies assessing the risks of cannabis use during pregnancy have small sample sizes and use different mechanisms to identify cannabis use and exposure (such as self-report versus urine drug screens). There are also challenges regarding methodology and quantifying the amount and potency of cannabis. The composition of

cannabis has changed over the years and the concentration of THC is much higher now than years earlier, which may limit the ability to compare outcomes over time [23]. Cannabis use frequently co-occurs with other illicit substances and tobacco use, psychiatric illness, and lower socioeconomic status that may further confound results regarding obstetric outcomes [3,24,25]. Despite these limitations, we will summarize currently available data regarding fetal and obstetric outcomes associated with perinatal cannabis use below and in Table 1.

Fetal malformations: In regards to fetal malformation, there are no clear data indicating an association between cannabis use and fetal malformations [30–32,34,50].

Stillbirth: There is a possible increased risk for stillbirth for patients using illicit substances and most commonly cannabis [15]. Varner and colleagues [15] completed a case report study looking at 663 stillbirths and assayed for illicit drug use and smoking during pregnancy. They found an association between cannabis use and stillbirth, though this finding may be confounded by concomitant tobacco use.

Preterm birth: Studies vary in regard to the risk of preterm birth and perinatal cannabis use. Two recent meta-analyses showed an association between cannabis use in pregnancy and pre-term birth [35,37] whereas two did not [34,38]. A 2016 meta-analysis by Conner and colleagues [38] initially found an association between preterm birth and cannabis use, but after controlling for tobacco use this was no longer significant.

TABLE 1
Outcomes Following Cannabis Use During Pregnancy[a]

Outcomes	Summary	Positive Association	No Association
Associated with malformation	No clear association [31]	• Cohort studies with increased risk for VSD [27], gastroschisis [28,29], and anencephaly [33] but significant limitations	• One meta-analysis [34] and multiple cohort [30,32,50] studies show no association
Stillbirth	Possible increased risk though major study did not control for tobacco use	• Case-control study with increased association [15]	
Preterm birth	Possible increased risk, though studies are mixed	• Multiple meta-analyses [35,37] and cohort studies [36,39] with a positive association	• Two meta-analyses [34,38] with no association after controlling for confounders
Low birth weight	Likely increased risk, unclear if clinically significant as the change in weight is small	• Multiple meta-analyses [34,35,37] and cohort studies [26,39,40,51] with positive association	• Meta-analysis with no association after controlling for cofounders [38]
NICU admission	Possible increased risk, though studies are mixed	• Multiple meta-analyses [34,37] and cohort studies [39,41,42] with a positive association	• Meta-analysis [38] and cohort study [26] with no association
Neuropsychiatric outcomes	Likely association but need additional studies	• Exaggerated startles, tremors, sleep deficits [43] • Differences in language, memory, attention, behavior, visual perception [44–47] • Increased risk of autism [36] • Increased vulnerability to psychopathology [48,49]	• No differences before age 4 [52]

[a] This is not a comprehensive or systematic review but a summary based on key articles.

Low birth weight: Although results are still mixed, there appears to be an association between low birth weight and prenatal cannabis use [34,35,37,38,51]. Notably, for Conner and colleagues [38] this association was only maintained for severe cannabis use after tobacco use was controlled for though more recent meta-analyses have demonstrated this association [35,37]. It is difficult to assess if this change in birth weight is clinically significant as it was estimated to be about 100 grams lower in exposed versus unexposed infants [34]. A study by El Marroun and colleagues [51] noted that low birth weight was dose-dependent.

Neonatal intensive care unit (NICU) admission: Two meta-analyses showed an increased rate of NICU admission for babies exposed to cannabis [34,37] though studies are mixed [26].

Neuropsychiatric outcomes: Three longitudinal studies examined long-term outcomes for infants and children after maternal cannabis exposure. The Ottawa Prenatal Prospective Study (OPPS) in Ottawa, Canada followed 698 women in the third trimester and children until ages 18 to 22, including about 200 women with perinatal cannabis, tobacco, and alcohol use. Initially after delivery for those with maternal cannabis use, infants were noted to have exaggerated startles, tremors, and sleep deficits [43] though no differences in neuropsychiatric outcomes before age 4 [52]. After age 4, differences were found in language, memory, attention, behavioral problems, and visual perception tasks [45]. The Maternal Health Practices and Child Development Study (MHPCD) followed a group of 1360 pregnant women and identified around 270 women who reported using cannabis during pregnancy in Pittsburgh, Pennsylvania. Children with fetal exposure to cannabis use showed more hyperactivity and impulsivity as well as impaired academic functioning [46,47]. The Generation R Study, the most recent cohort, is following 9778 pregnant women in the Netherlands, with 220 women reporting cannabis use during pregnancy. Results thus far indicate increased aggression and attention deficits for girls at 18 months old but these differences were not sustained over time [44]. No differences in language development or cognition were noted.

Two recent studies in the United States and Canada reviewed neuropsychiatric symptoms over time. A recent retrospective analysis of births in Ontario, Canada indicated an increased risk to develop autism with maternal cannabis exposure with a fully adjusted hazard ratio of 1.51 (95% confidence interval: 1.17 to 1.96), though noted possibility for residual confounding [53]. The ABCD study is a long-term study among 21 sites across the United States tracking development from adolescence into young adulthood among 11,880 children who were enrolled between 9 and 10 years old. Retrospective analyses identified 655 children exposed to cannabis in utero. Exposure to cannabis prenatally was associated with vulnerability to psychopathology in middle childhood and adolescence, specifically for participants exposed after maternal knowledge of pregnancy [48,49].

In general, based on the literature and noting the significant limitations of the current data, there appears to be some potential association between prenatal cannabis use and low birth weight, preterm birth, and adverse neuropsychiatric outcomes for children exposed in utero. More data are needed to control for other confounding exposures as well as improved quantification of the amount of cannabis and potency of THC. The increased rate of psychiatric comorbidities among patients using cannabis is difficult to fully control for as maternal psychiatric comorbidity is a risk factor for adverse neuropsychiatric outcomes in children; thus, it is challenging to determine if the longitudinal neuropsychiatric outcomes are related to cannabis use, maternal psychopathology, or both [54]. Genetic and environmental factors, both in utero and postnatally, may also impact these outcomes, and it is difficult to control for all of these factors[55].

Breastfeeding

THC levels in breastmilk are estimated to be about 0.8% of the weight-adjusted maternal dose and detectable in breastmilk samples up to 6 days after use [56]. One study indicated an impact on motor development at one year for infants exposed to cannabis in breastmilk, but this did not control for first-trimester exposure to cannabis [57], and another study showed no such association [58]. The Academy of Breastfeeding Medicine states that there is insufficient evidence at this time to recommend abstaining from breastfeeding if a mother is using cannabis [59]. They recommend counseling women to reduce cannabis use and discuss the lack of data regarding long-term outcomes as well as the data regarding neuropsychiatric outcomes following in utero exposure and weigh the potential risks versus benefits of breastfeeding for both mom and baby [59].

DISCUSSION

It is clear that rates of cannabis use and CUD are increasing throughout the United States, particularly among women of childbearing age. As legalization and decriminalization continue, we need to consider how this may impact our discussions regarding cannabis use with patients during the perinatal period. The increased rates indicate an important need to screen all patients for cannabis use, discuss how patients are using cannabis, and, perhaps most importantly, why they are using cannabis (as outlined in Box 1). Just as we ask all women about tobacco and alcohol, providers should normalize discussing cannabis use. Providers may be uncomfortable discussing cannabis because of the current political climate related to legalization, but this should not be a barrier to initiate these discussions and provide patients with available information regarding the risks. Patients may also be reluctant to report substance use due to mandatory reporting policies for providers. Reporting policies are state specific and so it is essential to be knowledgeable regarding mandatory reporting to ensure adherence to legal reporting standards while also maintaining patient privacy as able. Some women may feel that medical cannabis is safer than nonmedical cannabis, though ultimately this is not the case. There is no indication that medical cannabis is safer in pregnancy, except for less risk of contamination with other illicit drugs, and medical cannabis is not US Food and Drug Administration (FDA) regulated at this time.

There are significant limitations within the cannabis literature, both in the general and the perinatal population. In the general population, there are challenges for ongoing research due to regulatory barriers since cannabis remains a schedule I drug, including limited source production and lack of funding, which contributes to the lack of information regarding cannabis use in the general population [60]. In the perinatal patient population, all studies are observational studies and thus have confounding variables that must be controlled for, including comorbid substance use and psychiatric disorders. In much of the literature, women are self-reporting cannabis use and it is difficult to truly know the effect

of cannabis if we do not even understand exactly the formulation, quantity, timing, or method of use.

A risk-risk analysis is an important framework in reproductive psychiatry that can be used when discussing cannabis use. To complete a thorough risk-risk discussion, we must consider why the patient is using cannabis and what perceived benefit they receive from using cannabis. Patient-identified reasons for perinatal cannabis use include improvement in nausea, vomiting, stress, and mood [61]. The difficulty with the risk-risk discussion regarding cannabis is that we do not have data that cannabis actually alleviates these symptoms [62–64]. Cannabis use is associated with increased symptom severity longitudinally for patients with depression, bipolar disorder, and posttraumatic stress disorder (PTSD), although it is difficult to tease out the directionality of the relationship [65,66]. For those patients who are receiving medical cannabis for conditions such as PTSD and anxiety, there is a lack of sufficient data to suggest that medical cannabis is efficacious for these disorders [67]. The incongruence between perceived benefits from cannabis and lack of literature indicating benefits must be discussed with patients, including for medical cannabis. Alternative treatments for the management of nausea, vomiting, and mood symptoms should be discussed, as other treatments may have more evidence regarding efficacy and information about risks associated with use. Engaging in an open-ended conversation regarding the data may also be beneficial to provide information in a nonjudgmental way and allow patients themselves to weigh the potential risks [68]. Ideally, these discussions would begin before conception so that patients begin trialing other treatment options before pregnancy to reduce multiple exposures during pregnancy. We highlight some useful questions and statements during clinical evaluation to further guide this conversation in Table 2.

BOX 1
Guidelines for Clinicians When Discussing Perinatal Cannabis Use

Guidelines for clinicians:
1. Ask openly about substance use with patients
2. If cannabis use is identified, discuss frequency and route
3. Ask about why they use cannabis, and what symptoms it helps with (eg, anxiety, nausea, and insomnia)
4. Target these symptoms with psychotropic medications or alternate treatment options if applicable
5. Discuss the risks of cannabis use and limitations of current research
6. Encourage reduction of use or abstinence during pregnancy and when breastfeeding
7. Discuss breastfeeding plan and risks of cannabis use with breastfeeding
8. Continue to assess through pregnancy and postpartum

TABLE 2 Questions and Statements for Providers to Use When Discussing Cannabis Use	
Questions	**Statements**
Can you tell me about your cannabis use and how it makes you feel?	I understand that cannabis is helping to relieve some of your symptoms.
What symptoms does it help you with?	I want to hear how cannabis helps you as an individual and consider other treatments that may be beneficial.
Have you tried alternatives, such as medications or behavioral interventions, to help with those symptoms in the past?	Unfortunately, the evidence-based data for cannabis use is limited, even for medical cannabis. Perhaps we can discuss other options, including treatments with more safety data in pregnancy.
What are your concerns regarding cannabis use in pregnancy?	We can work together to identify resources and behavioral interventions to help decrease your cannabis use.

As the access to cannabis is changing, we need to consider how else to disseminate information about the risks of cannabis use during pregnancy. In some states where cannabis is legal, a government warning is required to inform people that cannabis use while pregnant or breastfeeding may cause harm. In Colorado statements are displayed in dispensaries regarding the risks of cannabis use in pregnancy and breastfeeding, though despite this a majority of cannabis dispensaries in Colorado recommended cannabis products for pregnant women with morning sickness, highlighting a gap in information for people who are providing cannabis to women [69]. Some states require all medical cannabis cards to contain a statement not to use medical cannabis during pregnancy and breastfeeding, and some require a physician to document a discussion regarding the risks of medical cannabis in pregnancy and breastfeeding, as well as a risk of being reported to child protection when issuing a medical cannabis card. At this time initiatives are state-dependent, which leads to varied requirements, labeling, and education. Increased education for physicians issuing medical cannabis cards as well as people who work at dispensaries are needed as both feel they have insufficient knowledge to counsel women [70]. Using a framework similar to that used for alcohol and tobacco may help to bridge this gap, to make clear that legality does not equate to safety in pregnancy [70].

SUMMARY

The prevalence of cannabis use in women of childbearing age is increasing drastically, likely related to increased legalization. Cannabis use during pregnancy is likely associated with preterm birth, low birth weight, and long-term neuropsychiatric outcomes, although data have significant limitations. Providers should screen for cannabis use and CUD regularly and counsel women about the known and unknown data regarding outcomes. It is important to identify co-occurring mental health disorders and ensure adequate treatment during pregnancy and postpartum. There is a significant need for more research into outcomes, treatment, and public health initiatives related to cannabis use in pregnancy and postpartum.

CLINICS CARE POINTS

- Cannabis use is becoming more common, especially for women of childbearing age
- Screen pregnant and postpartum patients routinely for cannabis use and use disorders
- Discuss why patients are using cannabis and identify other evidence-based treatment of their symptoms
- Discuss known adverse outcomes associated with cannabis use as well as the limitations of the literature
- Encourage abstinence or decreasing use during pregnancy and lactation

DISCLOSURE

The authors have nothing to disclose.

REFERENCES

[1] Substance Abuse and Mental Health Services Administration. Key substance use and mental health indicators in

the United States: results from the 2020 national survey on drug use and health, Center. In: for Behavioral Health Statistics and Quality, Substance Abuse and Mental. Rockville, MD: Health Services Administration; 2021.

[2] Volkow ND, Han B, Compton WM, et al. Self-reported medical and nonmedical cannabis use among pregnant women in the United States. JAMA 2019;322(2):167–9.

[3] Ko JY, Farr SL, Tong VT, et al. Prevalence and patterns of marijuana use among pregnant and nonpregnant women of reproductive age. Obstet Gynecol 2015; 213(2):201. e1–201. e10.

[4] Jarlenski M, Koma JW, Zank J, et al. Trends in perception of risk of regular marijuana use among US pregnant and nonpregnant reproductive-aged women. Am J Obstet Gynecol 2017;217(6):705–7.

[5] Mark K, Gryczynski J, Axenfeld E, et al. Pregnant women's current and intended cannabis use in relation to their views toward legalization and knowledge of potential harm. J Addiction Med 2017;11(3):211–6.

[6] Ng JH, Rice KK, Ananth CV, et al. Attitudes about marijuana use, potential risks, and legalization: a single-center survey of pregnant women. J Matern Fetal Neonatal Med 2020;35(24):4635–43.

[7] Jones JT, Baldwin A, Shu I. A comparison of meconium screening outcomes as an indicator of the impact of state-level relaxation of marijuana policy. Drug Alcohol Depend 2015;100(156):e104–5.

[8] Gnofam M, Allshouse AA, Stickrath EH, et al. Impact of marijuana legalization on prevalence of maternal marijuana use and perinatal outcomes. Am J Perinatol 2020;37(01):59.

[9] Ashton CH. Pharmacology and effects of cannabis: a brief review. Br J Psychiatry 2001;178(2):101–6.

[10] Young-Wolff KC, Adams SR, Brown QL, et al. Modes of cannabis administration in the year prior to conception among patients in Northern California. Addictive Behaviors Reports 2022;15:100416.

[11] McLaren J, Swift W, Dillon P, et al. Cannabis potency and contamination: a review of the literature. Addiction 2008;103(7):1100–9.

[12] Maia J, Fonseca BM, Teixeira N, et al. The fundamental role of the endocannabinoid system in endometrium and placenta: implications in pathophysiological aspects of uterine and pregnancy disorders. Hum Reprod Update 2020;26(4):586–602.

[13] Prewitt KC, Hayer S, Garg B, et al. Impact of prenatal cannabis use disorder on perinatal outcomes. J Addiction Med 2022.

[14] Coleman-Cowger VH, Oga EA, Peters EN, et al. Prevalence and associated birth outcomes of co-use of cannabis and tobacco cigarettes during pregnancy. Neurotoxicol Teratol 2018;68:84–90.

[15] Varner MW, Silver RM, Hogue CJR, et al. Association between stillbirth and illicit drug use and smoking during pregnancy. Obstet Gynecol 2014;123(1):113.

[16] Harkany T, Keimpema E, Barabás K, et al. Endocannabinoid functions controlling neuronal specification during brain development. Mol Cell Endocrinol 2008;286(1–2):S84–90.

[17] American Psychiatric Association. Diagnostic and statistical manual of mental disorders. 5th ed. Washington, DC: American Psychiatric Association; 2013.

[18] Livne O, Shmulewitz D, Lev-Ran S, et al. DSM-5 cannabis withdrawal syndrome: demographic and clinical correlates in US adults. Drug Alcohol Depend 2019;195: 170–7.

[19] Hasin DS, Saha TD, Kerridge BT, et al. Prevalence of marijuana use disorders in the United States between 2001-2002 and 2012-2013. JAMA Psychiatr 2015; 72(12):1235–42.

[20] Davis ML, Powers MB, Handelsman P, et al. Behavioral therapies for treatment-seeking cannabis users: a metaanalysis of randomized controlled trials. Eval Health Prof 2015;38(1):94–114.

[21] Connor JP, Stjepanovic D, Le Foll B, et al. Cannabis use and cannabis use disorder. Nat Rev Dis Prim 2021;7(1): 1–24.

[22] Nielsen S, Gowing L, Sabioni P, et al. Pharmacotherapies for cannabis dependence. Cochrane Database Syst Rev 2019;1:Q20 Q19.

[23] ElSohly MA, Chandra S, Radwan M, et al. A comprehensive review of cannabis potency in the United States in the last decade. Biol Psychiatr: Cognitive Neuroscience and Neuroimaging 2021;6(6):603–6.

[24] Goodwin RD, Zhu J, Heisler Z, et al. Cannabis use during pregnancy in the United States: the role of depression. Drug Alcohol Depend 2020;210:107881.

[25] Jeffers AM, Glantz S, Byers A, et al. Sociodemographic characteristics associated with and prevalence and frequency of cannabis use among adults in the US. JAMA Netw Open 2021;4(11):e2136571.

[26] Crume TL, Juhl AL, Brooks-Russell A, et al. Cannabis use during the perinatal period in a state with legalized recreational and medical marijuana. the association between maternal characteristics, breastfeeding patterns, and neonatal outcomes. J Pediatr 2018;197:90–6.

[27] Williams LJ, Correa A, Rasmussen S. Maternal lifestyle factors and risk for ventricular septal defects. Birth Defects Res Part A Clin Mol Teratol 2004;70(2):59–64.

[28] Torfs CP, Velie EM, Oechsli FW, et al. A population based study of gastroschisis: Demographic, pregnancy, and lifestyle risk factors. Teratology 1994;50(1):44–53.

[29] Forrester MB, Merz RD. Risk of selected birth defects with prenatal illicit drug use, Hawaii, 1986–2002. J Toxicol Environ Health, Part A 2006;70(1):7–18.

[30] Witter FR, Niebyl JR. Marijuana use in pregnancy and pregnancy outcome. Am J Perinatol 1990;7(01):36–8.

[31] Metz TD, Stickrath EH. Marijuana use in pregnancy and lactation: a review of the evidence. Obstet Gynecol 2015;213(6):761–78.

[32] Gibson GT, Baghurst PA, Colley DP. Maternal alcohol, tobacco and cannabis consumption and the outcome of pregnancy. Aust N Z J Obstet Gynaecol 1983;23(1): 15–9.

[33] van Gelder MM, Reefhuis J, Caton AR, et al. Maternal periconceptional illicit drug use and the risk of congenital malformations. Epidemiology 2009;20(1):60–6.

[34] Gunn J, Rosales CB, Center KE, et al. Prenatal exposure to cannabis and maternal and child health outcomes: a systematic review and meta-analysis. BMJ Open 2016;6(4): e009986.

[35] Baía I, Domingues RMSM. The effects of cannabis use during pregnancy on low birth weight and preterm birth: a systematic review and meta-analysis. Am J Perinatol 2022 (AAM).

[36] Corsi DJ, Walsh L, Weiss D, et al. Association between self-reported prenatal cannabis use and maternal, perinatal, and neonatal outcomes. JAMA 2019;322(2): 145–52.

[37] Marchand G, Masoud AT, Govindan M, et al. Birth outcomes of neonates exposed to marijuana in Utero: a systematic review and meta-analysis. JAMA Netw Open 2022;5(1):e2145653.

[38] Conner SN, Bedell V, Lipsey K, et al. Maternal marijuana use and adverse neonatal outcomes. Obstecot Gynecol 2016;128(4):713–23.

[39] Bailey BA, Wood DL, Shah D. Impact of pregnancy marijuana use on birth outcomes: results from two matched population-based cohorts. J Perinatol 2020;40(10): 1477–82.

[40] Roncero C, Valriberas-Herrero I, Mezzatesta-Gava M, et al. Cannabis use during pregnancy and its relationship with fetal developmental outcomes and psychiatric disorders. A systematic review. Reprod Health 2020;17(1): 1–9.

[41] Warshak CR, Regan J, Moore B, et al. Association between marijuana use and adverse obstetrical and neonatal outcomes. J Perinatol 2015;35(12):991–5.

[42] Metz TD, Allshouse AA, Hogue CJ, et al. Maternal marijuana use, adverse pregnancy outcomes, and neonatal morbidity. Obstet Gynecol 2017;217(4):478, e1–8.

[43] Fried PA. Marihuana use by pregnant women: neurobehavioral effects in neonates. Drug Alcohol Depend 1980;6(6):415–24.

[44] El Marroun H, Hudziak JJ, Tiemeier H, et al. Intrauterine cannabis exposure leads to more aggressive behavior and attention problems in 18-month-old girls. Drug Alcohol Depend 2011;118(2–3):470–4.

[45] Fried PA, Watkinson B, Gray R. Differential effects on cognitive functioning in 9-to 12-year olds prenatally exposed to cigarettes and marihuana. Neurotoxicol Teratol 1998;20(3):293–306.

[46] Goldschmidt L, Day NL, Richardson GA. Effects of prenatal marijuana exposure on child behavior problems at age 10. Neurotoxicol Teratol 2000;22(3):325–36.

[47] Goldschmidt L, Richardson GA, Cornelius MD, et al. Prenatal marijuana and alcohol exposure and academic achievement at age 10. Neurotoxicol Teratol 2004; 26(4):521–32.

[48] Paul SE, Hatoum AS, Fine JD, et al. Associations between prenatal cannabis exposure and childhood outcomes: results from the ABCD study. JAMA Psychiatr 2021; 78(1):64–76.

[49] Baranger DA, Paul SE, Colbert SM, et al. Association of mental health burden with prenatal cannabis exposure from childhood to early adolescence: longitudinal findings from the adolescent brain cognitive development (ABCD) study. JAMA pediatrics 2022;176(12):1261–5.

[50] Linn S, Schoenbaum SC, Monson RR, et al. The association of marijuana use with outcome of pregnancy. Am J Public Health 1983;73(10):1161–4.

[51] El Marroun H, Tiemeier H, Steegers EA, et al. Intrauterine cannabis exposure affects fetal growth trajectories: the Generation R Study. J Am Acad Child Adolesc Psychiatry 2009;48(12):1173–81.

[52] Fried PA. The Ottawa prenatal prospective study (OPPS): methodological issues and findings—it's easy to throw the baby out with the bath water. Life Sci 1995;56(23–24):2159–68.

[53] Corsi DJ, Donelle J, Sucha E, et al. Maternal cannabis use in pregnancy and child neurodevelopmental outcomes. Nat Med 2020;26(10):1536–40.

[54] Goodman SH, Rouse MH, Connell AM, et al. Maternal depression and child psychopathology: a meta-analytic review. Clin Child Fam Psychol Rev 2011;14(1):1–27.

[55] Molenaar NM, Tiemeier H, van Rossum EF, et al. Prenatal maternal psychopathology and stress and offspring HPA axis function at 6 years. Psychoneuroendocrinology 2019;99:120–7.

[56] Bertrand KA, Hanan NJ, Honerkamp-Smith G, et al. Marijuana use by breastfeeding mothers and cannabinoid concentrations in breast milk. Pediatrics 2018; 142(3).

[57] Astley SJ, Little RE. Maternal marijuana use during lactation and infant development at one year. Neurotoxicol Teratol 1990;12(2):161–8.

[58] Tennes K, Avitable N, Blackard C, et al. Marijuana: prenatal and postnatal exposure in the human. NIDA Res Monogr 1985;59:48–60.

[59] Reece-Stremtan S, Marinelli KA, Academy of Breastfeeding Medicine. ABM clinical protocol# 21: guidelines for breastfeeding and substance use or substance use disorder, revised 2015. Breastfeed Med 2015;10(3):135–41.

[60] Cooper ZD, Abrams DI, Gust S, et al. Challenges for clinical cannabis and cannabinoid research in the united states. J Natl Cancer Inst Monographs 2021;2021(58): 114–22.

[61] Chang JC, Tarr JA, Holland CL, et al. Beliefs and attitudes regarding prenatal marijuana use: perspectives of pregnant women who report use. Drug Alcohol Depend 2019;196:14–20.

[62] Turna J, Patterson B, Van Ameringen M. Is cannabis treatment for anxiety, mood, and related disorders ready for prime time? Depress Anxiety 2017;34(11):1006–17.

[63] Bahji A, Meyyappan AC, Hawken ER. Efficacy and acceptability of cannabinoids for anxiety disorders in adults: a systematic review & meta-analysis. J Psychiatr Res 2020; 129:257–64.

[64] Black N, Stockings E, Campbell G, et al. Cannabinoids for the treatment of mental disorders and symptoms of mental disorders: a systematic review and meta-analysis. Lancet Psychiatr 2019;6(12):995–1010.

[65] Kuhns L, Kroon E, Colyer-Patel K, et al. Associations between cannabis use, cannabis use disorder, and mood disorders: longitudinal, genetic, and neurocognitive evidence. Psychopharmacology (Berl) 2022;239(5): 1231–49.

[66] Mammen G, Rueda S, Roerecke M, et al. Association of cannabis with long-term clinical symptoms in anxiety and mood disorders: a systematic review of prospective studies. J Clin Psychiatry 2018;79(4):2248.

[67] Stanciu CN, Brunette MF, Teja N, et al. Evidence for use of cannabinoids in mood disorders, anxiety disorders, and PTSD: a systematic review. Psychiatr Serv 2021; 72(4):429–36.

[68] Weisbeck SJ, Bright KS, Ginn CS, et al. Perceptions about cannabis use during pregnancy: a rapid best-framework qualitative synthesis. Can J Public Health 2021;112(1): 49–59.

[69] Dickson B, Mansfield C, Guiahi M, et al. Recommendations from cannabis dispensaries about first-trimester cannabis use. Obstet Gynecol 2018;131(6): 1031.

[70] Barbosa-Leiker C, Brooks O, Smith CL, et al. Healthcare professionals' and budtenders' perceptions of perinatal cannabis use. Am J Drug Alcohol Abuse 2022;48(2): 186–94.

Advances in Psychiatry and Behavioral Health 3 (2023) 91–101

ADVANCES IN PSYCHIATRY AND BEHAVIORAL HEALTH

Polycystic Ovary Syndrome

A Guide for Psychiatric Providers

Lindsay R. Standeven, MD[a,b,*], Kelsey Hannan, BA[a,b], Bhuchitra Singh, MD, MPH, MS, MBA[c], Liisa Hantsoo, PhD[a,b]

[a]Department of Psychiatry and Behavioral Sciences, Johns Hopkins University School of Medicine, Baltimore, MD, USA; [b]The Johns Hopkins Reproductive Mental Health Center (RMHC), The Johns Hopkins University School of Medicine, 550 North Broadway, Suite 305, Baltimore, MD 21205, USA; [c]Department of Gynecology and Obstetrics, Division of Reproductive Sciences & Women's Health Research, Johns Hopkins University School of Medicine, 720 Rutland Avenue, Ross Research Building, Room 624, Baltimore, MD 21205, USA

KEYWORDS
• Anxiety • Depression • Mood • Polycystic ovary syndrome

KEY POINTS
• Women with polycystic ovary syndrome (PCOS) have high rates of psychiatric diseases.
• Psychiatric providers should be aware of the signs and symptoms of PCOS to facilitate multidisciplinary care.
• Disease and symptom-specific questionnaires can aide in the screening for PCOS and facilitate in targeted treatment to address the associated psychological sequela.

INTRODUCTION

Polycystic ovary syndrome (PCOS) is the most common endocrine disorder affecting reproductive-age women [1]. Depending on the cohort studied and diagnostic criteria used, PCOS has an estimated prevalence ranging from 6% to 20%. As PCOS is a diagnosis of exclusion, the large prevalence range results from the fact that there are several different sets of diagnostic criteria, which differ in stringency. In 2003, The European Society of Human Reproduction and Embryology and the American Society for Reproductive Medicine both endorsed diagnosis using at least two of the three Rotterdam Criteria: (1) evidence of oligo-anovulation (irregular menstrual cycles or anovulation), (2) polycystic ovaries (PCO) on ultrasonography, and (3) clinical or biochemical hyperandrogenism (elevated testosterone levels or hirsutism) [2]. At its essence, PCOS results from dysregulation of the hypothalamic–pituitary–gonadal (HPG) axis, with subsequent abnormalities in sex steroids (namely progesterone and

testosterone), which have diverse interactions with the metabolic, neurologic, reproductive, and immunologic systems, resulting in many medical comorbidities [3–8]. Women with PCOS also have higher odds of psychiatric diseases compared with controls, particularly depression, anxiety, bulimia, and bipolar disorders [4,5]. Given the elevated rate of psychiatric burden among women with PCOS and the high prevalence of PCOS in the general population, psychiatric providers are likely to encounter many women with PCOS in their practices. Although there has been a push for standardized screening of depression and anxiety symptoms at the time of PCOS diagnosis [1,6], many providers remain unaware of the increased psychiatric risks in this population [7]. Importantly, the risk of depression and anxiety also increases with a delay in PCOS diagnosis and treatment [8]. It is therefore important that psychiatric providers are aware of the basic clinical features, diagnosis, and medical comorbidities to aid in selecting treatments and facilitate

*Corresponding author. The Johns Hopkins Reproductive Mental Health Center (RMHC), The Johns Hopkins University School of Medicine, 550 North Broadway, Suite 305, Baltimore, MD 21205. *E-mail address:* lrothen2@jhmi.edu

https://doi.org/10.1016/j.ypsc.2023.03.014
2667-3827/23/

appropriate referrals to specialists. This review therefore presents an overview of recent research on the prevalence of comorbid psychiatric conditions and the effectiveness of current treatments in targeting psychiatric symptoms among PCOS women.

QUALITY OF LIFE AND PSYCHIATRIC COMORBIDITIES

Quality of Life

Until recently, most of the research on the mental health implications observed in women with PCOS focused on reduced quality of life (QoL) secondary to medical comorbidities. Health-related quality of life (HR-QoL) is the measurement of the impact of a disease or treatment on multiple domains of an individual's life (eg, physical, mental, and perceived functioning). As might be expected, struggles with infertility, hirsutism, menstrual cycle irregularities, and weight can contribute to significant psychosocial distress. Using validated measures (Table 1), researchers have found significant reductions in HR-QoL related to all these domains, though which symptom(s) affect women most has varied across studies, possibly related to sociocultural

differences [6,9–11]. Notably, in a meta-analysis by Bazarganipour and colleagues [12], hirsutism and menstruation irregularities were cited as the greatest contributors to reduced QoL. PCOS was found to impair QOL to the same degree as chronic conditions such as asthma, migraine, and rheumatoid arthritis. Addition of HR-QOL measures to the longitudinal psychiatric care of women with PCOS may improve awareness of the many life domains impacted by PCOS, as well as guide treatment (see Table 1 and "Treatment" section below) and medical referrals.

Depression

Most studies on psychiatric symptoms among women with PCOS have focused on depression using cross-sectional and symptom-specific measurements (eg, Bec Depression Inventory [BDI]) [13]. In a large meta-analysis of more than 3000 subjects, using only studies with stringent PCOS criteria and accounting for the severity of depressive symptoms, Cooney and colleagues [14] found that women with PCOS were more than twice as likely to have depressive symptoms (36% vs 14%) and had four-times higher odds of moderate to severe depression levels compared with non-PCOS

TABLE 1
Validated Polycystic Ovary Syndrome-Specific Symptom Screening and Tracking Questionnaires or Scales for Associated Medical Symptoms

Disease-Specific Quality of Life Questionnaires

Polycystic Ovary Syndrome Questionnaire (PCOSQ)	26-item questionnaire that contains the following domains: emotions (eight items), hirsutism (five items), weight (five items), infertility (four items), and menstrual disorders (four items).

Specific Symptom Tracking Questionnaires/Scales

Ferriman–Gallwey Score	Incorporates nine body regions (excludes legs and forearms) for the assessment of hair growth and is used to evaluate and quantify hirsutism in women.
Menstrual Symptom Trackers	Numerous trackers available can help to track menstrual cycle and ovulation. Recommend Daily Record of Severity of Problems (DRSP) that allows tracking of mood and neurovegetative symptoms.
Female Sexual Function Index (FSFI)	19 items multidimensional scale to assess female sexual function under 6 domains: desire; arousal; lubrication; orgasm; satisfaction; and pain
Rosenberg Self-Esteem Scale	10-item measures global self-worth by measuring both positive and negative feelings about the self.
Globalized Acne Grading Scale	6-item clinical tool to assess the severity of acne vulgaris
Eating Disorder Examination-Questionnaire (EDE-Q)	4 domains of disordered eating: restraint eating, eating concerns, shape concerns, and weight concerns, as well as behavioral symptoms

controls. Although most studies support elevated depressive symptoms, a comparative minority have used psychiatric interviews to diagnose depressive disorders, and even fewer have measured the course of depressive symptoms longitudinally. In one of the only longitudinal studies of the prevalence of psychiatric disorders among women with PCOS, Kerchner and colleagues [15] found that nearly 60% of subjects had a depressive disorder, with an additional 11 new cases diagnosed for the 2-year follow up. In a population of Taiwanese women with PCOS followed up to 10 years, women with PCOS developed depressive disorders at higher rates than matched controls, with most cases starting more than a year after PCOS diagnosis [16]. Notably, although some research has found associations between elevated rates of depression among women with PCOS and elevated body mass index (BMI), hirsutism, infertility, or acne [17], other studies support elevated depressive symptomology even after controlling for these comorbidities [15,18]. In a large Swedish registry comparing women with PCOS to unaffected female twins and to women without PCOS in the general population, Cesta and colleagues [9] found that PCOS-affected twins had the highest risk for depression, followed by a still elevated risk in their unaffected siblings, compared with the general population; 63% of the risk for depression was attributed to common genetic factors and the remainder contributed to PCOS-specific pathology.

Anxiety Disorders

Although not as widely studied as depression, research also supports elevated levels of anxiety among women with PCOS. A meta-analysis of over 50 studies found that women with PCOS have a significantly increased likelihood of having an anxiety disorder (odds ratio 1.37) or obsessive-compulsive disorder (odds ratio 2.75), compared with non-PCOS controls [5]. Yet another study showed increased rates of Generalized Anxiety Disorder and Social Phobia, but not obsessive-compulsive disorder [19]. The prevalence of anxiety symptoms among women with PCOS is even more robust than depressive symptoms; in a meta-analysis by Cooney and colleagues [20], PCOS women had 5-times higher odds of experiencing anxiety symptoms and nearly 6-times higher odds of moderate to severe levels of anxiety symptoms compared with non-PCOS controls. Like the literature on depression, although some studies support an association between anxiety symptomatology and elevated BMI, hirsutism, or free testosterone ([21–23]), others support an association across PCOS phenotypes [20].

Bipolar Disorder

Although anxiety and depression have been the most extensively studied in relation to PCOS, associations with other disorders have been posited. The meta-analysis by Brutocao and colleagues [1] found that 5% of women with PCOS in the included studies had bipolar disorder, a higher rate than controls. Chen and colleagues [7] found that women with PCOS in their sample were at higher risk of developing new incidence of bipolar disorder compared with controls. Other studies in different world regions have not found this association [16]. Consistent and robust studies into this association are needed.

Eating Disorders

In addition to the significant association between PCOS and obesity, women with PCOS also express greater body dissatisfaction than controls [24,25]. There is also research supporting a link between alterations in sex hormones (particularly elevated androgens) and excess hunger as well as reduced satiety signaling through alterations in the orexigenic hormone, ghrelin [26]. Combined with the increased risk for depressive disorders, it is perhaps not surprising that women with PCOS are at increased risk for not only disordered eating [16], but also pathologic eating disorders [4]. Lee and colleagues [27] found women with PCOS had significantly higher scores on the Eating Disorder Examination-Questionnaire (EDE-Q), as well as increased rates of bulimia nervosa and binge eating disorder, though the latter did not reach statistical significance. In one study, the prevalence of Binge Eating Disorder was found to be 12.6% in women with PCOS versus 1.9% in non-PCOS controls [18]. These findings were replicated in two meta-analyses confirming a higher likelihood for women with PCOS to have bulimia nervosa or binge eating disorder, particularly among women with PCOS with elevated BMIs or comorbid depression or anxiety [9,27]. Taken together, psychiatric providers should closely screen for eating disorders (see Table 1) in this population and treat comorbid depression and anxiety to further reduce this risk. Lastly, BMI and increased risk toward insulin resistance (noted in both overweight and lean women with PCOS) should be considered when selecting psychotropics with adverse metabolic side effects. Some studies have shown an improvement in disordered eating among women with PCOS treated with insulin-sensitizing agents, but it is not known if the same benefit will occur in women with PCOS and binge eating disorders [28].

Other Psychiatric Disorders and Psychological Traits

With expanding awareness of the increased rates of psychiatric comorbidity among women with PCOS, results from large cohort studies have been able to assess rates of other disorders, including less common psychiatric disorders. Cesta and colleagues [4], for example, found significantly increased rates of schizophrenia, personality disorders, autism spectrum disorders, and tic disorders. Several studies have also supported increased rates (up to twice as high) of sleep disorders, including obstructive sleep apnea and excessive daytime sleepiness, among women with PCOS, associations that remain significant after adjusting for BMI [16,29,30]. Given prior research supporting the bidirectional relationship between psychiatric symptoms and sleep disorders, these data reinforce the importance of assessing sleep quality in women with PCOS.

Suicidal Ideation

Of particular concern, recent studies have found a higher prevalence of suicidal ideation and suicide attempts among women with PCOS. Shockingly, one study found that suicide attempts were seven times more common in women with PCOS than in controls [12]. A more recent study estimated the risk of attempted suicide was 40% higher in women with PCOS than those without; however, this was no longer statistically significant when adjusting for comorbid psychiatric disorders [13]. This would suggest that the suicide risk may stem from the high rate of psychiatric comorbidities seen in PCOS. Williams and colleagues [31] examined potential pathways from PCOS to future suicidal intention and found that women with PCOS had higher rates of non-suicidal self-injury (NSSI), recent and future suicidal ideation, emotion dysregulation, and rumination.

DIAGNOSTIC MEASURES, SYMPTOM SCREENING, AND TRACKING

Most women with PCOS wait for at least 2 years before being diagnosed with PCOS and a minority receive information about PCOS and its medical and psychiatric comorbidities [32]. Delays in the treatment of PCOS symptoms have also been associated with worsening psychiatric symptomatology and QoL [23]. Psychiatrists can therefore play a critical role in screening for symptoms, ordering initial diagnostic labs, making appropriate referrals, and of course treating the psychiatric sequelae of PCOS. Without treatment, symptoms of anxiety and depression may otherwise prevent women with PCOS from engaging or sustaining the life-style changes and health care adherence needed to treat this multisystem illness. Perhaps one of the simplest and most powerful interventions in screening for PCOS is to ask patients for a brief gynecologic history, including the onset of first menstrual cycles (menstrual cycles may remain irregular within 2 years of onset) [32] and regularity of cycle (normal is 25 to 35 days) over the past 6 months. Because it is estimated that 20% to 60% of women experience a premenstrual exacerbation of psychiatric symptoms [33], menstrual tracking can provide additional insight into psychiatric symptom fluctuations. In addition to psychiatric symptom tracking, it may also be useful to track some of the key symptoms shown to impact QOL (see Table 1). Table 1 outlines validated PCOS symptom screening and tracking questionnaires for PCOS-specific and associated symptoms, including QOL, fatigue, menstrual regularity, hirsutism, acne, self-esteem, and sexual dysfunction. Table 2 provides the basic, signs, symptoms, and laboratory tests needed to diagnose PCOS according to Rotterdam Criteria [2].

TREATMENTS AND THERAPEUTIC INTERVENTIONS

Treatment for women with PCOS has traditionally focused on correcting endocrine abnormalities to restore menstrual cycling, improve fertility, and manage symptoms such as weight gain, insulin resistance, hirsutism, and acne [34]. Lifestyle interventions targeted at dietary modifications and exercise to promote weight loss (target 5% to 10% initial weight reduction) are used first line to combat insulin resistance and restore menstrual regularity. Pharmacologic treatments, such as insulin-sensitizing agents (eg, metformin), oral contraception (OCP), and anti-androgens (eg, spironolactone), are often used the second line for similar reasons and to control hirsutism.

As clinical research emerged supporting a link between the symptoms of PCOS and reduced QoL, researchers explored the impact of PCOS-specific treatments on QOL outcomes. Multiple randomized clinical trials have evaluated metformin, lifestyle modification, exercise, OCP, and counseling on pre- and post-treatment QOL scores and found particular improvement with the addition of metformin and OCP [35–38]. Far fewer studies, however, have evaluated the effect of PCOS-specific treatments on psychiatric outcomes, and a minority have measured biological correlates with the mood changes to help elucidate the underlying etiology of the marked association between

TABLE 2
Signs, Symptoms, and Laboratory Tests to Diagnose Polycystic Ovary Syndrome and Treat Each Symptom Domain

PCOS Signs and Symptoms (Two Out of Three Per Rotterdam Criteria)	Symptom Screening	Laboratory Tests	Treatment
Oligomenorrhea/anovulation	Menstrual symptoms tracking (see Table 1)	TSH/T4: Rule out thyroid disease HCG: rule out pregnancy	Oral contraception, weight loss (initial goal is 5% to 10%), Metformin
Hyperandrogenism	PCOSQ Ferriman–Gallwey (see Table 1)	Free testosterone, androstenedione, sex hormone-binding globulin (SHBG)	Cosmetic therapy (laser hair removal is first line), anti-androgen therapy (spironolactone or cyproterone acetate), OCPs
Polycystic ovaries		Transvaginal ultrasound showing 12 or more follicles in one or both ovaries and/or increased ovarian volume, that is, >10 mL.	

PCOS and psychiatric symptoms (Table 3). It therefore remains largely unknown whether women with PCOS will respond to traditional psychiatric treatments or if PCOS-specific treatments work independently or through augmentation to improve depression and anxiety. The following section outlines studies to date on psychiatric outcomes using PCOS-specific treatments (insulin-sensitizing agents and OCPs) and traditional treatments (psychotropic medications and psychotherapy) to help inform psychiatric practice and fuel research directions.

Insulin-Sensitizing Agents

Metformin is prescribed to women with PCOS to combat insulin resistance and metabolic sequelae [35]. Through its insulin-reducing properties, metformin also decreases circulating androgens (namely testosterone and androstenedione) and thereby improves menstrual cyclicity and chances of conceiving for women with PCOS struggling with infertility [39]. Because alterations in both testosterone levels and insulin resistance have been associated with higher rates of depression in the general population ([40–43]), and some studies support an association between elevated testosterone levels and higher rates of comorbid depression in women with PCOS [44,45], there has been growing interest in whether metformin might improve depression and anxiety symptoms among women with PCOS and whether any such changes might be mediated by reductions in testosterone or insulin resistance. Interestingly, Metformin was found to

significantly improve both QOL and depression and anxiety indices in two studies (Hahn and colleagues [46] and Erensoy and colleagues [47]) independent of testosterone, perhaps suggesting an alternative sex steroid mechanism of action (see full review on steroid alterations and mood in women with PCOS [13]). An alternative insulin-sensitizing agent, pioglitazone (previously associated with neuroprotective and anti-inflammatory effects and improvement in neuropsychiatric and affective disorders), has been shown to be superior to metformin in reducing depression and anxiety scores among women with PCOS independent of its insulin-sensitizing and androgen-reducing effects [48], and in conjunction with a reduction in inflammatory markers [49].

Oral Contraception

OCP is used in women with PCOS to control menstrual cycles, reduce acne and hirsutism, and provide progestin to reduce endometrial cancer risk from unopposed estrogen of anovulatory cycles [50]. In a randomized controlled trial among women with PCOS assigned to receive either continuous OCPs or lifestyle changes or both, OCPs significantly improved QOL and significantly reduced depressive (but not anxiety) symptoms. In another study, women with PCOS using an OCP with the anti-androgenic progestin, drospirenone, showed reduced testosterone and hirsutism and restored menstrual cycle regularity. Although the OCP significantly improved the emotional domain on the PCOS Quality of Life Scale (PCOSQ), it did not affect

TABLE 3
Select Studies Evaluating Polycystic Ovary Syndrome-Specific and Psychotropic Medication Treatment on Psychiatric Outcomes and Associated Biological Correlates in Women with Polycystic Ovary Syndrome

Intervention	Author, Year	Study Design	Psychiatric Outcome Measured	Biological Correlate to Mood Change	Result
Psychotropics	Karabacak et al.[59] 2004	16 women with PCOS; single-center two-arm parallel RCT comparing sibutramine vs fluoxetine.	None	None	No psychological outcomes reported—sibutramine was associated with reduced leptin levels. No differences in pre- and post-insulin levels between either group.
	Masoudi et al.[53] 2021	Parallel design RCT with N = 74 women with PCOS (38 with normal prolactin levels and 36 with high prolactin levels) assigned to sertraline 50 mg or placebo and assessed after 6 wk	HDRS	prolactin	Significant improvement in depression scores across groups and no changes in prolactin levels.
Insulin-sensitizing agents	Guo et al,[49] 2020	RCT, N = 75 women with PCOS randomly assigned to pioglitazone, metformin, or placebo.	Symptom checklist 90-R	Pioglitazone-associated reduction in inflammatory markers and total testosterone levels.	Pioglitazone reduced anxiety and depression symptoms over metformin or placebo.
	Erensoy et al,[47] 2019	N = 44 adolescents and adults with PCOS, trial of 1500 mg metformin/d, anxiety and depression measured after 90 d.	BAI BDI	Did not correlate mood change with a reduction in Homeostatic Model Assessment for Insulin Resistance (HOMA-IR) or insulin levels.	Modest but statistically significant decreases in BDI and BAI (3.3- and 3.4-point reduction, respectively)
	Kashini et al,[48] 2010	N = 50 women with PCOS and meeting DSM-IV-TR criteria for depression randomly assigned to pioglitazone (P) or metformin (M).	HDRS (weeks 0, 3, and 6)	HOMA-IR, testosterone, dehydroepiandrosterone-sulfate (DHEA-S), sex hormone binding globulin (SHBG)	P superior to M in reducing HDRS scores at the end of the study (38.3% vs 8.3%, $P < .001$), no correlation between HDRS reduction and follow-up hormone or HOMA-IR levels.

| Oral contraception | Dokras et al,[6] 2016 | Secondary analysis of RCT comparing lifestyle changes, continuous OCP-, and combination on HR-QoL and depression/anxiety outcomes after 16 wk. | PRIME-MD SF-36 | Testosterone | OCPs significantly reduced PRIME-MD depressive symptoms (13.3% vs 4.4%), whereas lifestyle changes improved anxiety symptoms (15.9% vs 4.7%). Reductions in testosterone were not associated with either. |
| | Cinar et al,[17] 2012 | Prospective study of $N = 36$ women with PCOS started on estradiol/drospirenone (EE/DRSP) oral contraception. | PCOSQ BDI STAI HADS | Testosterone, androstenedione, DHEA-S, SHBG, fasting insulin (FAI) | Reduced T, FAI, and DHEA-S, with an increase in SHBG. No changes on BDI or HADS. |

Abbreviations: BAI, beck anxiety inventory; BDI, beck depression inventory; HADS, hospital anxiety depression scale; HDRS, Hamilton depression rating scale; PRIME-MD, primary care evaluation of mental disorders; STAI, state trait anxiety inventory.

depression and anxiety symptoms, though the small sample size may have limited the ability to detect such an effect [17]. Given the literature on the intersection of OCPs and mood symptoms [51], and that OCPs remain the first-line treatment for women with PCOS, more research is needed to assess the psychiatric outcomes related to treatment with OCPs in this population. Additional research observing changes in the hormonal profiles of women with PCOS as they remain on OCPs longitudinally and in correlation with mood symptoms may additionally shed light on the etiology of psychiatric symptoms. It may be that women with PCOS respond better to certain types of progestins (perhaps those that are more anti-androgenic), as has been observed among some women [51] and certain subpopulations of women with premenstrual mood changes (eg, Premenstrual Dysphoric Disorder) [52], although to date there are no data supporting the use of any particular OCP among women with PCOS.

Psychotropics

Despite the high prevalence of comorbid psychiatric symptoms, particularly depression, and anxiety, little research has evaluated the efficacy of psychotropics in reducing affective symptoms among women with PCOS. In a Cochrane review by Zhuang and colleagues [53], only one study was identified; it compared how fluoxetine versus sibutramine affected various biological factors, but did not assess baseline or outcome psychiatric symptoms. In a recent study, sertraline at 50 mg significantly decreased depression symptoms in PCOS women irrespective of and without effect on baseline prolactin levels. To date, there is not sufficient data to suggest modifying dosages or preference for antidepressants among women with PCOS. However, given the correlation between BMI and QOL, selecting psychotropics that are weight neutral or weight-loss inducing may be preferred. Women with PCOS on mood stabilizers or neuroleptics may require co-treatment with metformin sooner. Overall, however, additional research is needed to evaluate if women with PCOS metabolize and respond to psychotropics the same as non-PCOS women. Future studies assessing the utility of the co-administration of metformin and/or OCPs with psychotropics on psychiatric outcomes are needed to inform the psychiatric care of this unique population.

Psychotherapy Interventions

Psychotherapy, alone or in conjunction with psychotropic medication, can be beneficial for managing affective symptoms that occur with PCOS. Regular meetings with a therapist may also provide structure and accountability for affective symptom tracking across the menstrual cycle, and support for sustaining lifestyle changes long-term. Cognitive-behavioral therapy (CBT) is a well-established, empirically supported intervention for affective disorders, and has been trialed in women with PCOS who have depression or anxiety. CBT tools for managing affective symptoms occurring in the context of PCOS can include, for instance, behavioral activation and restructuring negative cognitions. Studies of CBT in PCOS have typically provided treatment for 30 to 60 min per week over 8 weeks [54,55]. Two recent meta-analyses examined CBT treatment of affective symptoms in PCOS. A high-quality meta-analysis found that, across four randomized controlled trials, there was a large effect size for CBT interventions decreasing depressive symptoms compared with a control condition [56]. A second, less rigorous meta-analysis of four studies found that CBT significantly improved anxiety symptoms and QoL in PCOS, but did not significantly improve depressive symptoms [57]. Overall, given the beneficial effects of CBT on affective symptoms in PCOS, psychiatric providers may consider adding CBT to the treatment plan for women with PCOS or referring patients to a CBT-trained provider. Mindfulness-based therapy may be another useful intervention. A mindfulness-based stress management program over 8 weeks significantly reduced stress, depressive symptoms, and anxiety symptoms, while improving life satisfaction and QoL in women with PCOS, compared with a control condition [58]. More research is needed on mindfulness-based interventions for affective symptoms in PCOS, but these initial results are promising.

DISCUSSION

For too long PCOS treatment has been siloed under gynecology, primary care, and reproductive medicine, with little attention paid to the disproportionate psychiatric comorbidity. Psychiatric providers are in a unique position to act as one of the first medical contacts to screen for and provide education to patients about PCOS. Like many medical conditions with high rates of psychiatric comorbidity (eg, multiple sclerosis, cardiovascular disease, and diabetes), psychiatric providers are uniquely qualified to address the psychological and behavioral aspects of PCOS, which may act as additional barriers in improving QOL for this population. Although the past decade of research has confirmed a relationship between PCOS and psychiatric conditions, longitudinal studies are needed to characterize psychiatric symptoms over time. Additionally, studies evaluating the biological etiology of psychiatric symptoms remain limited, with theories ranging from proposed alterations in neurosteroids (though this data has focused almost exclusively on testosterone) to inflammatory contributors. Indeed, longitudinal studies evaluating psychiatric symptoms in conjunction with biological correlates will help elucidate the etiology of PCOS, inform future research, and tailor treatment targets. For example, does metformin significantly improve depression and anxiety symptoms, and is this benefit conferred through an alternative biological process outside of insulin-sensitizing? Does metformin in combination with antidepressant agents provide additional benefit to mood symptom improvement among women with PCOS? Do women with PCOS experience a remission of psychiatric symptoms following menopause when the HPG-axis reverts to a non-cyclical state, or do their psychiatric symptoms persist at higher levels than age-matched controls? Psychiatrists can play a key role in answering these and other research questions, as well as, advocating for women with PCOS by helping to facilitate diagnoses, referrals, and working as part of the multidisciplinary team caring for these medically complicated and too-often psychiatrically neglected women.

CLINICS CARE POINTS

- Women with polycystic ovary syndrome (PCOS) have higher rates of psychiatric diseases compared with controls, particularly depression, anxiety, bulimia, and bipolar disorders.
- Addition of health-related quality of life (HR-QOL) measures to the psychiatric care of women with PCOS may improve awareness of the many life domains affected by PCOS and target care.
- A first step in screening for PCOS is to ask patients for a brief gynecologic history, including the onset of first menstrual cycles (menstrual cycles may remain irregular within 2 years of onset), and regularity of cycle (normal is 25 to 35 days). Menstrual cycle tracking will also aid in the diagnosis and evaluation of premenstrual symptoms.
- To date, there are not sufficient data to suggest modifying dosages or preference for antidepressants among women with PCOS. However, given the correlation between body mass index and QOL, selecting psychotropics that are weight neutral or weight-loss inducing may be preferred.

FUNDING
Work was supported by JHMI gift funds K12HD085845 (PI-Standeven); R21MH125936(PI-Hantsoo).

DISCLOSURE
The authors have nothing to disclose.

REFERENCES

[1] Teede HJ, Misso ML, Deeks AA, et al. Assessment and management of polycystic ovary syndrome: summary of an evidence-based guideline. Med J Aust 2011;195: S65–112.

[2] Rotterdam ESHRE/ASRM-Sponsored PCOS Consensus Workshop Group. Revised 2003 consensus on diagnostic criteria and long-term health risks related to polycystic ovary syndrome. Fertil Steril 2004;81:19–25.

[3] Norman RJ, Dewailly D, Legro RS, et al. Polycystic ovary syndrome. Lancet 2007;370:685–97.

[4] Cesta CE, Månsson M, Palm C, et al. Polycystic ovary syndrome and psychiatric disorders: Co-morbidity and heritability in a nationwide Swedish cohort. Psychoneuroendocrinology 2016;73:196–203.

[5] Brutocao C, Zaiem F, Alsawas M, et al. Psychiatric disorders in women with polycystic ovary syndrome: a systematic review and meta-analysis. Endocrine 2018;62: 318–25.

[6] Dokras A, Stener-Victorin E, Yildiz BO, et al. Androgen excess- polycystic ovary syndrome society: position statement on depression, anxiety, quality of life, and eating disorders in polycystic ovary syndrome. Fertil Steril 2018;109:888–99.

[7] Dokras A, Saini S, Gibson-Helm M, et al. Gaps in knowledge among physicians regarding diagnostic criteria and management of polycystic ovary syndrome. Fertil Steril 2017;107:1380–6.e1.

[8] Moulana M. Persistent risk: psychological comorbidity in polycystic ovary syndrome. Endocrinology&Metabolism International Journal 2020;8:139–41.

[9] Thannickal A, Brutocao C, Alsawas M, et al. Eating, sleeping and sexual function disorders in women with polycystic ovary syndrome (PCOS): a systematic review and meta-analysis. Clin Endocrinol (Oxf) 2020. https://doi.org/10.1111/cen.14153.

[10] Alur-Gupta S, Lee I, Chemerinski A, et al. Racial differences in anxiety, depression, and quality of life in women with polycystic ovary syndrome. F S Rep 2021;2:230–7.

[11] Elsenbruch S, Hahn S, Kowalsky D, et al. Quality of life, psychosocial well-being, and sexual satisfaction in women with polycystic ovary syndrome. J Clin Endocrinol Metab 2003;88:5801–7.

[12] Karjula S, Morin-Papunen L, Franks S, et al. Population-based Data at Ages 31 and 46 Show Decreased HRQoL and Life Satisfaction in Women with PCOS Symptoms. J Clin Endocrinol Metab 2020;105:1814–26.

[13] Standeven LR, Olson E, Leistikow N, et al. Polycystic ovary syndrome, affective symptoms, and neuroactive steroids: a focus on allopregnanolone. Curr Psychiatry Rep 2021;23:36.

[14] Cooney LG, Lee I, Sammel MD, et al. High prevalence of moderate and severe depressive and anxiety symptoms in polycystic ovary syndrome: a systematic review and meta-analysis. Hum Reprod 2017;32:1075–91.

[15] Kerchner A, Lester W, Stuart SP, et al. Risk of depression and other mental health disorders in women with polycystic ovary syndrome: a longitudinal study. Fertil Steril 2009;91:207–12.

[16] Hung JH, Hu LY, Tsai SJ, et al. Risk of psychiatric disorders following polycystic ovary syndrome: a nationwide population-based cohort study. PLoS One 2014;9: e97041.

[17] Cinar N, Kizilarslanoglu MC, Harmanci A, et al. Depression, anxiety and cardiometabolic risk in polycystic ovary syndrome. Hum Reprod 2011;26:3339–45.

[18] Hollinrake E, Abreu A, Maifeld M, et al. Increased risk of depressive disorders in women with polycystic ovary syndrome. Fertil Steril 2007;87:1369–76.

[19] Månsson M, Holte J, Landin-Wilhelmsen K, et al. Women with polycystic ovary syndrome are often depressed or anxious—A case control study. Psychoneuroendocrinology 2008;33:1132–8.

[20] Cooney LG, Dokras A. Depression and anxiety in polycystic ovary syndrome: etiology and treatment. Curr Psychiatry Rep 2017;19:83.

[21] Jedel E, Waern M, Gustafson D, et al. Anxiety and depression symptoms in women with polycystic ovary syndrome compared with controls matched for body mass index. Human Reproduction (Oxford, England) 2010;25:450–6.

[22] Barry JA, Hardiman PJ, Saxby BK, et al. Testosterone and mood dysfunction in women with polycystic ovarian syndrome compared to subfertile controls. J Psychosom Obstet Gynaecol 2011;32:104–11.

[23] Annagur BB, Tazegul A, Akbaba N. Body image, self-esteem and depressive symptomatology in women with polycystic ovary syndrome. Noro Psikiyatr Ars 2014;51: 129–32.

[24] Himelein MJ, Thatcher SS. Depression and body image among women with polycystic ovary syndrome. J Health Psychol 2006;11:613–25.

[25] Karacan E, Caglar GS, Gürsoy AY, et al. Body satisfaction and eating attitudes among girls and young women with and without polycystic ovary syndrome. J Pediatr Adolesc Gynecol 2014;27:72–7.

[26] Moran LJ, Noakes M, Clifton PM, et al. Postprandial ghrelin, cholecystokinin, peptide YY, and appetite before and after weight loss in overweight women with and without polycystic ovary syndrome. Am J Clin Nutr 2007;86:1603–10.

[27] Lee I, Cooney LG, Saini S, et al. Increased odds of disordered eating in polycystic ovary syndrome: a systematic review and meta-analysis. Eat Weight Disord 2019;24: 787–97.

[28] Jensterle M, Kocjan T, Kravos NA, et al. Short-term intervention with liraglutide improved eating behavior in obese women with polycystic ovary syndrome. Endocr Res 2015;40:133–8.

[29] Lin T-Y, Lin P-Y, Su T-P, et al. Risk of developing obstructive sleep apnea among women with polycystic ovarian syndrome: a nationwide longitudinal follow-up study. Sleep Med 2017;36:165–9.

[30] Fernandez RC, Moore VM, Van Ryswyk EM, et al. Sleep disturbances in women with polycystic ovary syndrome: prevalence, pathophysiology, impact and management strategies. Nat Sci Sleep 2018;10:45–64.

[31] Williams S, Fido D, Sheffield D. Polycystic ovary syndrome (PCOS) and non-suicidal self-injury (NSSI): a community-based study. Healthcare (Basel) 2022;10: 1118.

[32] Hoeger KM, Dokras A, Piltonen T. Update on PCOS: Consequences, Challenges, and Guiding Treatment. J Clin Endocrinol Metab 2021;106:e1071–83.

[33] Hsiao M-C, Hsiao C-C, Liu C-Y. Premenstrual symptoms and premenstrual exacerbation in patients with psychiatric disorders. Psychiatr Clin Neurosci 2004;58:186–90.

[34] Goodman NF, Cobin RH, Futterweit W, et al. American association of clinical endocrinologists, american college of endocrinology, and androgen excess and pcos society disease state clinical review: guide to the best practices in the evaluation and treatment of polycystic ovary syndrome–part 1. Endocr Pract 2015;21:1291–300.

[35] AlHussain F, AlRuthia Y, Al-Mandeel H, et al. Metformin improves the depression symptoms of women with polycystic ovary syndrome in a lifestyle modification program. Patient Prefer Adherence 2020;14:737–46.

[36] Moiz A, Mohammad I, Shehroz K. Effects of metformin on symptoms of polycystic ovarian syndrome among women of reproductive age. Cureus 2018;10(8):e3203.

[37] Hahn S, Janssen OE, Tan S, et al. Clinical and psychological correlates of quality-of-life in polycystic ovary syndrome. Eur J Endocrinol 2005;153:853–60.

[38] Altinok ML, Ravn P, Andersen M, et al. Effect of 12-month treatment with metformin and/or oral contraceptives on health-related quality of life in polycystic ovary syndrome. Gynecol Endocrinol 2018;34:859–63.

[39] Kurzthaler D, Hadziomerovic-Pekic D, Wildt L, et al. Metformin induces a prompt decrease in LH-stimulated testosterone response in women with PCOS independent of its insulin-sensitizing effects. Reprod Biol Endocrinol 2014;12:98.

[40] Barry JA, Qu F, Hardiman PJ. An exploration of the hypothesis that testosterone is implicated in the psychological functioning of women with polycystic ovary syndrome (PCOS). Med Hypotheses 2018;110:42–5.

[41] Maharjan DT, Syed AAS, Lin GN, et al. testosterone in female depression: a meta-analysis and mendelian randomization study. Biomolecules 2021;11:409.

[42] Ethirajulu A, Alkasabera A, Onyali CB, et al. Insulin resistance, hyperandrogenism, and its associated symptoms are the precipitating factors for depression in women

with polycystic ovarian syndrome. Cureus 2021;13: e18013.

[43] Lawlor DA, Smith GD, Ebrahim S, British Women's Heart, Health Study. Association of insulin resistance with depression: cross sectional findings from the British Women's Heart and Health Study. BMJ 2003;327: 1383–4.

[44] Weiner CL, Primeau M, Ehrmann DA. Androgens and mood dysfunction in women: comparison of women with polycystic ovarian syndrome to healthy controls. Psychosom Med 2004;66:356–62.

[45] Jedel E, Gustafson D, Waern M, et al. Sex steroids, insulin sensitivity and sympathetic nerve activity in relation to affective symptoms in women with polycystic ovary syndrome. Psychoneuroendocrinology 2011;36:1470–9.

[46] Hahn S, Benson S, Elsenbruch S, et al. Metformin treatment of polycystic ovary syndrome improves health-related quality-of-life, emotional distress and sexuality. Hum Reprod 2006;21:1925–34.

[47] Erensoy H, Niafar M, Ghafarzadeh S, et al. A pilot trial of metformin for insulin resistance and mood disturbances in adolescent and adult women with polycystic ovary syndrome. Gynecol Endocrinol 2019;35:72–5.

[48] Kashani L, Omidvar T, Farazmand B, et al. Does pioglitazone improve depression through insulin-sensitization? Results of a randomized double-blind metformin-controlled trial in patients with polycystic ovarian syndrome and comorbid depression. Psychoneuroendocrinology 2013;38:767–76.

[49] Guo Q-J, Shan J, Xu Y-F, et al. Pioglitazone metformin complex improves polycystic ovary syndrome comorbid psychological distress via inhibiting NLRP3 inflammasome activation: a prospective clinical study. Mediators Inflamm 2020;2020:3050487.

[50] Ignatov A, Ortmann O. Endocrine risk factors of endometrial cancer: polycystic ovary syndrome, oral contraceptives, infertility. Tamoxifen. Cancers (Basel) 2020; 12;1766

[51] Standeven LR, McEvoy KO, Osborne LM. Progesterone, reproduction, and psychiatric illness. Best Pract Res Clin Obstet Gynaecol 2020;69:108–26.

[52] Hantsoo L, Epperson CN. Premenstrual dysphoric disorder: epidemiology and treatment. Curr Psychiatry Rep 2015;17:87.

[53] Masoudi M, Ansari S, Kashani L, et al. Effect of sertraline on depression severity and prolactin levels in women with polycystic ovary syndrome: a placebo-controlled randomized trial. Int Clin Psychopharmacol 2021;36: 238–43.

[54] Cooney LG, Milman LW, Hantsoo L, et al. Cognitive-behavioral therapy improves weight loss and quality of life in women with polycystic ovary syndrome: a pilot randomized clinical trial. Fertil Steril 2018;110: 161–71.e1.

[55] Abdollahi L, Mirghafourvand M, Babapour JK, et al. Effectiveness of cognitive-behavioral therapy (CBT) in improving the quality of life and psychological fatigue in women with polycystic ovarian syndrome: a randomized controlled clinical trial. J Psychosom Obstet Gynecol 2019;40:283–93.

[56] Jiskoot G, van der Kooi A-L, Busschbach J, et al. Cognitive behavioural therapy for depression in women with PCOS: systematic review and meta-analysis. Reprod Biomed Online 2022;45:599–607.

[57] Tang R, Yang J, Yu Y, et al. The effects of cognitive behavioral therapy in women with polycystic ovary syndrome: A meta-analysis. Front Psychol 2022;13:796594.

[58] Stefanaki C, Bacopoulou F, Livadas S, et al. Impact of a mindfulness stress management program on stress, anxiety, depression and quality of life in women with polycystic ovary syndrome: a randomized controlled trial. Stress 2015;18:57–66.

[59] Karabacak IYNI, Karabacak O, Törüner FB, et al. Treatment effect of sibutramine compared to fluoxetine on leptin levels in polycystic ovary disease. Gynecol Endocrinol 2004;19(4):196–201.

Advances in Psychiatry and Behavioral Health 3 (2023) 103–113

ADVANCES IN PSYCHIATRY AND BEHAVIORAL HEALTH

Intimate Partner Violence and Women's Mental Health Across the Life Course: A Clinical Review

Armaan A. Rowther, MD, PhD[a],*, Obianuju O. Berry, MD, MPH[b], Elizabeth M. Fitelson, MD[c]

[a]Department of International Health, Johns Hopkins University Bloomberg School of Public Health, 1830 East Monument Street, Ste 2-300, Baltimore, MD 21205, USA; [b]Hassenfeld Children's Hospital at NYU Langone, Department of Child and Adolescent Psychiatry, Child Study Center, One Park Avenue, Room 7-223, New York, NY 10016, USA; [c]CUIMC/Neurological Institute of New York, 710 West 168th Street, New York, NY 10032, USA

KEYWORDS
• Intimate partner violence • Domestic violence • Women's mental health • Life course

KEY POINTS
• Physical, sexual, and psychological violence by an intimate partner is a public health problem that disproportionately and asymmetrically affects women and girls in prevalence and severity.
• Exposure to intimate partner violence (IPV), when not lethal, has both direct and indirect effects on women's mental health that increases risk of experiencing anxiety, depression, post-traumatic stress disorder, substance use disorder, self-harm, and suicide across their lifespan.
• Owing to the interrelatedness between mental health and IPV, mental health assessments should routinely include screening by trained health care providers for women's experiences of violence with intimate partners or others, and pregnant women should be routinely screened for IPV exposure.
• Opportunities for intervention and prevention of IPV and its effects on women's mental health exist across stages of the life course, including programs that foster multisectoral or interdisciplinary collaboration to also address social and structural factors of IPVs impact on mental health.

CASE VIGNETTE PANEL 1

Anna is a 27-year-old divorced, remarried mother of 4 children (ages: 14, 9, 4, and 2 years) living with her husband and three youngest children. She is undocumented, unemployed, and financially supported by her second husband. She came to the Family Justice Center—a walk-in center that offers social and legal services to help survivors of domestic violence, elder abuse, and sex trafficking—seeking legal services as she was trying to locate her 14-year-old child, who to her knowledge was living in another state with her

ex-husband. She was referred by her attorney to mental health services as she expressed significant distress in the process of providing information to apply for a nonimmigrant status "U visa."

Introduction

Intimate partner violence (IPV) is a key public health challenge that affects the mortality, health, and financial and social stability of millions of families worldwide [1,2]. Despite growing awareness of the prevalence and impact of trauma, the true extent of harm caused by

---

*Corresponding author. 1830 East Monument Street, Suite 2-300, Baltimore, MD 21205-1832. E-mail address: armaan.rowther@jhu.edu

https://doi.org/10.1016/j.ypsc.2023.03.004
2667-3827/23/

IPV to individuals and societies is often hidden from view as abuse and violence occurs behind closed doors. Because IPV has historically been framed as a social problem for survivors or a criminal justice problem for those who cause harm, the importance of its mental health antecedents and consequences has only recently been recognized in conventional psychiatric care. IPV, such as the depressive and anxiety disorders that often accompany it, disproportionately impacts women of childbearing and childrearing age. The combined stigma and structural barriers of victimhood and its mental health consequences for women create additional challenges to achieving safety and recovery. Moreover, the mental health impact of this violence can span generations for the women, children, and families exposed. This article provides a narrative review of the impact of IPV on women's mental health across the life course. The authors provide an IPV case narrative drawn from their patient experiences with a mental health program colocated in advocacy settings in New York City to highlight the ways in which IPV intersects with mental health from a clinical perspective, how mental health interventions can help move survivors toward safety and recovery, and the need for innovative solutions to the structural barriers to care for those most in need of it. The overall objective of the article is to bring awareness to mental health clinicians of the prevalence of IPV across the life course, the gendered dynamics of IPV and mental health, and some of the interventions available to target the mental health effects of IPV across sectors and stages of the life course.

Definitions

The terms "Domestic Violence" and "Intimate Partner Violence" are often used interchangeably in both the lay press and medical literature. However, it is important to understand the commonly used terms to discuss the impact and opportunities for intervention (Table 1) [3,4]. Although all forms of violence in intimate relationships can cause harm, most experts and advocates consider coercive physical, sexual, and psychological tactics exerted to establish a fixed imbalance of power and control to be the hallmarks of IPV.

Prevalence

The global prevalence of physical and/or sexual IPV among ever-partnered women is 30% [5]. In the United States, one in four women and one in ten men experience physical or sexual violence or stalking by a current or former intimate partner during their lifetime, and over one-third of women (43.5 million) report lifetime psychological aggression by a partner [6]. Certain

TABLE 1
Intimate partner violence-related terms, categories, and definitions

Term	Definition
Intimate partner violence (IPV)	Physical violence, sexual violence, stalking, and psychological aggression (including coercive tactics) by a current or former intimate partner (ie, spouse ,boyfriend/girlfriend, dating partner, or ongoing sexual partner)[6]
Domestic violence (DV)	Encompasses a larger scope of family violence, including IPV and child abuse
Gender-based violence (GBV)	Any harmful act that is perpetrated against a person's will and that is based on socially ascribed gender differences, including violence committed with the explicit purpose of reinforcing gender inequitable norms of masculinity and femininity.
Psychological aggression	Use of verbal and nonverbal communication with the intent to (a) harm another person mentally or emotionally and/or (b) exert control over another person.
Intimate terrorism	An attempt to dominate one's partner and to exert general control over the relationship
Stalking	A pattern of repeated, unwanted, attention and contact that causes fear or concern for one's own safety or the safety of someone else (eg, family member, close friend).
Sexual violence	A sexual act that is committed or attempted by another person without freely given consent of the victim or against someone who is unable to consent or refuse.
Sexual trafficking	The recruitment, hairboring, transportation, provision, or obtaining of a person for the purpose of commercial sex act.

groups are at higher risk for both IPV incidence and health sequelae, including young adults (ages 18–24); those identifying as sexual or gender minorities [7]; multiracial, American Indian, Alaska Native, or Black women [8]; immigrants [9]; and those with lower financial mobility. The World Health Organization advocates understanding IPV through an ecological model involving the interaction of individual, relationship, community, and societal factors (Fig. 1) [10].

Gender and Intimate Partner Violence

The term "domestic violence" and its recognition as a serious societal and legal problem in the United States, rather than a "family matter" best left behind closed doors, emerged out of the feminist movement of the 1970s. The 1994 Violence Against Women Act created a legal structure with criminal penalties for perpetrators of IPV and directed resources for survivors [11]. However, the relationship between IPV and gender is more complex than stereotyped heteronormative characterizations of male perpetrators and female victims. Lesbian, gay, bisexual, transgender, and genderqueer individuals report higher rates of IPV victimization in some (but not all) studies, with perpetration both between and across genders [12]. In one survey, 5.8% of men and 5.6% of women reported violence in an intimate relationship in the previous 12 months, with women being more likely to experience severe physical violence, significant injury, or rape [13]. Women are also more likely to be killed by a current or former partner [14]. Both

structural gender disparities (eg, laws disadvantaging women in their access to land and financial resources) and inequitable gender norms are correlated with higher rates of IPV for women [15]. Limitations by gender norms are even more pronounced for women who are racially/ethnically marginalized. Data demonstrate that the types and contexts of violence in intimate relationships vary, those who identify as women are disproportionately affected by severe abuse. Situational couple violence also differs in scope and consequences from the coercive tactics of power and control that characterize intimate partner terrorism in which violence is an instrument of control over the woman [16].

CASE VIGNETTE PANEL 2

On evaluation by the mental health team, Anna exhibited symptoms of both major depressive disorder (MDD) and post-traumatic stress disorder (PTSD), including low self-esteem, insomnia, irritability, anger, anhedonia and sadness, as well as hyperarousal, reexperiencing symptoms, and avoidance behaviors. She expressed passive suicidal ideation but denied active ideation and had strong protective factors.

MENTAL HEALTH CONSEQUENCES ACROSS THE LIFE COURSE

Adverse health effects of IPV are well-documented, highly morbid, and very widespread. These include

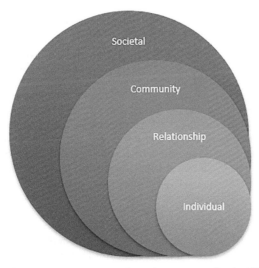

Societal – sociocultural norms, public policies that support or oppose use of violence, socioeconomic inequalities

Community – places of work, study, or residence where social relationship and violence is embedded

Relationship – social circle of family, peers, and partners that shape one's behaviours, including perpetration or victimhood to violence

Individual – personal history, biological factors affecting likelihood to become a victim or perpetrator such as one's age, education, income, or history of abuse

FIG. 1 Social-ecological model for violence prevention by WHO. (*From* Calton JM, Cattaneo LB, Gebhard KT. Barriers to Help Seeking for Lesbian, Gay, Bisexual, Transgender, and Queer Survivors of Intimate Partner Violence. Trauma Violence Abuse. Dec 2016;17(5):585 - 600; with permission.)

physical injury, cardiovascular, neurologic and urologic conditions, sexual and reproductive health problems, sexually transmitted infections (STIs), and death [17,18]. IPV is also associated with health risk behaviors such as unsafe sex, poor nutrition, substance use, and increased health care system utilization [19]. Beyond the short- and long-term direct effects of physical and sexual violence, trauma can impact health through complex environmental, physiological, and behavioral stress pathways. These include poor coping and health behaviors [20], immune and neuroendocrine dysregulation [21], alterations in brain structure and connectivity [22], telomere shortening [23], and epigenetic modification of gene expression [24]. These pathways of toxic stress intersect with the impact of other social determinants of health, including racial inequities, housing and economic insecurity, environmental exposures, and lack of access to health promoting resources [25], which are also risk factors for emotional distress and psychiatric disorders. Mental health outcomes in women survivors of IPV are inseparable from the violence they experience but cannot be understood as solely a direct consequence of this violence. Women survivors are often over-pathologized (eg, as "masochistic" in older psychotherapeutic literature [26]) or stigmatized for remaining in relationships involving IPV. Their mental health needs may simultaneously be dismissed as a "social" issue in medical settings (ie, "Who wouldn't be depressed when trapped in a violent relationship?"). Understanding the mental health consequences of IPV across the life course can help contextualize psychiatric suffering in survivors as both a manifestation of longitudinal trauma and a risk factor for its perpetuation.

CASE VIGNETTE PANEL 3

Anna was fearful of allowing her children out of her sight. At home, she kept the window shades down at all times, and her children did not engage in any extracurricular activities or play dates without her presence. The older child at home was starting to act out in school, with frequent fights and falling grades, and was recommended by the school counselor for mental health evaluation.

Childhood Exposure and Mental Health

Psychological harm to children who are exposed to IPV includes the effects of witnessing violence as well as effects from compromised parenting or responsiveness. Children under the age of 5 predominantly bear the burden. In a nationally representative survey of US children, 17.2% of children aged 5 years or younger were exposed to verbal, physical, or psychological violence involving a caregiver [27]. In early childhood, exposure to IPV in caregivers is associated with development of insecure attachment styles [28], disrupting primary attachment relationships as the child may perceive threat to the caregiver or instability in the caregiver's ability to meet the primary needs of nurturance and protection. Such instability may be exacerbated by depression, anxiety, or other mental health sequelae in affected caregivers. Insecure attachment styles in children are associated with later difficulties in adult relationships, internalizing symptoms, externalizing behaviors, and emotion dysregulation [29]. Recent research suggests that witnessing IPV confers similar harm to children's mental health and learning as some forms of direct child abuse [30]. These risks, including risk for major depression and other disorders, persist into adulthood [31]. Children exposed to IPV are also at higher risk of victimization and perpetration of violence in childhood and adulthood, including experiencing or committing IPV [32,33].

CASE VIGNETTE PANEL 4

Anna revealed a history of significant physical and sexual abuse as well as witnessed IPV in her home. She was raped at age 12 and married to the rapist at age 13. She had her first child soon after. She was later trafficked to the United States for hard physical labor. She escaped that situation and moved to New York City, where she met her now husband.

Adolescent Girls, Teen Dating Violence, and Mental Health

Relationship violence in adolescent girls, or teen dating violence (TDV), is common and predicts IPV victimization in adult women. Around one in four ever-partnered adolescent girls has experienced physical violence, sexual violence, or both from a partner [2]. In the 2013 Youth Risk Survey among students who dated, 20.9% of female students and 10.4% of male students experienced some form of TDV during the prior 12 months [34]. Female students who experienced sexual TDV were more likely to get in a physical fight, carry a weapon, be electronically bullied, and report current alcohol use and binge drinking. Youth who reported relationship violence were almost twice as likely to experience suicidal ideation and 2.4 times as likely to make a suicide attempt [35]. Most of the women who report lifetime experience of sexual or physical violence or stalking by an intimate partner first experienced these or other forms of violence before age 25 years, and a quarter of those first experienced IPV before age 18 years [6]. Revictimization is common; in one survey of college women, those who reported sexual violence pre-college were three times more likely to report sexual assault on campus [36]. Revictimized young women and girls are 4 to 8 times as likely as non-victimized individuals to meet criteria for PTSD [37].

CASE VIGNETTE PANEL 5

The psychiatrist started Anna on a low-dose selective serotonin reuptake inhibitor (SSRI), which helped with her low mood, sleep, and reduced some of her hypervigilance symptoms and panic. She began working with the psychotherapist on the team. It became clear that the process of telling the story of her early life trauma and trafficking to the United States to the legal team for her U visa application had triggered an exacerbation of her trauma symptoms, leading her to use alcohol to cope.

Intimate Partner Violence in Adult Women and Mental Health

Mental health sequelae of IPV in adult women can be seen as both an outcome and a reinforcer of the systems of coercive control that maintain a fixed imbalance of power. Preexisting mental illness confers vulnerability for IPV, as mental illness may in turn be exploited by an abusive partner to maintain control (ie, using isolation from psychosocial supports, control over access to care, threats to child custody, and exaggeration or minimization of psychiatric symptoms). Individuals with severe mental illness are more vulnerable to violent victimization; they are 11 times more likely to be victims of any violent crime than the general population [38]. In one systematic review, lifetime prevalence of severe domestic violence among psychiatric inpatients ranged from 30% to 60%, with rates higher in women compared with men [39]. There is significantly higher lifetime risk of IPV among women with depressive disorders (odds ratio [OR] 2.77 [95% CI 1.96–3.92]), anxiety disorders (OR 4.08 [95% CI 2.39–6.97]), and PTSD (OR 7.34 [95% CI 4.50–11.98]) compared with women without mental disorders [40]. IPV has also been associated with higher rates of alcohol and illicit substance use [41] as well as eating disorders, psychosis, bipolar disorder, sleep disturbances, suicidal ideation, and self-harm [42]. In a chart review of treatment-seeking IPV survivors in an advocacy setting, 40% reported a prior suicide attempt, and most reported no or only brief previous contact with mental health care

providers, highlighting both the severity of illness in this population and limited access to care [43].

The bidirectional correlation between IPV and mental health disorders such as depression, anxiety, substance use disorder, and particularly PTSD makes intuitive sense; for women with prior traumatic exposure and psychiatric symptoms, the trauma of violence and coercion creates conditions for the emergence of demoralization, hopelessness, fear, and avoidance-based coping. There is also increasing evidence suggesting that IPV can be a precipitating factor for the emergence of psychiatric diagnoses. Among individuals without prior mental illness in one survey, IPV exposure in the prior year was a risk factor for new onset of almost any psychiatric diagnosis (22.5% vs 9.7% in unexposed), including psychotic disorders and bipolar disorder [13]. Significantly, women with both childhood abuse and IPV were four to seven times more likely to experience depression [44].

Traumatic brain injury (TBI) and nonfatal strangulation in the context of IPV are common and signal a high risk of femicide and severe morbidity (such as carotid dissection). Repeated anoxic injury from strangulation, such as TBI, can cause cognitive problems, difficulty with attention, and memory deficits that overlap with and may be conflated with psychiatric symptoms and dissociative phenomena [45].

Intimate Partner Violence and Women's Reproductive Mental Health

IPV has profound effects on women's reproductive and sexual health. In the United States, an estimated 2.8 million women have contracted an STI as a result of sexual violence in an intimate relationship, and 2.9 million women have become pregnant as a result of intimate partner rape [46,47]. In addition to acts of sexual violence, abusive partners may exert reproductive control over their female partners, including contraceptive sabotage, intentional exposure to STI, pressuring her to become pregnant against her will, and coercing a woman to either carry a pregnancy to term or to have an abortion [48]. Reproductive control and sexual abuse are associated with chronic pain conditions generally and pelvic pain syndromes specifically [45].

Sexual abuse and life stress is correlated with higher rates of clinically significant premenstrual mood symptoms and higher rates of premenstrual dysphoric disorder (PMDD) [49]. In women with PMDD, histories of physical or sexual abuse are associated with stronger mood and anxiety response to ovarian hormone fluctuations, implicating the role of such abuse in dysregulating the stress response system and altering the modulating role of ovarian hormones such as allopreg-nanolone [50].

IPV in pregnancy is associated with multiple adverse perinatal outcomes, including preterm birth, low birth weight, miscarriage, premature rupture of membranes, and perinatal death [51]. Homicide is a leading cause of pregnancy-associated maternal mortality, more common than death by eclampsia or hemorrhage. In a study using the National Violent Deaths Reporting System data, 45% of maternal deaths by homicide were committed by a current or former intimate partner. In the same study, IPV was noted in 53% of maternal suicides, the second leading cause of maternal death [52].

The presence of IPV increases the risk for perinatal mood and anxiety disorders. In one study of nulliparous women followed through pregnancy and postpartum, 29% reported IPV in the first 4 years of motherhood [53]. Both childhood abuse and IPV in this study were independently associated with the increased risk of poor mental and physical health in mothers through pregnancy and the first year postpartum, with the highest risk in the cohort that experienced both childhood abuse and IPV. Psychological aggression and physical abuse by partners are both associated with post-traumatic stress (PTS) in the postpartum period, particularly in women with histories of childhood sexual abuse [54]. One systematic review of longitudinal studies found a significant relationship between any form of lifetime and perinatal IPV exposure and perinatal depression and PTS, particularly with more recent IPV, and suggested a bidirectional relationship between maternal mental health outcomes and IPV risk [55].

Mothers remain at risk for IPV and related mental health sequelae well after the perinatal period, with consequences for both their health and child wellbeing. Poor maternal mental health is associated with emotional and behavioral problems in children, with IPV impacting children both directly through witnessed abuse and indirectly through impact on mothers' mental health and parenting [56]. Mothers' cumulative exposure to violence and poor mental health both independently increased the odds of emotional and behavioral problems in their children [53]. In the Avon Longitudinal Study of Parents and Children cohort study, antenatal IPV was associated with both poor maternal mental health and adverse child behavioral outcomes at 42 months follow-up [57].

Intimate Partner Violence in Older Women

There is a paucity of data about the long-term impact of IPV in women after childbearing years. A recent systematic review identified evidence of increased risk for multiple chronic health conditions in women affected by IPV, including hypertension, obesity, heart disease, diabetes, headaches, chronic pain, and general poor health. Women experiencing IPV were also more likely to acquire human immunodeficiency virus (HIV) and have poorer health outcomes [58]. Gibsen and colleagues evaluated the associations between IPV, sexual assault, and PTSD symptoms with menopause symptoms [59]. Women in this study with current symptoms of PTSD had higher rates of sleep dysregulation, vasomotor symptoms, and vaginal dryness, whereas a history of physical IPV was associated with night sweats and sexual assault with vaginal symptoms.

IPV in older adults has often been categorized as a form of elder abuse without explicit attention to the unique needs or gendered power dynamics among older adults [60–62]. Although the prevalence of physical and sexual violence seem to decline in late life, nonphysical IPV often persists and may even increase in frequency or severity, suggesting increased psychological vulnerability for partnered women as they age [63]. IPV prevalence in older women ranges from 10% to 13% for sexual and physical violence and 24% to 36% for psychological violence [64]. A review of qualitative studies highlighted the centrality of gender norms in older women's experiences of violence and particular barriers (eg, disability, dependence on their partner) to accessing help for IPV, which was the most frequent form of violence against older women reported [65]. Factors behind escalating IPV included changing relationship dynamics from aging such as a spouse or intimate partner's retirement, children leaving home, and diagnoses of chronic or terminal illness.

MENTAL HEALTH CARE BARRIERS AND INTERVENTIONS ACROSS THE LIFE COURSE

IPV is common among patients who access mental health resources, but services rarely address mental health needs in ways that are gender- and IPV-sensitive [66,67]. This reflects not only the dominance of a medical model of care, focused on symptomatology of diagnostic categories, but also the deficit in training and knowledge about IPV dynamics and sequelae for women's mental health among health care professionals [68–70]. Tending to a survivor's mental health is essential for achieving both physical and psychological safety. Further, improving women's mental health is a critical component of preventing

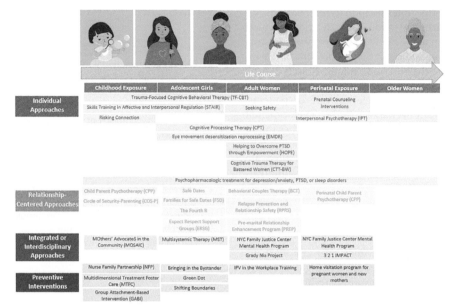

FIG. 2 Approaches and interventions to prevent IPV or support the mental health of women survivors.

future IPV and mitigating its impact across generations. Unfortunately, many of the factors that lead to perpetuation of IPV in relationships and revictimization also create barriers to effective engagement with mental health treatment. As such, screening for IPV and trauma-informed approaches to care are important for all patients in mental health care contexts or those presenting with symptoms of depression/anxiety, PTSD, or attempts of suicide or self-harm. In addition to general health screenings, IPV survivors should be evaluated for safety risks from suicide or homicide, history of substance misuse, and social support. Previously validated tools for assessing the risk of women being killed by their intimate partner include The Danger Assessment and The Danger Assessment-Revised for women in same-sex relationships [71,72].

Individual-level barriers to reporting include self-blame or fears of complications and consequences from disclosure (including reports to Child Protective Services). Systemic factors also prevent survivors from accessing mental health care such as lack of stable housing or transportation, financial mobility, access to health insurance that is not tied to their abuser, language barriers, insecure immigration status, and mistrust of law enforcement or the medical establishment [73]. Moreover, the effects of IPV may pervade women's lives through paths that intersect with social participation, employment, and housing [74–76]. These obstacles are especially pronounced for minority

women, who in the United States are less likely than white women to seek help from various formal and informal sources [77,78]. The *Lancet Psychiatry Commission* on IPV highlights risk factors and targets for intervention across the life course by emphasizing structural systems that are responsible for interventions such as policy and politics, welfare services, health and social services, and education [17].

Although both trauma-focused and non-trauma-focused psychotherapy have been shown to provide benefit in cases of IPV, no single approach is appropriate or sufficient to address the diverse needs of all IPV survivors [79]. In addition to PTSD and the immediate concerns for safety and support, IPV-related stressors that psychotherapy can help address include those related to social isolation, loss of a relationship, or parenting challenges. Another review of evidence for the effects of advocacy-based interventions—those aiming to empower women to improve their situation or reduce abuse through safety planning and access to other services beyond counseling—found benefits on the mental health among IPV survivors in lowering risk of depression as well as reducing severity of abuse in the short term [80].

In Fig. 2, the authors summarize key mental health care approaches and examples of interventions to prevent IPV or support the mental health of women survivors. These include not only individual-level therapy (pharmacologic and/or psychological) but also the integration of either interdisciplinary or relationship-centered approaches to address social and structural pathways relevant to the safety and recovery of survivors across the lifespan. Although the full breadth of IPV interventions across the life course is not within the scope of this article, our aim is to highlight key interventions and themes relevant to the clinical care or patients. There is a significant overlap across the developmental age window as the impact of IPV and approaches for interventions can be directed at multiple time points over the life course. However, as previously stated, there are fewer interventions targeted for women past childrearing age.

CASE VIGNETTE PANEL 6

The therapist worked with Anna over the next 10 months, initially in skills-based work using the Seeking Safety model, and later using exposure techniques. A reported significant improvement in all depressive and PTSD symptoms as well as in her ability to function as a parent. She began attending financial empowerment groups, and subsequently dropped out of treatment after she found part-time employment.

SUMMARY

IPV is a prevalent form of violence and major contributor to trauma and short- and long-term negative mental health impacts on women that span life course stages, from prenatal exposures through older age. In addition to overcoming significant barriers to accessing care, IPV survivors often face highly medicalized models of care that assign them psychiatric diagnoses without sensitivity to gender- or trauma-related needs. The care of women survivors requires not only empathic acknowledgment and nonjudgmental clinical care but also collaborative and culturally sensitive approaches to appropriately assess for risk of suicide or homicide, psychological distress, general health concerns, psychiatric disorders, and substance misuse. Moreover, many women survivors, whether ready to leave a violent partner or not, are in need of referral to and connection with multidisciplinary resources such as legal services, safe shelter, financial assistance, and support through community-based organizations. Interconnectedness of social service needs and mental health needs among women survivors represents a key challenge necessitating further development and expansion of integrated programs that address both social systems and mental health concerns.

CLINICS CARE POINTS

- Given the bidirectional relationship between IPV and mental health disorders, women presenting with symptoms of derpession, anxiety, PTSD, etc., should be screened for exposure to IPV.
- Many of the factors that lead to perpetuation of IPV also function as barriers to effective engagement with mental health treatment, making IPV-sensitive and trauma-informed approaches to care important for all patients.
- The experience and sequelae of IPV can vary across across stages of the life course, and helping survivors move toward safety and recovery requires not only effective safety screenings but also addressing unique risk factors for women by life stage and their structural barriers to care.

REFERENCES

[1] Leight J. Intimate partner violence against women: a persistent and urgent challenge. Lancet 2022; 399(10327):770–1.

[2] Sardinha L, Maheu-Giroux M, Stöckl H, et al. Global, regional, and national prevalence estimates of physical or sexual, or both, intimate partner violence against women in 2018. Lancet 2022;399(10327):803–13.

[3] Intimate partner violence surveillance: uniform definitions and recommended data elements, Version 2.0 (2015).

[4] Stark L, Seff I, Reis C. Gender-based violence against adolescent girls in humanitarian settings: a review of the evidence. Lancet Child Adolesc Health 2020. https://doi.org/10.1016/s2352-4642(20)30245-5.

[5] WHO, Global and Regional estimates of violence against women: prevalence and health effects of intimate partner violence and non-partner sexual violence, Organization WH, Italy, 2013 Available at: https://www.who.int/publications/i/item/9789241564625.

[6] Smith SG, Zhang X, Basile KC, et al. The national intimate partner and sexual violence survey (NISVS): 2015 data brief - updated release, Control NCfIPa. Atlanta, Georgia; 2018.

[7] Kim C. Assessment of Research on Intimate Partner Violence (IPV) Among Sexual Minorities in the United States. Trauma Violence Abuse 2019;2019. https://doi.org/10.1177/1524838019881732.

[8] Petrosky E, Blair JM, Betz CJ, et al. Racial and Ethnic Differences in Homicides of Adult Women and the Role of Intimate Partner Violence - United States, 2003-2014. MMWR Morb Mortal Wkly Rep 2017;66(28):741–6.

[9] Menjivar CSO. Immigrant Women and Domestic Violence: common experiences in different countries. Gend Soc 2002;16(6):898–920.

[10] Krug EG, Mercy JA, Dahlberg LL, et al. The world report on violence and health. Lancet 2002;360(9339): 1083–8.

[11] Lehrner A, Allen NE. Still a movement after all these years? Current tensions in the domestic violence movement. Violence Against Women 2009;15(6):656–77.

[12] Calton JM, Cattaneo LB, Gebhard KT. Barriers to Help Seeking for Lesbian, Gay, Bisexual, Transgender, and Queer Survivors of Intimate Partner Violence. Trauma Violence Abuse 2016;17(5):585–600.

[13] Okuda M, Olfson M, Hasin D, et al. Mental health of victims of intimate partner violence: results from a national epidemiologic survey. Psychiatr Serv 2011;62(8):959–62.

[14] Stöckl H, Devries K, Rotstein A, et al. The global prevalence of intimate partner homicide: a systematic review. Lancet 2013;382(9895):859–65.

[15] Heise LL, Kotsadam A. Cross-national and multilevel correlates of partner violence: an analysis of data from population-based surveys. Lancet Glob Health 2015; 3(6):e332–40.

[16] Johnson MP, Leone JM. The Differential Effects of Intimate Terrorism and Situational Couple Violence:Findings From the National Violence Against Women Survey. J Fam Issues 2005;26(3):322–49.

[17] Oram S, Fisher HL, Minnis H, et al. The Lancet Psychiatry Commission on intimate partner violence and mental health: advancing mental health services, research, and policy. Lancet Psychiatr 2022;9(6):487–524.

[18] Coker AL, Davis KE, Arias I, et al. Physical and mental health effects of intimate partner violence for men and women. Am J Prev Med 2002;23(4):260–8.

[19] Niolon PH, Kearns M, Dills J, et al. Preventing intimate partner violence across the lifespan: a technical package of programs, policies, and practices, Control NCfIPa. Atlanta, Georgia; 2017.

[20] Finkelhor D, Ormrod RK, Turner HA. Polyvictimization and trauma in a national longitudinal cohort. Dev Psychopathol. Winter 2007;19(1):149 66.

[21] Altemus M, Cloitre M, Dhabhar FS. Enhanced cellular immune response in women with PTSD related to childhood abuse. Am J Psychiatry 2003;160(9):1705–7.

[22] Logue MW. Smaller Hippocampal Volume in Posttraumatic Stress Disorder: A Multisite ENIGMA-PGC Study: Subcortical Volumetry Results From Posttraumatic Stress Disorder Consortia. Biol Psychiatr 2018 2018;83(3): 244–53.

[23] Anda RF, Felitti VJ, Bremner JD, et al. The enduring effects of abuse and related adverse experiences in childhood. A convergence of evidence from neurobiology and epidemiology. Eur Arch Psychiatry Clin Neurosci 2006;256(3):174–86.

[24] Champagne FA, Francis DD, Mar A, et al. Variations in maternal care in the rat as a mediating influence for the effects of environment on development. Physiol Behav 2003;79(3):359–71.

[25] Beck AF, Cohen AJ, Colvin JD, et al. Perspectives from the Society for Pediatric Research: interventions targeting social needs in pediatric clinical care. Pediatr Res 2018; 84(1):10–21.

[26] Symonds A. Violence against women–the myth of masochism. Am J Psychother 1979;33(2):161–73.

[27] Hamby S, Finkelhor D, Turner H, et al. Children's exposure to intimate partner violence and other family violence (2011). 2016;

[28] Noonan CB, Pilkington PD. Intimate partner violence and child attachment: A systematic review and meta-analysis. Child Abuse & Neglect 2020;109:104765.

[29] Levendosky AA, Lannert B, Yalch M. The effects of intimate partner violence on women and child survivors: an attachment perspective. Psychodyn Psychiatry 2012; 40(3):397–433.

[30] MacMillan HL, Wathen CN. Children's Exposure to Intimate Partner Violence. Child and Adolescent Psychiatric Clinics of North America 2014;23(2):295–308.

[31] Roland N, Leon C, du Roscoat E, et al. Witnessing interparental violence in childhood and symptoms of depression in adulthood: data from the 2017 French Health Barometer. Fam Pract 2020. https://doi.org/10.1093/fampra/cmaa127.

[32] Ehrensaft MK, Cohen P, Brown J, et al. Intergenerational transmission of partner violence: a 20-year prospective study. J Consult Clin Psychol 2003;71(4):741–53.

[33] Whitfield CL, Anda RF, Dube SR, et al. Violent Childhood Experiences and the Risk of Intimate Partner Violence in Adults:Assessment in a Large Health Maintenance Organization. J Interpers Violence 2003;18(2): 166–85.

[34] Vagi KJ, O'Malley Olsen E, Basile KC, et al. Teen Dating Violence (Physical and Sexual) Among US High School Students: Findings From the 2013 National Youth Risk Behavior Survey. JAMA Pediatr 2015;169(5):474–82.

[35] Baiden P, Mengo C, Small E. History of Physical Teen Dating Violence and Its Association With Suicidal Behaviors Among Adolescent High School Students: Results From the 2015 Youth Risk Behavior Survey. J Interpers Violence 2019. https://doi.org/10.1177/0886260519860087 886260519860087.

[36] Mellins CA, Walsh K, Sarvet AL, et al. Sexual assault incidents among college undergraduates: Prevalence and factors associated with risk. PLoS One 2017;12(11): e0186471.

[37] Walsh K, Danielson CK, McCauley JL, et al. National prevalence of posttraumatic stress disorder among sexually revictimized adolescent, college, and adult household-residing women. Arch Gen Psychiatry 2012; 69(9):935–42.

[38] Teplin LA, McClelland GM, Abram KM, et al. Crime Victimization in Adults With Severe Mental Illness: Comparison With the National Crime Victimization Survey. Arch Gen Psychiatr 2005;62(8):911–21.

[39] Howard LM, Trevillion K, Khalifeh H, et al. Domestic violence and severe psychiatric disorders: prevalence and interventions. Psychol Med 2010;40(6):881–93.

[40] Trevillion K, Oram S, Feder G, et al. Experiences of domestic violence and mental disorders: a systematic review and meta-analysis. PLoS One 2012;7(12): e51740.

[41] Salom CL, Williams GM, Najman JM, et al. Substance use and mental health disorders are linked to different forms of intimate partner violence victimisation. Drug Alcohol Depend 2015;151:121–7.

[42] Stewart DE, Vigod SN. Update on Mental Health Aspects of Intimate Partner Violence. Med Clin 2019;103(4): 735–49.

[43] Weiss M, Benavides MO, Fitelson E, et al. The Domestic Violence Initiative: A Private-Public Partnership Providing Psychiatric Care in a Nontraditional Setting. Psychiatr Serv 2017;68(2):212.

[44] Ouellet-Morin I, Fisher HL, York-Smith M, et al. Intimate partner violence and new-onset depression: a longitudinal study of women's childhood and adult histories of abuse. Depress Anxiety 2015;32(5):316–24.

[45] Lutgendorf MA. Intimate Partner Violence and Women's Health. Obstetrics and gynecology (New York 1953) 2019;134(3):470–80.

[46] Basile KC, Smith SG, Chen J, et al. Chronic Diseases, Health Conditions, and Other Impacts Associated With Rape Victimization of U.S. Women. J Interpers Violence 2021;36(23–24):Np12504–20.

[47] Basile KC, Smith SG, Liu Y, et al. Rape-Related Pregnancy and Association With Reproductive Coercion in the U.S. Am J Prev Med 2018;55(6):770–6.

[48] Hasstedt K RA. Understanding intimate partner violence as a sexual and reproductive health and rights issue in the United States. Guttmacher Institute. 2021. Available at: https://www.guttmacher.org/gpr/2016/07/understanding-intimate-partner-violence-sexual-and-reproductive-health-and-rights-issue. Accessed January, 20 2021

[49] Ross LE, Steiner M. A biopsychosocial approach to premenstrual dysphoric disorder. Psychiatr Clin North Am 2003;26(3):529–46.

[50] Eisenlohr-Moul TA, Rubinow DR, Schiller CE, et al. Histories of abuse predict stronger within-person covariation of ovarian steroids and mood symptoms in women with menstrually related mood disorder. Psychoneuroendocrinology 2016;67:142–52.

[51] Pastor-Moreno G, Ruiz-Pérez I, Henares-Montiel J, et al. Intimate partner violence and perinatal health: a systematic review. Bjog 2020;127(5):537–47.

[52] Palladino CL, Singh V, Campbell J, et al. Homicide and suicide during the perinatal period: findings from the National Violent Death Reporting System. Obstet Gynecol 2011;118(5):1056–63.

[53] Gartland D. Intergenerational Impacts of Family Violence - Mothers and Children in a Large Prospective Pregnancy Cohort Study. EClinicalMedicine 2019;15: 51–61.

[54] Oliveira AGESd. Childhood sexual abuse, intimate partner violence during pregnancy, and posttraumatic stress symptoms following childbirth: a path analysis. Arch Wom Ment Health 2017;20(2):297–309.

[55] Paulson JL. Intimate Partner Violence and Perinatal Post-Traumatic Stress and Depression Symptoms: A Systematic Review of Findings in Longitudinal Studies. Trauma Violence Abuse 2020. https://doi.org/10.1177/1524838020976098.

[56] Wickramaratne P, Gameroff MJ, Pilowsky DJ, et al. Children of depressed mothers 1 year after remission of maternal depression: findings from the STAR*D-Child study. Am J Psychiatry 2011;168(6):593–602.

[57] Flach C. Antenatal domestic violence, maternal mental health and subsequent child behaviour: a cohort study. BJOG An Int J Obstet Gynaecol 2011;118(11):1383–91.

[58] Stubbs A, Szoeke C. The Effect of Intimate Partner Violence on the Physical Health and Health-Related Behaviors of Women: A Systematic Review of the Literature. Trauma Violence Abuse 2021;5. https://doi.org/10.1177/1524838020985541:1524838020985541.

[59] Gibson CJ. Associations of Intimate Partner Violence, Sexual Assault, and Posttraumatic Stress Disorder With Menopause Symptoms Among Midlife and Older Women. JAMA Intern Med 2019;179(1):80–7.

[60] Penhale B. Bruises on the soul: older women, domestic violence and elder abuse. Bold 1998;8(2):16–30.

[61] McGarry J, Simpson C, Hinchliff-Smith K. The impact of domestic abuse for older women: a review of the literature. Health Soc Care Community 2011;19(1): 3–14.

[62] Brownell P. A reflection on gender issues in elder abuse research: Brazil and Portugal. Cien Saude Colet 2016; 21(11):3323–30.

[63] Roberto KA, McPherson MC, Brossoie N. Intimate partner violence in late life: a review of the empirical literature. Violence Against Women 2013;19(12):1538–58.

[64] Warmling D, Lindner SR, Coelho EBS. Intimate partner violence prevalence in the elderly and associated factors: systematic review. Cien Saude Colet 2017;22(9): 3111–25. https://doi.org/10.1590/1413-81232017229.12312017, Prevalência de violência por parceiro íntimo em idosos e fatores associados: revisão sistemática.

[65] Meyer SR, Lasater ME, García-Moreno C. Violence against older women: A systematic review of qualitative literature. PLoS One 2020;15(9):e0239560.

[66] Oram S, Trevillion K, Feder G, et al. Prevalence of experiences of domestic violence among psychiatric patients: systematic review. Br J Psychiatry 2013;202:94–9.

[67] Oram S, Khalifeh H, Howard LM. Violence against women and mental health. Lancet Psychiatry 2017; 4(2):159–70.

[68] Warshaw C. Limitations of the medical model in the care of battered women. Gend Soc 1989;3(4):506–17.

[69] O'Dwyer C, Tarzia L, Fernbacher S, et al. Health professionals' perceptions of how gender sensitive care is enacted across acute psychiatric inpatient units for women who are survivors of sexual violence. BMC Health Serv Res 2019;19(1):990.

[70] Stewart DE, Chandra PS. WPA International Competency-Based Curriculum for Mental Health Providers on Intimate Partner Violence and Sexual Violence Against Women. World Psychiatr 2017;16(2):223–4.

[71] Campbell JC, Webster DW, Glass N. The danger assessment: validation of a lethality risk assessment instrument for intimate partner femicide. J Interpers Violence. Apr 2009;24(4):653–74.

[72] Glass N, Perrin N, Hanson G, et al. Risk for reassault in abusive female same-sex relationships. Am J Public Health 2008;98(6):1021–7.

[73] Mason C. Intimate partner violence in the healthcare setting. Intimate partner violence. Los Angeles, CA: Springer; 2021. p. 7–15.

[74] Mburia-Mwalili A, Clements-Nolle K, Lee W, et al. Intimate partner violence and depression in a population-based sample of women: can social support help? J Interpers Violence 2010;25(12):2258–78.

[75] Baker CK, Niolon PH, Oliphant H. A descriptive analysis of transitional housing programs for survivors of intimate partner violence in the United States. Violence Against Women 2009;15(4):460–81.

[76] Moulding N, Franzway S, Wendt S, et al. Rethinking Women's Mental Health After Intimate Partner Violence. Violence Against Women 2021;27(8):1064–90.

[77] Lipsky S, Caetano R, Field CA, et al. The role of intimate partner violence, race, and ethnicity in help-seeking behaviors. Ethn Health 2006;11(1):81–100.

[78] Rodriguez M, Valentine JM, Son JB, et al. Intimate partner violence and barriers to mental health care for ethnically diverse populations of women. Trauma Violence Abuse 2009;10(4):358–74.

[79] Hameed M, O'Doherty L, Gilchrist G, et al. Psychological therapies for women who experience intimate partner violence. Cochrane Database Syst Rev 2020;7(7): Cd013017.

[80] Rivas C, Ramsay J, Sadowski L, et al. Advocacy interventions to reduce or eliminate violence and promote the physical and psychosocial well-being of women who experience intimate partner abuse. Cochrane Database Syst Rev 2015;2015(12):Cd005043.

Child and Adolescent

Advances in Psychiatry and Behavioral Health 3 (2023) 115–128

ADVANCES IN PSYCHIATRY AND BEHAVIORAL HEALTH

Alcohol Use Among Latino Adolescents

Current State and Directions for Future Research and Practice

Erika S. Trent, MA[a], Abbas Karim, BS[b], Andres G. Viana, PhD, ABPP[a,c],*

[a]Department of Psychology, University of Houston, Health and Biomedical Sciences Building 1, 4849 Calhoun Road, Houston, TX 77204, USA; [b]University of Texas Medical Branch (UTMB), John Sealy School of Medicine, 301 University Boulevard, Galveston, TX 77555, USA; [c]Texas Institute of Measurement, Evaluation, & Statistics, University of Houston, Health and Biomedical Sciences Building 1, 4849 Calhoun Road, Houston, TX 77204, USA

KEYWORDS

• Latino • Hispanic • Alcohol • Drinking • Substance use • Adolescence • Prevention • Intervention

KEY POINTS

• Latino adolescents in the United States are at a heightened risk of problematic alcohol use and its associated physical and mental health consequences.

• Problematic alcohol use among Latino adolescents is influenced by risk and protective factors across multiple developmental contexts, including individual, family, peer, school, community, and sociocultural contexts.

• Family-based programs, such as *Familias Unidas,* currently have the strongest evidence base for preventing alcohol use problems in Latino adolescents.

• To best serve this historically underserved and heterogenous population, clinicians should familiarize themselves with the myriad cultural factors related to alcohol use among Latino adolescents.

• Future research should expand on intervention efforts and examine clinically relevant therapist variables that may influence alcohol treatment approaches among Latino youth.

INTRODUCTION/BACKGROUND

Underage drinking (ie, alcohol use among youth under the legal drinking age of 21) is a significant public health issue in the United States. Between 75% and 87% of high schoolers report that alcohol is easily attainable, making it the most widely accessible substance in this age group [1]. Adolescent alcohol use is linked to a plethora of negative consequences, including accidental injuries and deaths, academic impairments, and mental health problems [2]. Underage drinking is particularly prevalent among Latino[a] adolescents. Indeed, research has found that Latino eighth graders are more likely to consume alcohol and binge drink than their non-Latino White (hereafter "White") or Black counterparts [3]. Given that Latino youth are the largest and fastest-growing ethnic minority group of youth in the United States [4] and expected to make up one-third of all youth by 2050 [4], it is paramount that health service professionals understand the risk and protective factors associated with problematic alcohol use in this population.

The goal of this narrative review is to provide an updated summary of research from the past 20 years on alcohol use among Latino adolescents in the United

---

*Corresponding author, *E-mail address:* agviana@uh.edu

[a]Throughout this article, we use the term Latinos to refer to individuals of Latin American and/or Hispanic descent.

https://doi.org/10.1016/j.ypsc.2023.03.015
2667-3827/23/   © 2023 Elsevier Inc. All rights reserved.

States. Such a review is critical for several reasons. First, alcohol is more prevalent and accessible in comparison to other substances [1], and thus, it is important to examine alcohol specifically (cf, other substances). Second, Latino adolescents in the United States face unique stressors, including racial discrimination, acculturative stress, and socioeconomic disadvantages [5], which make them particularly vulnerable to alcohol use and its negative consequences [6]. Understanding unique risk and protective factors can inform intervention and prevention efforts for this group. Third, adolescence (ages 13–21 years), compared with adulthood, involves distinct risk and protective factors such as peer, school, and family influences. Fourth, the literature on alcohol use problems in Latino youth contains mixed findings. An updated review that reconciles such mixed findings and identifies remaining gaps in the literature is needed. In this review, the authors focus on the following domains of relevance to the adolescent Latino population: prevalence of alcohol use, consequences of alcohol use, risk and protective factors, and prevention and intervention efforts. The authors conclude with recommendations for clinical practice and directions for future research.

CURRENT EVIDENCE
Prevalence of Drinking Among Latino Youth
Between 14% and 25% of Latino students in grades 7 to 12 report alcohol use in the past month [6,7] and 8% report binge drinking in the past month [7]. Rates of lifetime alcohol use, past-month alcohol use, and past-2-week binge drinking for Latino youth are higher compared with their White or Black peers [3]. The literature on gender differences in drinking prevalence among Latino youth is mixed, with studies finding higher rates in male students [6], higher rates in female students [8], or no gender differences [9,10]. These mixed findings may be partially attributed to characteristics of the sample (eg, age, country of origin, type of alcohol use).

Latino youth, on average, begin drinking at 16 years of age (cf, age 17 years in White youth) [11]. Problematic alcohol use and heavy drinking gradually increase in adolescence, peak between ages 18 and 25, and decrease in one's 30s [12]. There may be an age-crossover effect in alcohol use among Latino youth. In preadolescence (ages 11–13), Latino youth are more likely to endorse alcohol use and heavy drinking than White youth [13]. Conversely, in adolescence, Latino youth are less likely to drink than White youth,

but their alcohol use continues to increase in their 20s and "catches up" to White youth by their 30s, closing the racial gap [13].

Drinking patterns in Latino youth have changed over the past decades. Between 1975 and 2019, the prevalence of past-month alcohol use among Latino adolescents decreased from 60% to 20% and the prevalence of 2-week binge drinking decreased from 40% to 10% [14]. Younger cohorts of Latino boys delayed their peak alcohol use compared with older cohorts [15]. However, younger cohorts of Latina girls drank more heavily than older cohorts [15]. Mixed findings in the literature may be influenced by definitions of heavy drinking and data collection methods (eg, paper-and-pencil vs computerized surveys). Overall, underage drinking has decreased across all ethnicities, although this decrease may be less consistent for Latino youth [14,16].

Consequences of Drinking Among Latino Youth
Latino youth are particularly vulnerable to problems related to alcohol [6]. In this review, the authors focus on polysubstance use, academic problems, mental health problems, violence perpetration and victimization, risky sexual behaviors, and other risk-taking behaviors.

Polysubstance use
Latino adolescents who endorse past-month alcohol use are 2.5 to 3.5 times more likely to also endorse past-month cigarette use, marijuana use, and hard drug use [17]. A longitudinal study of youth ages 10 to 15 years found that alcohol use in the fall semester predicted the onset of cigarette use in the spring, suggesting a "gateway" effect; however, this trend was not unique to Latinos [18].

Academic problems
Latino youth ages 12 to 14 years who endorse past-month alcohol use are twice as likely to report truancy than their nondrinking peers [17]. Latino middle schoolers and high schoolers who drank larger amounts in the past 12 months concurrently reported more frequent truancy and poorer academic grades [19]. Longitudinally, Latino youth who drink more in middle school later report greater academic unpreparedness in high school [20]. Moreover, truancy and grades do not longitudinally predict alcohol use 1 year later [19], suggesting that these academic problems are a result—and not a cause—of alcohol use.

Mental health problems

Latino adolescents are more likely than non-Latinos to experience comorbid mental health problems as a result of alcohol use [21]. The combination of alcohol use and other risk factors is associated with suicidality [22]. For example, among 9th to 12th grade girls, alcohol use mediated the relationship between experience of forced sexual intercourse and suicidality for all ethnicities/races; however, the proportion of variance in suicidality explained by alcohol use was largest among Latina girls [23].

Violence victimization/perpetration

Alcohol use is associated with both victimization and perpetration of violence, and this association is stronger in Latino youth. Latino adolescents who frequently drink heavily are more likely to engage in physical fights than White or Black adolescents [24]. Latinos ages 12 to 14 years who drank alcohol in the past 30 days are 2.4 times more likely to have been in a physical fight in the past year compared with abstinent Latinos [17]. The association between past-month alcohol use and past-year physical fighting is stronger in Latino students than in White students [25]. Alcohol use in 10th grade Latina girls also longitudinally predicts both perpetration and victimization of psychological intimate partner violence in early adulthood [26].

Risky sexual behaviors

Alcohol use is associated with risky sexual behaviors in youth, although this relationship may be weaker among Latino youth than non-Latino youth [27]. Earlier alcohol use initiation is associated with an earlier age of first sexual encounter across all racial/ethnic groups, including Latinos [27]. Latino boys report similar rates of alcohol-related risky sexual behaviors as White boys; yet, Latina girls are less likely than White girls to report unplanned sex or unprotected sex after drinking [27].

Other risk-taking behaviors

Latino youth perceive drinking while driving as less dangerous than White youth [28]. Compared with non-Latinos, Latino youth are more likely to drive while intoxicated [29]. Latino adolescents who drank at school within the past month are seven times more likely to carry a weapon and nearly 11 times more likely to carry a gun specifically [30]. Among Latino adolescents, recent alcohol use and binge drinking predicted involvement with the legal system [31]. Latino adolescents in grades 7 to 12 who drank (vs did not drink) in the past month more frequently got in trouble at school, got in trouble with the police, participated in gang-related activities, and attended parties in which alcohol or marijuana was available [6].

Risk Factors and Protective Factors for Alcohol Use

The ecodevelopmental framework of substance use [32] combines Bronfenbrenner's bioecological model and developmental theory. The ecodevelopmental framework conceptualizes adolescent substance use as the result of interactions across multiple developmental systems in which an adolescent is embedded, including both proximal (eg, individual, family) and distal contexts (eg, community, culture). Consistent with this framework, the authors examine individual, family, peer, school, community, and sociocultural risk and protective factors for alcohol use in Latino youth (Fig. 1).

Individual factors

Attitudes and beliefs about alcohol. Latino youth who have more positive attitudes toward alcohol use are more likely to initiate alcohol use at earlier ages [11]. On the other hand, negative expectancies about alcohol use are associated with later alcohol initiation, less binge drinking, and less drunk driving [33]. Adolescents' confidence in resisting offers of alcohol also protects against alcohol initiation and binge drinking [34].

Other substance use. Cigarette and e-cigarette use may act as a "gateway drug" toward alcohol use among Latino youth [35]. Although the prevalence of cigarette or e-cigarette use is lower among Latino youth than non-Latino youth, Latino youth who use these nicotine products are at increased odds of alcohol use [35].

Trauma. Adverse childhood experiences (ACEs; ie, abuse, neglect, and household challenges such as family incarceration or family substance use) place Latino youth at an increased risk of alcohol use [36]. Latino ninth graders who experienced an ACE reported greater past-30-day alcohol use, and the prevalence of alcohol use steeply inclined with every additional ACE experienced [36]. Compared with their peers who experienced no ACEs, Latino youth who experienced household challenges in childhood were 1.2 times more likely to drink heavily, and Latino youth who experienced (vs did not experience) childhood abuse were 11 times more likely to drink heavily [37]. A separate study also found that sexual abuse predicted early alcohol

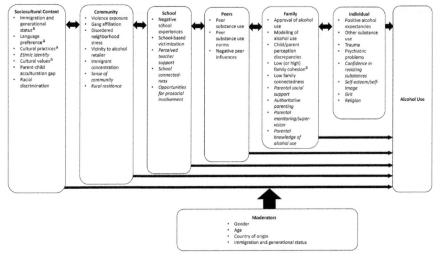

FIG. 1 A conceptual model of risk and protective factors that contribute to problematic alcohol use in Latino adolescents in the United States, organized within an ecodevelopmental framework. Specific variables within each category are based on findings in the literature from the past two decades as reviewed in this manuscript. *Protective factors are italicized.* [a]Factors with an asterisk are those with mixed findings in the literature.

initiation among Latino—but not Black or White—seventh graders [38].

Among justice-involved Latino youth, those with a history of trauma exposure are more likely to use alcohol [39]. In one study, experience of physical victimization increased alcohol use among Latino and Black youth, but not Whites [40]. Furthermore, having had a family member detained or deported in the past year longitudinally increases Latino adolescents' odds of alcohol use by nearly threefold [41].

Psychiatric problems. Psychiatric problems have been implicated in the initiation and frequency of alcohol use in Latino youth. Compared with Latino adolescents with a substance use disorder alone, those with a comorbid externalizing disorder were four times more likely to have drank in the past month [42]. Latino youth with severe depressive symptoms are 1.7 times more likely to drink than those with moderate depressive symptoms [43]. Although internalizing symptoms and alcohol use showed reciprocal relations longitudinally between ages 14 and 16 [44], depression may precede alcohol use [45].

Protective intraindividual factors. Self-esteem protects Latino youth from alcohol use [46]. Latino adolescents with a stronger sense of identity are also less likely to initiate alcohol use compared with those

who struggle with identity confusion [47]. In a sample of majority Latino adolescents, those high in grit (ie, "perseverance… despite failure and adversity" [48] [p280]) were less likely to endorse past-30-day alcohol use than those low in grit [48]. Finally, Latino adolescents who considered religion to be "very" important or attended religious events at least weekly were at lower odds of past-30-day alcohol use—a protective effect that was stronger among Latinos than Whites [49].

Family factors

Family attitudes and behaviors surrounding substance use. Latino youth whose parents do not disapprove of alcohol use are 3.5 times more likely to use alcohol than those whose parents disapprove of alcohol use [50]. Observing a same-sex family member drinking contributes to beliefs about the acceptability of drinking, which leads to greater alcohol use [51]. This effect was not found in White youth, suggesting that family influences may be stronger among Latinos. Latino youth whose siblings use substances were nearly four times as likely to drink than Latino youth without sibling substance use [52].

Parental support and involvement. Among Latino youth, negative parent–adolescent interactions predicted earlier alcohol initiation, whereas parental social support predicted later alcohol initiation [53].

Similarly, compared with Latino youth reporting high authoritative parenting (generally considered the optimal parenting style), those who reported low authoritative parenting were more likely to endorse recent alcohol use and binge drinking [54]. Greater discrepancies between child- and parent-perceived parental involvement and parent–adolescent communication were also linked with greater alcohol use [55].

Family cohesion. Findings on the influence of family cohesion on problematic alcohol use in Latino adolescents are mixed. Low family cohesion was associated with greater alcohol use problems, mediated through psychological distress, poor school connectedness, and negative peer influence [56]. Likewise, youth with low family connectedness were nearly twice as likely to report alcohol use than youth with high family connectedness [50]. However, a separate investigation found that *high* family cohesion was associated with greater alcohol use [57]. In a study of Mexican-heritage adolescents, both high *and* low levels of family cohesion (vs average levels) increased alcohol use [10]. Others have found that family cohesion was significantly associated with alcohol-related problems among White youth, but not Latino youth [58]. These inconsistencies in the literature have been ascribed to variability in the functional outcomes of family cohesion. In some families, low family cohesion may contribute to other factors that increase risk for alcohol use (eg, distress, low support); in other families, high family cohesion may increase adolescents' exposure to family contexts in which alcohol use is normalized (eg, *quinceañeras*, Barbeques) [57].

Parental monitoring of alcohol use. Latino youth with high (vs low) parental monitoring are less likely to initiate alcohol use [38] and drink less frequently [59]. Youth who have family dinners and parental support are less likely to endorse past-year alcohol use [60]. Adolescents whose parents know about their substance use are less likely to associate with substance-using peers, which leads to lower substance use [61]. Conversely, youth with low parental supervision are three times more likely to endorse alcohol use [50]. Adolescents of parents who did not accurately know their alcohol use were more likely to endorse lifetime alcohol use [55]. However, one study found that family monitoring and family connectedness did not directly influence alcohol use among Latino adolescents, whereas peer and school factors did [62]; thus, the contributions of nonfamilial factors also warrant attention.

Peer factors
Although peer influences on alcohol use seem to be weaker in Latino youth than in White youth [63], Latino youth whose peers use alcohol or other substances are more likely to initiate alcohol use at an earlier age [38] and endorse past-30-day alcohol use [64]. Peer substance use increases adolescent alcohol use by promoting positive beliefs about the acceptability of drinking [51], alcohol expectancies [65], and the social benefits of drinking [66]. Indeed, peer norms [62] and negative peer influences (ie, how strongly an adolescent feels influenced by their peers) [56] are associated with Latino adolescents' alcohol use. Influences of same-sex peers are especially strong [51]. However, the influence of peer substance use may decrease over time; for example, peer alcohol use in 11th grade did not predict alcohol initiation in adulthood [67].

School-level factors
Latino youth who have had negative school experiences (eg, school-based victimization) are more likely to endorse recent alcohol use and binge drinking compared with their peers who have had positive school experiences [68]. However, greater perceived teacher support attenuates this association—a protective effect that is stronger for Latino youth than for White youth [69]. Poor school connectedness is associated with greater alcohol use via the mediating effects of psychological distress and negative peer influence [56]. On the other hand, opportunities for prosocial involvement protect against alcohol use [64].

Communal factors
Exposure to community and gang violence. Exposure to community and gang violence is linked with earlier initiation [38] and greater frequency of alcohol use, above and beyond the impact of other relevant factors such as socioeconomic stress and discrimination-related stress [70]. Moreover, 30% of Latino youth who maintain gang affiliation report weekly alcohol use (cf, 12% of nonaffiliated youth) [71].

Neighborhood characteristics. Latino youth who perceived greater (vs lower) disordered neighborhood stress (eg, poor neighborhood environment, low community trust, graffiti, and alcohol and drug activity) were more likely to endorse past-month alcohol use [72]. Living nearby an alcohol retailer is also associated with increased alcohol use in Latino adolescents, even after controlling for other predictors (eg, parental discipline, acculturation, peer substance use) [73]. Conversely, immigrant concentration and social cohesion may protect against underage drinking. For example, Latino adolescents who live in neighborhoods with a higher (vs lower) concentration of immigrants are less likely to drink [74]. However, this protective effect is weaker among adolescents in neighborhoods whose residents frequently visit other neighborhoods of varying immigrant concentrations for routine activities (eg, school, grocery shopping, health care) [74]. A separate investigation found that Latino adolescents who perceived a sense of community were protected from the deleterious effects of social disorganization and violent-deviant behavior on substance use [75].

Residence in urban versus rural areas. Compared with Latino youth in urban areas, those in rural areas face unique stressors that increase the risk of alcohol use (eg, prejudice, discrimination, language barriers, parent immigration-related stress) [76]. This may be because Latino youth in urban areas have the option to move into neighborhoods with a large, stable, and homogenous ethnic enclave that promotes social cohesion—cf, Latino youth in rural areas who may reside in less cohesive communities composed of multiple Latino national backgrounds [76].

Sociocultural considerations

Distal acculturation-related factors. Acculturation is defined as the process by which a member of a minority group adopts the cultural practices of the majority group [77]. One distal, acculturation-related factor with relevance to alcohol use among Latino youth is generational status; however, findings are mixed. US-born Latino youth engage in more frequent alcohol use and drunk driving than their foreign-born counterparts [29]. US-born Latinos with immigrant parents (ie, second-generation) are 2.3 times more likely to engage in problematic alcohol use than foreign-born youth (ie, first-generation) [78]. US-born youth with US-born parents (ie, third-generation and beyond) are 3.3 times more likely to engage in problematic alcohol use than foreign-born youth [78]. However, one study found that third-generation Latinas were *less likely* to endorse alcohol use (but more likely to endorse greater *intentions to use*) than first- or second-generation Latinas [79]. Another study also found that first-generation Latino youth were more susceptible to alcohol use than second-generation youth and beyond, where alcohol use susceptibility was defined as either past-30-day alcohol use, intentions to try alcohol within the next year, or willingness to try alcohol if offered [80].

Several explanations for these mixed findings have been put forward. First, the effects of immigration and generational status on alcohol use may vary by nationality [81]. Second, the effects of generational status on drinking may be stronger for female Latina youth [8]. Different conceptualizations of alcohol use are also notable (eg, lifetime use, recent use frequency, intentions to drink, susceptibility to use). The mechanisms underlying immigrant generation and alcohol use are another important consideration. For instance, erosion of family closeness [9], family functioning [80], associations with substance-using peers [9], and more proximal indicators of acculturation [8,80,81], which are discussed further below, may better explain associations between generational status and alcohol use patterns.

Proximal acculturation-related factors. Language preference is a well-studied proximal indicator of acculturation [82–84]. Across Latino adolescents of various generational statuses, those who prefer to speak English (vs Spanish) use alcohol more frequently [59]. Greater English-speaking proficiency is associated with greater risk of both lifetime and recent alcohol use [82]. However, a longitudinal study found complex relations between language preference, years in the United States, lifetime alcohol use, and binge drinking [83]. Specifically, among first-generation Latino youth who had never tried alcohol at baseline, neither language preference nor years in the United States influenced odds of binge drinking. Among youth who had already experimented with alcohol at baseline, odds of binge drinking were highest among Spanish-preferring youth who were new to the United States *and* youth who had many years of exposure to the United States (regardless of language preference). After 12 years in the United States, both Spanish-preferring and English-preferring youth (who had experimented with alcohol) had similar odds of binge drinking [83].

One study of Latino adolescents who recently immigrated to the United States within the past 5 years examined the influence of broader cultural practices (eg, language preference, food preference, associations with Latino vs American friends) on alcohol use. Among girls, adherence to US cultural practices increased alcohol use frequency and amount [84]. However, among boys, adherence to Latino cultural practices increased alcohol use frequency [84]. One potential explanation for this gender difference is that Latino boys in this sample may have used alcohol to express aspects of *machismo*, a cultural value that can include the ability to "hold one's drink." [84].

There is also evidence that some Latino cultural values may have a protective effect against alcohol use. Latinos with stronger collectivist values perceive greater disapproval of drinking, which in turn lowers alcohol use [85]. *Simpatía* (ie, valuing interpersonal harmony) emerged in one study as the cultural value that protected most strongly against alcohol use [86]. On the other hand, the association between *familismo* (ie, valuing family connectedness and obligation [87]) and alcohol use is weaker. One study found that decreased *familismo* predicted greater alcohol use among US-born Latino middle schoolers [88]. However, a more recent study found that neither *familismo* nor parental respect was associated with alcohol initiation among Latino youth [87].

Strong ethnic identity among Latino youth is associated with lower alcohol susceptibility [80]. In contrast, identity confusion is longitudinally associated with positive alcohol expectancies, which in turn predicts more frequent drunkenness [89]. Another study found that Latino youth with greater ethnic pride perceive fewer benefits of cigarettes and are more confident in their ability to avoid cigarettes, which in turn, predicts lower cigarette *and* alcohol use [90].

Parent–child acculturation gap. The parent–child acculturation gap is associated with higher risk of alcohol use both cross-sectionally and prospectively [91,92]. Mediators that underlie the association between the parent–child acculturation gap and problematic alcohol use include greater parent–child conflict [92], poorer parent–child communication [93], lower parental involvement in schooling [91], and poorer family cohesion [94].

Racial discrimination. Experiences of racial discrimination are associated with both lifetime and past-30-day alcohol use among Latino adolescents [95]. Adolescents who experience greater discrimination report fewer positive peer affiliations, which in turn, leads to greater alcohol use [96]. Ethnic-biased bullying (ie, bullying based on race, ethnicity, or national origin) indirectly influenced alcohol use via increased depressive symptoms [97]. Parents' own context of reception (ie, the degree of welcomeness felt from receiving communities) also influences Latino adolescents' drinking behaviors. In particular, parents who felt unwelcome in their community tended to have poorer communication with their adolescents, which predicted greater adolescent binge drinking and alcohol use frequency [93].

Intervention Efforts Targeting Drinking Among Latino Youth

Substance use programs developed for Latino youth thus far are largely preventive in nature, family-focused, and culturally grounded. Most of the family-focused programs are based in the ecodevelopmental framework and target risk factors across multiple developmental contexts.

Family-focused programs based on the ecodevelopmental framework

Familias Unidas is an evidence-based preventive intervention program that aims to prevent substance use and risky sexual behaviors among Latino adolescents. It consists of (1) eight parent-only group sessions, in which parents learn their role in protecting their adolescent from risky behaviors and acquire parenting skills and (2) four family sessions, in which parents put their skills into practice [98]. The efficacy of *Familias Unidas* has been established in multiple randomized controlled trials (RCTs) in research environments [98]. Recently, an effectiveness study demonstrated that *Familias Unidas* can also be delivered by non-research personnel in school settings [99]. In an RCT, evaluating *Familias Unidas* delivered by trained school personnel (eg, social workers, mental health counselors) to Latino eighth graders, *Familias Unidas* prevented increases in alcohol use as compared with prevention as usual—an effect that was maintained 30 months post-baseline [99]. Although *Familias Unidas* improved family functioning and parental monitoring of peers, those factors did not serve as mediators of alcohol use outcomes [99,100].

Moderation analyses suggest that *Familias Unidas* may be more effective for families with parents who had low social support at baseline [101]. Specifically, compared with community practice, youth who underwent *Familias Unidas* were more likely to no longer meet criteria for alcohol dependence *only if* their parents had low social support at baseline [101]. The intervention effects of *Familias Unidas* on adolescent alcohol use may also vary by nativity status [102]. *Familias Unidas* effectively prevented and reduced alcohol use among US-born youth; however, it was not effective for foreign-born youth [102].

Unidos Se Puede! is a family-based intervention that strengthens family involvement in adolescents' schooling and promotes adolescents' personal agency and positive peer affiliations. This is accomplished through family workshops, individual youth coaching, and youth groups [103]. Adolescents who received

Unidos Se Puede! demonstrated a nonsignificant difference in alcohol use from pre- to post-intervention, compared with a nonequivalent control group of Latino adolescents which showed significant *increases* in probability and frequency of alcohol use [103].

Sembrando Salud is a community-based tobacco and alcohol use prevention program for migrant youth. It involves parental communication skills training and adolescent problem-solving skills training. An RCT found that *Sembrando Salud* was not efficacious in preventing alcohol consumption: there were no statistically significant differences between the intervention group and the attention control group with regard to past-30-day drinking or drinking susceptibility (ie, intentions to drink in the future) at any study timepoint (ie, baseline, post-intervention, follow-up) [104]. In the intervention group and attention control group, the prevalence of recent drinking remained comparably low across all study timepoints (ie, 5%–9% reported past-30-day drinking). However, the intervention showed a dose–response effect: adolescents who completed more (vs fewer) sessions and homework assignments demonstrated lower alcohol susceptibility post-intervention. Thus, the intervention effects may have been masked by low levels of drinking at baseline and by a dose–response effect [104].

Bridges/Puentes is a 9-week, family-focused universal middle school prevention program aimed at preventing substance abuse and increasing school engagement [105]. It includes workshops focused on adolescent coping, parenting skills, and family strengthening. In an RCT conducted in English and Spanish among Mexican American middle schoolers and their families, *Bridges/Puentes* reduced the likelihood of developing an alcohol use disorder 5 years later [105]. The program's effects on drinking outcomes (ie, frequency of drinking and of drunkenness) were significant among early initiators of substances, but not among early abstainers [105].

Family-focused programs based on other theoretical frameworks

Several family-focused substance use programs are based on theoretical frameworks outside of the ecodevelopmental model. For example, the Brief Systemic Family Therapy (BSFT), based on structural family systems theory, has been adapted for treating substance use problems in Latino adolescents [106]. Latino adolescents with behavior problems were randomized into a control condition (ie, group treatment providing support, education, and problem-solving skills) or BSFT, which involved 20 weekly hour-long family sessions to address maladaptive family interaction patterns. Compared with the control group, adolescents of families who received BSFT showed meaningful decreases in conduct problems and marijuana, but not alcohol use [106].

Nuestras Familias is a culturally adapted variant of parent management training (PMT) that addresses substance use problems in Latino adolescents in immigrant families [107]. It includes 12 weekly group-based family sessions that deliver core PMT components (eg, parental warmth, effective discipline) through presentations, discussions, and role-plays. Compared with youth in the no-treatment control group, youth who received *Nuestras Familias* were less likely to use tobacco or illicit drugs and marginally less likely to use alcohol [107].

Familias Preparando la Nueva Generación (FPNG) [108] is a culturally specific prevention intervention for Latino immigrant families. It was developed from the principles of the school-based Keepin' it REAL (kiR) program (see Youth-focused programs section). FPNG helps parents support their adolescent in resisting substance use by using the same skillset taught in kiR and helps parents improve family communication and problem-solving. In an RCT of recent Latino immigrant families, the parent-only program (FPNG only) showed better alcohol use outcomes than the parent–youth combined program (FPNG + kiR) [109]. The stronger effect of the parent-only program may be explained by its emphasis on empowering parents to be the primary supporter for their child (cf, relying on the teachers who deliver kiR to students) [109]. Furthermore, the underlying mechanism of change for these programs seems to be positive changes in antidrug norms [108].

Youth-focused programs

kiR is a culturally grounded, evidence-based substance use prevention program for middle school youth [108]. It is recognized by the Substance Abuse and Mental Health Services Administration as being effective for Latino youth in preventing substance use and increasing confidence to refuse substances if offered [108]. The Alcohol Treatment Targeting Adolescents in Need (ATTAIN) is a version of guided self-change intervention (ie, a skill-based, motivational cognitive behavioral intervention for alcohol use problems) that is adapted to be developmentally and culturally appropriate for multiethnic justice-involved youth. ATTAIN significantly reduced alcohol use among Latino justice-involved youth, with US-born but low-acculturated Latino youth (ie, strong ethnic orientation and ethnic pride) showing greater reductions in alcohol use after completing ATTAIN [88].

Innovations in treatment delivery

Familias Unidas has been adapted to Internet-based delivery, known as eHealth *Familias Unidas*. In an RCT, evaluating eHealth *Familias Unidas* delivered online in community settings (ie, by trained mental health professionals) versus prevention as usual, eHealth *Familias Unidas* was more efficacious in reducing non-alcohol substance use, but not alcohol use [100]. A separate RCT evaluated the effectiveness of a smartphone app (*Vamos*) designed to provide a tailored, skill-based content to prevent substance use [110]. Adolescents who used the app demonstrated a smaller increase in alcohol use from baseline to 2-year follow-up, compared with youth in the control condition (who showed a larger increase in alcohol use) [110]. Additional benefits of using the app included improved skills to refuse offers of alcohol [110].

SUMMARY AND RECOMMENDATIONS FOR FUTURE RESEARCH

This narrative review uses an ecodevelopmental framework to highlight the complex nature of alcohol use among Latino adolescents. As reflected in the literature reviewed, alcohol use among Latino adolescents results from complex individual–environment transactions occurring at multiple levels over time. Alcohol use in this population is related to a plethora of negative consequences, including polysubstance use, academic problems, mental health problems, violence perpetration and victimization, risky sexual behaviors, and other risk-taking behaviors. Moreover, alcohol use among Latino youth seems to be best explained by considering multiple risks and protective factors, including yet not limited to attitudes and beliefs about alcohol, traumatic experiences, psychiatric comorbidity, family attitudes, parental support and involvement, and family cohesion. Association with substance-using peers, negative school experiences, and negative neighborhood characteristics also play an important role in increasing risk for alcohol consumption. Finally, sociocultural processes, including language preferences, nativity and generational status, experiences of racial discrimination, and Latino-specific cultural values (eg, *simpatía*, *machismo*) exert important effects on alcohol use among Latino youth (see Fig. 1).

Considering the current state of the literature, the authors offer the following recommendations to researchers and clinicians working with Latino adolescents. First, to provide personalized client care, clinicians should recognize that there are multiple risk and protective factors that influence alcohol use among Latino adolescents. Second, to best serve this historically underserved and heterogenous population, clinicians should be cognizant of cultural factors that influence alcohol use while also recognizing that Latinos are not a monolithic group. As evidenced in the literature, there is variability in alcohol use prevalence, risk factors, protective factors, and treatment outcomes as a function of several variables, including nativity, immigration status, family factors, age, and gender, among others. Sample heterogeneity (eg, age, country of origin, level of acculturation), variability in the alcohol-related outcomes that are evaluated (eg, lifetime use, past-30-day use, frequency of use, amount of use, severity of problems related to alcohol use, intentions to drink), and variability in the conceptualization of independent variables (eg, how acculturation is defined and measured) may be partially responsible for inconsistent findings across studies. Future research should make concerted efforts to report detailed demographic breakdowns (eg, country of origin) on the sample studied, and where possible, assess subgroup differences. To facilitate replication, future research should also clearly operationalize alcohol-related outcomes and the independent variables purported to be associated with those outcomes.

Third, although (largely correlational) past work has been essential to our understanding of factors related to alcohol use in this population, one promising line of research pertains to examining the specific mechanisms responsible for differential outcomes in alcohol use among Latino youth. For example, what mechanisms explain why low and high levels of family cohesion (but not average levels) are related to increased alcohol use among Latino youth? What mechanisms explain the inconsistent findings regarding generational status and alcohol use in this population? What mechanisms explain the finding that among Latinas, adherence to US cultural practices is related to increased alcohol use, but among Latinos, it is adherence to *Latino* cultural practices that relate to higher alcohol use? Although several theory-driven hypotheses have been put forth for these and other findings, more mechanistic research is needed for a comprehensive understanding of alcohol use patterns in this growing population.

Fourth, researchers and clinicians should be familiar with evidence-based approaches to address alcohol use problems in this population. Based on the current state of the field, family-based approaches have the strongest evidence base for preventing alcohol use problems in Latino adolescents. In particular, family-focused programs that are based in ecodevelopmental frameworks, such as *Familias Unidas*, have the strongest empirical support. Most intervention studies to date have focused on *preventing* alcohol use by aiming to minimize developmentally expected increases in alcohol use during middle school. Research evaluating *intervention* efforts with older adolescents (eg, treating alcohol use disorders) is less common. Moreover, currently available evidence-based treatments are largely based on parenting skill-based frameworks. Treatment efforts that integrate other evidence-based approaches to substance use treatment (eg, motivational interviewing, cognitive behavioral therapy) may provide additional avenues for progress. Likewise, continued research on moderators of treatment outcomes may improve personalized intervention efforts to address the needs of each adolescent and their family.

Finally, there is a surprising dearth of research studies examining clinically relevant therapist variables that may influence alcohol treatment approaches among Latino youth. Our search of the literature identified one such study, which examined techniques used by therapists working with youth seeking treatment for problematic alcohol use [111]. The study found that therapists tend to use less motivational interviewing skills with Latino patients than with non-Latino patients, which predicted poorer treatment outcomes for Latinos in terms of alcohol-related problems [111]. Additional research on clinically relevant therapist variables (eg, specific skills, cultural humility, ethnic matching, rapport) may help clinicians work more effectively with these populations.

SUMMARY

Latino youth are the largest and fastest-growing ethnic minority group in the United States, and they face unique stressors that heighten their vulnerability to problematic alcohol use. Alcohol use is highly prevalent in this group, and the negative consequences of problematic alcohol use are far-reaching. Consistent with the ecodevelopmental framework, problematic alcohol use in Latino adolescents is influenced by risk and protective factors across multiple developmental contexts, including individual, family, peer, school, community, and sociocultural contexts. Intervention and prevention efforts, while having made strides in the past two decades, are lagging behind treatment research for other ethnic groups. In summary, clinicians and researchers working with this population should be cognizant of the role cultural factors in alcohol use while also recognizing that Latinos are a heterogeneous group. Future research should elucidate discrepancies in

the literature by conducting mechanism-oriented investigations, expand on intervention efforts, and examine clinically relevant therapist variables that may influence alcohol use treatment in this population.

CLINICS CARE POINTS

- Latino adolescents in the United States are at a heightened risk of alcohol use and related problems.
- Recognizing the multiple risk and protective factors (individual, family, peer, school, community, sociocultural) related to alcohol use among Latino adolescents will facilitate personalized client care.
- The family-based approaches currently have the strongest evidence base for prevention of alcohol use and related problems in Latino adolescents.

DISCLOSURE

A.G. Viana receives honoraria from Springer and Elsevier and is supported by the National Institute on Alcohol Abuse and Alcoholism, United States of the National Institutes of Health under Awards 1K23AA025920-01A1 and 1R01AA029807-01. The content is solely the responsibility of the authors and does not necessarily represent the official views of the National Institutes of Health, United States. The other authors have nothing to disclose.

REFERENCES

[1] Johnston LD, O'Malley PM, Miech RA, et al. Monitoring the future national survey results on drug use, 1975-2015: overview, key findings on adolescent drug use, Institute for Social Research. Ann Arbor, MI: The University of Michigan; 2016.

[2] Office of Juvenile Justice, Delinquency Prevention. Effects and consequences of underage drinking. Washington, D.C: U.S. Department of Justice; 2012.

[3] Johnston LD, O'Malley PM, Miech RA, et al. Demographic subgroup trends among adolescents in the use of various licit and illicit drugs, 1975–2015, Institute for Social Research. Ann Arbor, MI: The University of Michigan; 2016.

[4] Murphey D, Guzman L, Torres A. America's Hispanic Children. Child Trends 2014;36.

[5] Lawton KE, Gerdes AC. Acculturation and Latino Adolescent Mental Health: Integration of Individual, Environmental, and Family Influences. Clin Child Fam Psychol Rev 2014;17(4):385–98.

[6] King KA, Vidourek RA. Psychosocial factors associated with recent alcohol use among hispanic youth. Hisp J Behav Sci 2010;32(3):470–85.

[7] King KA, Vidourek RA, Merianos AL, et al. Psychosocial Factors Associated with Alcohol Use Among Hispanic Youth. J Immigr Minor Health 2017;19(5):1035–41.

[8] Wahl AMG, Eitle TM. Gender, acculturation and alcohol use among Latina/o adolescents: a multi-ethnic comparison. J Immigr Minor Health 2010; 12(2):153–65.

[9] Bacio GA, Mays VM, Lau AS. Drinking initiation and problematic drinking among Latino adolescents: explanations of the immigrant paradox. Psychol Addict Behav J Soc Psychol Addict Behav 2013;27(1):14–22.

[10] Marsiglia FF, Kulis S, Parsai M, et al. Cohesion and conflict: family influences on adolescent alcohol use in immigrant Latino families. J Ethn Subst Abuse 2009; 8(4):400–12.

[11] Chartier KG, Hesselbrock MN, Hesselbrock VM. Ethnicity and adolescent pathways to alcohol use. J Stud Alcohol Drugs 2009;70(3):337–45.

[12] Niño MD, Cai T, Mota-Back X, et al. Gender differences in trajectories of alcohol use from ages 13 to 33 across Latina/o ethnic groups. Drug Alcohol Depend 2017; 180:113–20.

[13] Chen P, Jacobson KC. Developmental trajectories of substance use from early adolescence to young adulthood: gender and racial/ethnic differences. J Adolesc Health 2012;50(2):154–63.

[14] L.D. Johnston, R.A. Miech, P.M. O'Malley, et al., Demographic subgroup trends among adolescents in the use of various licit and illicit drugs, 1975–2019, Institute for Social Research, The University of Michigan, Ann Arbor, MI, 2020.

[15] Williams E, Mulia N, Karriker-Jaffe KJ, et al. Changing Racial/Ethnic Disparities in Heavy Drinking Trajectories Through Young Adulthood: A Comparative Cohort Study. Alcohol Clin Exp Res 2018;42(1):135–43.

[16] Keyes KM, Miech R. Age, period, and cohort effects in heavy episodic drinking in the US from 1985 to 2009. Drug Alcohol Depend 2013;132(1–2):140–8.

[17] Salas-Wright CP, Hernandez L, Maynard B R, et al. Alcohol use among Hispanic early adolescents in the United States: An examination of behavioral risk and protective profiles. Subst Use Misuse 2014;49(7):864–77.

[18] D'Amico EJ, McCarthy DM. Escalation and initiation of younger adolescents' substance use: the impact of perceived peer use. J Adolesc Health 2006;39(4):481–7.

[19] Vaughan EL, Martinez S, Escobar OS, et al. School Factors and Alcohol Use: The Moderating Effect of Nativity in a National Sample of Latino Adolescents. Subst Use Misuse 2016;51(6):742–51.

[20] D'Amico EJ, Tucker JS, Miles JNV, et al. Alcohol and marijuana use trajectories in a diverse longitudinal sample of adolescents: examining use patterns from age 11 to 17 years. Addict Abingdon Engl 2016;111(10): 1825–35.

[21] Miech RA, Johnston LD, O'Malley PM, Bachman JG, Schulenberg JE. Monitoring the Future National Survey Results on Drug Use, 1975–2015: Volume I, Secondary School Students. Institute for Social Research, The University of Michigan; 2016. Available at: http:// monitoringthefuture.org/pubs.html#monographs.

[22] Giano Z, O'Neil AM, Stowe M, et al. Examining Profiles of Latinx Sexual Minority Adolescents Associated with Suicide Risk. J Immigr Minor Health 2021;23(3):452–62.

[23] Le YCL, Behnken MP, Markham CM, et al. Alcohol use as a potential mediator of forced sexual intercourse and suicidality among African American, Caucasian, and Hispanic high school girls. J Adolesc Health 2011;49(4):437–9.

[24] Khan MR, Cleland CM, Scheidell JD, et al. Gender and racial/ethnic differences in patterns of adolescent alcohol use and associations with adolescent and adult illicit drug use. Am J Drug Alcohol Abuse 2014;40(3): 213–24.

[25] Mercado-Crespo MC, Mbah AK. Race and Ethnicity, Substance Use, and Physical Aggression Among U.S. High School Students. J Interpers Violence 2013; 28(7):1367–84.

[26] Grest CV, Amaro H, Unger J. Longitudinal Predictors of Intimate Partner Violence Perpetration and Victimization in Latino Emerging Adults. J Youth Adolesc 2018; 47(3):560–74.

[27] Rothman EF, Wise LA, Bernstein E, et al. The timing of alcohol use and sexual initiation among a sample of Black, Hispanic, and White adolescents. J Ethn Subst Abuse 2009;8(2):129–45.

[28] Ginsburg KR, Winston FK, Senserrick TM, et al. National Young-Driver Survey: Teen Perspective and Experience With Factors That Affect Driving Safety. Pediatrics 2008;121(5):e1391–403.

[29] Maldonado-Molina MM, Reingle JM, Jennings WG, et al. Drinking and driving among immigrant and US-born Hispanic young adults: Results from a longitudinal and nationally representative study. Addict Behav 2011;36(4):381–8.

[30] Khubchandani J, Price JH. Violence Related Behaviors and Weapon Carrying Among Hispanic Adolescents: Results from the National Youth Risk Behavior Survey, 2001-2015. J Community Health 2018;43(2):391–9.

[31] Vidourek RA, King KA, Merianos AL, et al. Risk factors for legal involvement among a nationally representative sample of Hispanic adolescents. Vulnerable Child Youth Stud 2016;11(2):115–26.

[32] Szapocznik J, Coatsworth JD. An ecodevelopmental framework for organizing the influences on drug abuse: A developmental model of risk and protection. In: Glantz MD, Hartel CR, editors. Drug abuse: Origins & interventions. Washington, D.C: American Psychological Association; 1999. p. 331–66.

[33] Shih RA, V Miles JN, Tucker JS, et al. Racial/Ethnic Differences in Adolescent Substance Use: Mediation by Individual, Family, and School Factors. J Stud Alcohol Drugs 2010;71:640–51.

[34] Siqueira LM, Crandall LA. Risk and protective factors for binge drinking among hispanic subgroups in Florida. J Ethn Subst Abuse 2008;7(1):81–92.

[35] Wong DN, Fan W. Ethnic and sex differences in E-cigarette use and relation to alcohol use in California adolescents: the California Health Interview Survey. Publ Health 2018;157:147–52.

[36] Rogers CJ, Forster M, Grigsby TJ, et al. The impact of childhood trauma on substance use trajectories from adolescence to adulthood: Findings from a longitudinal Hispanic cohort study. Child Abuse Negl 2021;120(July 2020):105200.

[37] Lee RD, Chen J. Adverse childhood experiences, mental health, and excessive alcohol use: Examination of race/ethnicity and sex differences. Child Abuse Negl 2017;69(March):40–8.

[38] Bossarte RM, Swahn MH. Interactions between race/ethnicity and psychosocial correlates of preteen alcohol use initiation among seventh grade students in an urban setting. J Stud Alcohol Drugs 2008;69(5):660–5.

[39] Hoskins D, Marshall BDL, Koinis-Mitchell D, et al. Latinx Youth in First Contact with the Justice System: Trauma and Associated Behavioral Health Needs. Child Psychiatry Hum Dev 2019;50(3):459–72.

[40] Steele JL. Race and General Strain Theory: Examining the Impact of Racial Discrimination and Fear on Adolescent Marijuana and Alcohol Use. Subst Use Misuse 2016;51(12):1637–48.

[41] Roche KM, White RMB, Rivera MI, et al. Recent immigration actions and news and the adjustment of US Latino/a adolescents. Cultur Divers Ethnic Minor Psychol 2020. https://doi.org/10.1037/cdp0000330 Published online August 6.

[42] Gattamorta KA, Mena MP, Ainsley JB, et al. The Comorbidity of Psychiatric and Substance Use Disorders Among Hispanic Adolescents. J Dual Diagn 2017;13(4):254–63.

[43] Merianos AL, Swoboda CM, Oluwoye OA, et al. Depression and Alcohol Use in a National Sample of Hispanic Adolescents. Subst Use Misuse 2018;53(5):716–23.

[44] Parrish DE, von Sternberg K, Benjamins LJ, et al. CHOICES-TEEN: Reducing substance-exposed pregnancy and HIV among juvenile justice adolescent females. Res Soc Work Pract 2019;29(6):618–27.

[45] Birkley EL, Zapolski TCB, Smith GT. Racial differences in the transactional relationship between depression and alcohol use from elementary school to middle school. J Stud Alcohol Drugs 2015;76(5):799–808.

[46] Zamboanga BL, Schwartz SJ, Jarvis LH, et al. Acculturation and substance use among Hispanic early adolescents: Investigating the mediating roles of acculturative stress and self-esteem. J Prim Prev 2009;30(3–4):315–33.

[47] Schwartz SJ, Mason CA, Pantin H, et al. Effects of family functioning and identity confusion on substance use and sexual behavior in Hispanic immigrant early adolescents. Identity 2008;8(2):107–24.

[48] Guerrero LR, Dudovitz R, Chung PJ, et al. Grit: A Potential Protective Factor Against Substance Use and Other Risk Behaviors among Latino Adolescents. Acad Pediatr 2016;16(3):275–81.

[49] Wallace JM, Delva J, O'Malley PM, et al. Race/Ethnicity, religiosity and adolescent alcohol, cigarette and marijuana use. Soc Work Public Health 2008;23(2–3):193–213.

[50] Sale E, Sambrano S, Springer JF, et al. Family protection and prevention of alcohol use among Hispanic youth at high risk. Am J Community Psychol 2005;36(3–4):195–205.

[51] Corbin WR, Vaughan EL, Fromme K. Ethnic differences and the closing of the sex gap in alcohol use among college-bound students. Psychol Addict Behav J Soc Psychol Addict Behav 2008;22(2):240–8.

[52] Rogers CJ, Forster M, Valente TW, et al. Associations between network-level acculturation, individual-level acculturation, and substance use among Hispanic adolescents. J Ethn Subst Abuse 2022;21(2):439–56.

[53] Moreno O, Janssen T, Cox MJ, et al. Parent-adolescent relationships in Hispanic versus Caucasian families: Associations with alcohol and marijuana use onset. Addict Behav 2017;74:74–81.

[54] Merianos AL, King KA, Vidourek RA, et al. Recent Alcohol Use and Binge Drinking Based on Authoritative Parenting Among Hispanic Youth Nationwide. J Child Fam Stud 2015;24(7):1966–76.

[55] Cordova D, Huang S, Lally M, et al. Do parent-adolescent discrepancies in family functioning increase the risk of Hispanic adolescent HIV risk behaviors? Fam Process 2014;53(2):348–63.

[56] Chun H, Devall E, Sandau-Beckler P. Psychoecological model of alcohol use in Mexican American adolescents. J Prim Prev 2013;34(3):119–34.

[57] Forster M, Dyal SR, Baezconde-Garbanati L, et al. Bullying victimization as a mediator of associations between cultural/familial variables, substance use, and depressive symptoms among Hispanic youth. Ethn Health 2013;18(4):415–32.

[58] Reeb BT, Chan SYS, Conger KJ, et al. Prospective Effects of Family Cohesion on Alcohol-Related Problems in Adolescence: Similarities and Differences by Race/Ethnicity. J Youth Adolesc 2015;44(10):1941–53.

[59] McCoy SI, Jewell NP, Hubbard A, et al. A trajectory analysis of alcohol and marijuana use among Latino adolescents in San Francisco, California. J Adolesc Health 2010;47(6):564–74.

[60] Constante K, Huntley ED, Si Y, et al. Conceptualizing protective family context and its effect on substance use: Comparisons across diverse ethnic-racial youth. Subst Abuse 2021;42(4):796–805.

[61] Wang J, Simons-Morton BG, Farhat T, et al. Socio-demographic variability in adolescent substance use: mediation by parents and peers. Prev Sci 2009;10(4):387–96.

[62] Yan FA, Beck KH, Howard D, et al. A structural model of alcohol use pathways among Latino youth. Am J Health Behav 2008;32(2):209–19.

[63] Bersamin M, Paschall MJ, Flewelling RL. Ethnic differences in relationships between risk factors and adolescent binge drinking: a national study. Prev Sci 2005; 6(2):127–37.

[64] Saint-Jean G, Crandall LA. Ethnic differences in the salience of risk and protective factors for alcohol and marijuana: Findings from a statewide survey. J Ethn Subst Abuse 2004;3(1):11–27.

[65] Segura YL, Page MC, Neighbors BD, et al. The Importance of Peers in Alcohol Use among Latino Adolescents: The Role of Alcohol Expectancies and Acculturation. J Ethn Subst Abuse 2003;2(3):31–49.

[66] Gattamorta KA, Varela A, McCabe BE, et al. Psychiatric Symptoms, Parental Attachment, and Reasons for Use as Correlates of Heavy Substance Use Among Treatment-Seeking Hispanic Adolescents. Subst Use Misuse 2017;52(3):392–400.

[67] Grigsby TJ, Forster M, Meca A, et al. Cultural stressors, identity development, and substance use attitudes among Hispanic immigrant adolescents. J Community Psychol 2018;46(1):117–32.

[68] Merianos AL, Vidourek RA, Nabors LA, et al. School Experiences Associated With Alcohol Use Among Hispanic Youth. J Sch Health 2015;85(9):621–8.

[69] Watson RJ, Fish JN, Poteat VP, et al. Teacher Support, Victimization, and Alcohol Use Among Sexual and Gender Minority Youth: Considering Ethnoracial Identity. Prev Sci 2021;22(5):590–601.

[70] Goldbach JT, Berger Cardoso J, Cervantes RC, et al. The Relation Between Stress and Alcohol Use Among Hispanic Adolescents. Psychol Addict Behav 2015;29(4):960–8.

[71] van Dommelen-Gonzalez E, Deardorff J, Herd D, et al. Homies with Aspirations and Positive Peer Network Ties: Associations with Reduced Frequent Substance Use among Gang-Affiliated Latino Youth. J Urban Health 2015;92(2):322–37.

[72] Valdez ES, Valdez L, Korchmaros J, et al. Socioenvironmental Risk Factors for Adolescent Marijuana Use in a United States-Mexico Border Community. Am J Health Promot 2021;35(1):20–7.

[73] West JH, Blumberg EJ, Kelley NJ, et al. Does proximity to retailers influence alcohol and tobacco use among Latino adolescents? J Immigr Minor Health 2010; 12(5):626–33.

[74] Jackson AL, Browning CR, Krivo LJ, et al. The Role of Immigrant Concentration Within and Beyond Residential Neighborhoods in Adolescent Alcohol Use. J Youth Adolesc 2016;45(1):17–34.

[75] DTJr Lardier, Barrios VR, Garcia-Reid P, et al. Preventing substance use among Hispanic urban youth: Valuing the role of family, social support networks, school importance, and community engagement. J Child Adolesc Subst Abuse 2018;27(5–6):251–63.

[76] Torres Stone RA, Meyler D. Identifying potential risk and protective factors among non-metropolitan Latino youth: Cultural implications for substance use research. J Immigr Minor Health 2007;9(2):95–107.

[77] Warner TD, Fishbein DH, Krebs CP. The risk of assimilating? Alcohol use among immigrant and U.S.-born Mexican youth. Soc Sci Res 2010;39(1):176–86.

[78] Peña JB, Wyman PA, Brown CH, et al. Immigration generation status and its association with suicide attempts, substance use, and depressive symptoms among Latino adolescents in the USA. Prev Sci 2008;9(4):299–310.

[79] Martin-Gutierrez G, Wallander JL, Song AV, et al. Health-Related Issues in Latina Youth: Racial/Ethnic, Gender, and Generational Status Differences. J Adolesc Health 2017;61(4):478–85.

[80] Perreira KM, Marchante AN, Schwartz SJ, et al. Stress and Resilience: Key Correlates of Mental Health and Substance Use in the Hispanic Community Health Study of Latino Youth. J Immigr Minor Health 2019; 21(1):4–13.

[81] Eitle TMN, Wahl AMG, Aranda E. Immigrant generation, selective acculturation, and alcohol use among Latina/o adolescents. Soc Sci Res 2009;38(3):732–42.

[82] Myers R, Chou CP, Sussman S, et al. Acculturation and substance use: Social influence as a mediator among Hispanic alternative high school youth. J Health Soc Behav 2009;50(2):164–79.

[83] Guilamo-Ramos V, Johansson M, Jaccard J, et al. Binge drinking among Latino youth: Role of acculturation-related variables. Psychol Addict Behav 2004;18(2): 135–42.

[84] Schwartz SJ, Unger JB, Des Rosiers SE, et al. Domains of Acculturation and Their Effects on Substance Use and Sexual Behavior in Recent Hispanic Immigrant Adolescents. Prev Sci 2014;15(3):385–96.

[85] Lorenzo-Blanco EI, Schwartz SJ, Unger JB, et al. Alcohol use among recent immigrant Latino/a youth: acculturation, gender, and the Theory of Reasoned Action. Ethn Health 2016;21(6):609–27.

[86] Ma M, Malcolm LR, Díaz-Albertini K, et al. Cultural Assets and Substance Use Among Hispanic Adolescents. Health Educ Behav 2017;44(2):326–31.

[87] Shih RA, Miles JNV, Tucker JS, et al. Racial/ethnic differences in the influence of cultural values, alcohol resistance self-efficacy, and alcohol expectancies on risk for alcohol initiation. Psychol Addict Behav J Soc Psychol Addict Behav 2012;26(3):460–70.

[88] Gil AG, Wagner EF, Tubman JG. Culturally sensitive substance abuse intervention for Hispanic and African American adolescents: empirical examples from the Alcohol Treatment Targeting Adolescents in Need (ATTAIN) Project. Addict Abingdon Engl 2004; 99(Suppl 2):140–50.

[89] Oshri A, Schwartz SJ, Unger JB, et al. Bicultural stress, identity formation, and alcohol expectancies and misuse in Hispanic adolescents: a developmental approach. J Youth Adolesc 2014;43(12):2054–68.

[90] Castro FG, Stein JA, Bentler PM. Ethnic pride, traditional family values, and acculturation in early cigarette and alcohol use among Latino adolescents. J Prim Prev 2009;30(3–4):265–92.

[91] Cox RBJ, Roblyer MZ, Merten MJ, et al. Do parent-child acculturation gaps affect early adolescent Latino alcohol use? A study of the probability and extent of use. Subst Abuse Treat Prev Policy 2013;8:4.

[92] Nair RL, Roche KM, White RMB. Acculturation Gap Distress among Latino Youth: Prospective Links to Family Processes and Youth Depressive Symptoms, Alcohol Use, and Academic Performance. J Youth Adolesc 2018; 47(1):105–20.

[93] Schwartz SJ, Unger JB, Rosiers SED, et al. Substance use and sexual behavior among recent Hispanic immigrant adolescents: Effects of parent-adolescent differential acculturation and communication. Drug Alcohol Depend 2012;125(SUPPL.1). https://doi.org/10.1016/j.drugalcdep.2012.05.020.

[94] Unger JB, Ritt-Olson A, Soto DW, et al. Parent-child acculturation discrepancies as a risk factor for substance use among Hispanic adolescents in Southern California. J Immigr Minor Health 2009;11(3):149–57.

[95] Okamoto J, Ritt-Olson A, Soto D, et al. Perceived discrimination and substance use among Latino adolescents. Am J Health Behav 2009;33(6):718–27.

[96] Acosta SL, Hospital MM, Graziano JN, et al. Pathways to Drinking among Hispanic/Latino Adolescents: Perceived Discrimination, Ethnic Identity, and Peer Affiliations. J Ethn Subst Abuse 2015;14(3):270–86.

[97] Cardoso JB, Szlyk HS, Goldbach J, et al. General and Ethnic-Biased Bullying Among Latino Students: Exploring Risks of Depression, Suicidal Ideation, and Substance Use. J Immigr Minor Health 2018;20(4): 816–22.

[98] Pantin H, Prado G, Lopez B, et al. A randomized controlled trial of Familias Unidas for Hispanic adolescents with behavior problems. Psychosom Med 2009; 71(9):987.

[99] Estrada Y, Lee TK, Huang S, et al. Parent-centered prevention of risky behaviors among hispanic youths in Florida. Am J Public Health 2017;107(4):607–13.

[100] Estrada Y, Lee TK, Wagstaff R, et al. eHealth Familias Unidas: Efficacy Trial of an Evidence-Based Intervention Adapted for Use on the Internet with Hispanic Families. Prev Sci 2019;20(1):68–77.

[101] Prado G, Cordova D, Huang S, et al. The efficacy of Familias Unidas on drug and alcohol outcomes for Hispanic delinquent youth: main effects and interaction effects by parental stress and social support. Drug Alcohol Depend 2012;125(Suppl 1):S18–25.

[102] Cordova D, Huang S, Pantin H, et al. Do the effects of a family intervention on alcohol and drug use vary by nativity status? Psychol Addict Behav 2012;26(3):655–60.

[103] Cox RB, Washburn I, Greder K, et al. Preventing substance use among Latino youth: Initial results from a multistate family-based program focused on youth academic success. Am J Drug Alcohol Abuse 2022;48(1): 69–77.

[104] Elder JP, Litrownik AJ, Slymen DJ, et al. Tobacco and alcohol use-prevention program for Hispanic migrant adolescents. Am J Prev Med 2002;23(4):269–75.

[105] Gonzales NA, Jensen M, Tein JY, et al. Effect of middle school interventions on alcohol misuse and abuse in Mexican American high school adolescents five-year follow-up of a randomized clinical trial. JAMA Psychiatr 2018;75(5):429–37.

[106] Santisteban DA, Coatsworth JD, Perez-Vidal A, et al. Efficacy of brief strategic family therapy in modifying Hispanic adolescent behavior problems and substance use. J Fam Psychol 2003;17(1):121.

[107] Martinez CR Jr, Eddy JM, McClure HH, et al. Promoting Strong Latino Families Within an Emerging Immigration Context: Results of a Replication and Extension Trial of a Culturally Adapted Preventive Intervention. Prev Sci 2022;23(2):283–94.

[108] Marsiglia FF, Ayers SL, Baldwin-White A, et al. Changing Latino Adolescents' Substance Use Norms and Behaviors: The Effects of Synchronized Youth and Parent Drug Use Prevention Interventions. Prev Sci 2016; 17(1):1–12.

[109] Marsiglia FF, Ayers SL, Han SY, et al. The Role of Culture of Origin on the Effectiveness of a Parents-Involved Intervention to Prevent Substance Use Among Latino Middle School Youth: Results of a Cluster Randomized Controlled Trial. Prev Sci 2019;20(5):643–54.

[110] Schwinn TM, Fang L, Hopkins J, et al. Longitudinal outcomes of a smartphone application to prevent drug use among Hispanic youth. J Stud Alcohol Drugs 2021; 82(5):668–77.

[111] Feldstein Ewing SW, Gaume J, Ernst DB, et al. Do therapist behaviors differ with Hispanic youth? A brief look at within-session therapist behaviors and youth treatment response. Psychol Addict Behav 2015;29(3): 779–86.

Advances in Psychiatry and Behavioral Health 3 (2023) 129–138

ADVANCES IN PSYCHIATRY AND BEHAVIORAL HEALTH

Digital Single-Session Interventions for Child and Adolescent Mental Health

Evidence and Potential for Dissemination Across Low- and Middle-Income Countries

Arka Ghosh, PhD*, Riley McDanal, MA, Jessica L. Schleider, PhD

Department of Psychology, Stony Brook University, Psychology B Building, Stony Brook, NY 11794-2500, USA

KEYWORDS
- Single-session interventions • Children • Adolescents • Depression • Anxiety • Self-harm
- Digital mental health

KEY POINTS
- Globally, 10% of children and adolescents experience a mental health disorder.
- Structural barriers, knowledge barriers, and attitudinal barriers restrict treatment access for children and adolescents in high-income countries (HICs) leading to a huge treatment gap.
- The treatment gap is much worse in low-resource settings in HICs and in low- and middle-income countries where the treatment gap is mainly due to a lack of qualified mental health professionals.
- Single-session interventions, which are designed to impart maximum therapeutic impact in one session, have been shown to be effective for mental health problems in children and adolescents.
- Digital single-session interventions provide a scalable treatment approach that, by complementing and extending existing systems of care, has the potential to reduce the treatment gap to some extent.

INTRODUCTION

Prevalence of Depression, Anxiety, and Self-Harm in Children and Adolescents

Globally, 10% of children and adolescents experience a mental health disorder [1]. A meta-analysis of over 280,408 participants found that the lifetime prevalence of self-harm among 12- to 18-year-olds is 16.9% [2]. According to the data from the 2016 to 2019 survey years of the National Survey of Children's Health conducted in the United States, 4.4% of children and adolescents aged 3 to 17 years ever had a diagnosis of depression, and 9.4% of them have ever received a diagnosis of anxiety problems with point prevalence rates being 3.4% and 7.8%, respectively [3]. A recent meta-analysis among 10- to 19-year-olds found that the point prevalence of major depressive disorder and dysthymia were 8% and 4%, respectively [4]. They also found that elevated depressive symptoms were higher among female adolescents and were higher among adolescents from Middle Eastern, Asian, and African countries [4]. Among pre-pubertal children aged ≤ 12 years, the prevalence of major depression was 0.61%, with boys being significantly more likely to meet the diagnostic criteria than girls [5]. A recent report based on the Global

---

*Corresponding author, *E-mail address:* arka.ghosh@stonybrook.edu

https://doi.org/10.1016/j.ypsc.2023.03.016

School-based Student Health Survey found the prevalence of anxiety to be 9% among 12- to 17-year-olds [6]. During the coronavirus disease-2019 (COVID-19) pandemic, the global estimates of clinically elevated symptoms of depression and anxiety were 25.2% and 20.5%, respectively [7].

Treatment Gap due to Treatment Barriers in High-Income Countries and Low- and Middle-Income Countries

Despite the availability of evidence-based therapies, the treatment gap in high-income countries (HICs) is high with one estimate reporting that 70% to 80% of young people do not seek professional mental health care [8]. Even when they do seek help, only a small percentage of them receive minimally adequate treatment [9]. The major treatment barriers can be categorized into structural barriers, knowledge barriers, and attitudinal barriers. The major structural barriers include complex administrative processes to access treatment [10], high costs [10,11], and long waiting times [10]. Knowledge barriers included lack of information about available services [10,11], and difficulty identifying those in need because the instruments developed for adults do not translate to children and adolescents [12]. Attitudinal barriers include the inclination to self-manage the problems [11], youth and caregiver's negative perceptions of mental health professionals [10], and caregiver's perception of the child's mental health disorder [13]. Racial and ethnic minorities in HICs face additional barriers to accessing treatment including lack of mental health literacy [14], stigma and shame [15], provider mistrust [14,15], and fear of negative consequences [14,15]. The problem is worse in low- and middle-income countries (LMICs). In LMICs, 75% to 90% of all individuals get no mental health care [16,17]. The treatment gap for children and adolescents is expected to be even higher [18]. The major reason for this treatment gap in LMICs is the lack of mental health professionals trained to deal with child and adolescent mental health problems. Although the LMICs are home to about 90% of the world's children and adolescent population [19], 95% of professionals specializing in children and adolescent mental health are located in HICs [18]. The state of California has more child psychiatrists than the whole continent of Africa [18]. Apart from the lack of trained professionals, other barriers include the lack of evidence-based treatment guidelines for LMICs [18], limited budget for mental health problems [16], and societal stigma [16].

Ultimately, eliminating the treatment gap will require systematic efforts to address multilevel barriers to care. But one immediately-actionable step toward reducing this gap involves *increasing the availability of evidence-based treatments designed to maximize accessibility*, such as brief interventions, that are deliverable online, and those that are free to use. Treatments with these characteristics may circumvent structural barriers to care, offering access to support for the many young people who would otherwise receive no treatment at all. *Here, we introduce one especially scalable treatment option, single-session interventions, and overview its potential utility for narrowing treatment gaps worldwide.*

SINGLE-SESSION INTERVENTIONS AS A PATH TOWARD NARROWING THE TREATMENT GAP

What Are Single-Session Interventions?

Single-session interventions (SSIs) are defined as "specific, structured programs that *intentionally* [emphasis added] involve just one visit or encounter with a clinic, provider, or program" [20]. SSIs are designed to deliver the active ingredients of a treatment approach in a single session. However, SSIs might involve more than one session over time if the client deems it necessary. SSIs are not dependent on any single treatment approach but have been developed based on multiple treatment approaches including solution-focused, cognitive-behavioral, and psychodynamic techniques [20]. The flexibility offered by SSIs makes them suitable for delivery in a variety of settings, including clinics, schools, community centers [21], and online [22–24]. SSIs can also be used in conjunction with ongoing treatment, and are intended to complement, rather than replace, existing health care systems.

The need for single-session interventions and the existing evidence base

Even among the US youth who begin therapy, the mean number of sessions attended are 3.9 [25], and the modal number of treatments accessed by US youth is one [26]. This indicates that multi-session psychological interventions might not be the preferred treatment modality for US youth. So, SSIs provide a complementary treatment approach that maximizes the therapeutic impact that can be imparted within the short period of time available. SSIs have been shown to be effective for multiple mental health conditions including specific phobias [27,28], poor body image [29], conduct disorder [30], general mental health problems [31], and day-to-day social-evaluative stress [32]. An SSI has also been shown to increase hope [33].

SSIs targeting depression have been shown to be effective in reducing depression at 3-month [23], 4-month [34], and 9-month follow-up [35]. However, other SSIs have shown mixed results [36] or no significant results [37,38].

For anxiety symptoms, a values-based SSI showed greater reductions in anxiety symptoms compared with an active control teaching study skills among school students. The same study reported that both values-based and growth-based SSIs showed greater reductions in anxiety symptoms, compared with a study-skills control, among a clinical sub-sample of the school students at a 2-week follow-up [38]. Another SSI targeting growth mindset and stress-can-be-enhancing mindset synergistically was able to reduce anxiety symptoms during COVID-19 lockdowns [32]. A parent-directed SSI was found to be more effective in reducing the risk of their offspring developing anxiety disorders at one-year follow-up [39]. Other SSIs, however, failed to report significant effects on anxiety symptoms in adolescents [34,35,37,40].

The effect of SSIs on self-harm is more humbling, with one review reporting no improvement in self-harming behavior in three different studies evaluating parent-targeting SSIs [41] and another study finding no significant effects on the likelihood of future nonsuicidal self-injury or 3-month frequencies of non-suicidal self-injury [22]. They did, however, find a short-term improvement in self-hatred and desire to self-harm in the future.

A major meta-analysis showed a significant beneficial effect of SSIs for youth psychiatric problems that is only slightly smaller than multisession youth psychotherapy [21]. They reported a medium effect size ($g = 0.58$) for anxiety and a small effect size ($g = 0.21$) for depression. A significant finding of this meta-analysis was that there were no significant differences between therapist-administered and self-administered SSIs. SSIs have also been shown to be acceptable to diverse populations even before community-specific tailoring [42].

SSIs and other brief interventions have also been used in LMICs and low-resource settings with varying degrees of success. One parent-targeted SSI in Panama found that parent-reported behavioral difficulties of their children decreased at 2 weeks, 3 months, and 6 months compared with a no-intervention control [30]. Another SSI tested in Kenya, Shamiri-Digital, reported medium effects ($d = 0.50$) on adolescents with depressive symptoms and strong effects ($d = 0.83$) on the adolescent subsample with moderate to severe depressive symptoms [43]. They found no significant

effects on anxiety, well-being, or happiness. Another study tested three SSIs based on growth mindset, gratitude, and value affirmation against a study-skill active control group among secondary school students in Kenya [38]. The value affirmation-based SSI showed significant effects versus the active control in the total sample. Both the value affirmation SSI and the growth-mindset-based SSI showed significant reductions on anxiety on a clinical subsample. They found no effects on depression.

The unique promise of digital single-session interventions and the existing evidence base

With the advent of the Internet, a majority of adolescents and young adults seek information or help online for their mental health [44,45]. Online help-seeking is especially attractive as it provides a non-stigmatizing space, especially for marginalized populations, and supports the youth's need for self-reliance [46]. Moreover, digital SSIs (several of which are freely available online [24]) may be more easily accessible for adolescents with marginalized identities than are traditional face-to-face therapies (which require parent knowledge, involvement, and ongoing support). Lesbian, gay, bisexual, transgender, and queer (LGBTQ+) youths, for example, frequently indicate that a lack of parental permission serves as a key barrier to their ability to access in-person therapeutic support [47,48]. Parental permission may be difficult or impossible to obtain for youths whose parents are unsupportive of their gender identity and/or sexual orientation or unaware of their mental health struggles [49]. On the contrary, self-directed digital SSIs can be safely accessed without parent involvement [23,24], and they therefore have the potential to reach youths who are currently without therapeutic support [24]. In addition to their accessibility, digital SSIs have been shown to be acceptable [22,50–52] among youths across multiple countries. Digital SSIs have been successfully delivered in research settings [22,23,32,35,53], in school settings [34,43], and in real-world settings [24,50]. Delivering mental health care using digital SSIs is a relatively new approach and is an active area of research. The largest online study of digital SSIs evaluated two experimental SSIs—one behavioral activation SSI and one SSI teaching that traits are changeable—against an active control [23]. They found that the experimental SSIs reduced depressive symptoms at 3 months, decreased post-intervention and 3-month hopelessness, increased post-intervention agency, and reduced 3-month restrictive eating. Other studies reported digital SSIs to be effective in reducing depression [23,34,35] and anxiety

[32]. The evidence for the effectiveness of self-harm is limited [22]. Nevertheless, delivering mental health care using digital SSIs is a promising area due to its potential for scalability and warrants more research.

B.E.S.T. PRINCIPLES FOR DESIGNING DIGITAL SINGLE-SESSION INTERVENTIONS FOR YOUTH MENTAL HEALTH

Schleider and colleagues [20] have proposed that four scientifically-informed principles may helpfully guide the development of evidence-based, digital SSIs for youth mental health problems.

1. B: Brain science to normalize concepts in the program
2. E: Empower youths to a "helper" or "expert" role
3. S: Saying-is-believing exercises to solidify learning
4. T: Testimonials and evidence from valued others

These "B.E.S.T." principles are drawn from combining basic research in social psychology [54] with promising qualities common to self-administered SSIs [20]. These elements aim to increase SSI buy-in from and utility for adolescents by providing normalization, empowerment, engagement, and reassurance.

CASE EXAMPLES: TRIALS OF B.E.S.T.-ALIGNED SINGLE-SESSION INTERVENTIONS IN THE UNITED STATES AND KENYA

The "Action Brings Change" Project

The Action Brings Change (ABC) Project is a 20 to 30 min online, self-guided SSI developed to alleviate depressive symptoms (freely available at www.schleiderlab.org/yes). In particular, the ABC Project aims to enhance *agency*, which here refers to a youth's perceived ability to set behavioral goals and exert motivation toward those goals [55]. The process for increasing this agency, termed behavioral activation [56], encourages adolescents to take positive action *even without* having the preexisting motivation to take that action. In the ensuing cycle, participating in desired activities improves mood, improved mood leads to increased motivation, and increased motivation then leads to more engagement in enjoyable activities. When experiencing low mood, creating that initial positive behavioral change—especially with a lack of motivation—can be the hardest part. To help kickstart this process, the ABC Project helps adolescents identify and make a plan to engage in incremental, actionable steps toward

behavioral goals. Through leveraging B.E.S.T. principles, this program has led to significant reductions in depressive symptoms, reductions in hopelessness, and increases in the perceived agency from pre-to-post-intervention relative to a supportive control [23,24].

The B.E.S.T. principles, as applied in the development of the ABC Project, have aimed to increase buy-in from and utility for adolescents.

Brain science to normalize concepts in the program

Scientists and practitioners can use brain science to normalize and validate adolescent struggles, as well as to correspondingly show teens that change is possible. Accordingly, the ABC Project offers neuroscientific and evolutionary explanations behind common struggles, followed by evidence-backed techniques that help respond to these neuroscientific and evolutionary motivators when they go awry. For example, the ABC Project states that:

The human brain is designed to respond to stress by avoiding danger ... For early humans, this part of our brain helped us stay safe ... Sometimes, it still does protect us from danger. But other times, our brain can get things wrong. It can stay in 'must-avoid!' mode for longer than we need—even after the 'danger,' or stressful event, is long gone.

After enlisting teens to select and self-generate steps they can take to help combat such avoidance, the ABC Project further uses brain science to address barriers that can arise when working toward these steps:

Sometimes, it takes your brain some time to 'catch up' to the helpful actions you decide to do.

The ABC Project offers examples of strategies to combat this problem, such as breaking the activity into smaller pieces or planning out activities for the most feasible times for execution.

Empower youths to a "helper" or "expert" role

Elevating youths to a role above "participant" level not only improves teen engagement, but also in itself aims to increase teen perceived agency and competence [57]. Empowering youths to perceive themselves as an active agent of their own change, rather than a passive intervention recipient, might be especially useful for interventions self-directed by the adolescent themself. Throughout the ABC Project, the program emphasizes the importance of the teen's role not only in helping themselves but also in helping others:

Other teens have told us that they have found this activity interesting and helpful. But we need your help explaining it in a better way to help more kids like you.

The better you get at taking action, the more you can support others in coping with challenges, too.

You are the expert on what getting support should look like for you.

Saying-is-believing exercises to solidify learning

"Saying-is-believing" activities use self-persuasive writing exercises to encourage internalization of ideas [58], a strategy which works well for adolescent educational interventions [59]. Using information learned in a given intervention, adolescents are asked to identify and self-articulate their own perspective on how a given difficulty or barrier could be combated. In the ABC Project, after the participating teen begins to develop their own action plan for their own struggle, they are asked to identify a potential roadblock that might impede their ability to work toward their goal. The teen self-describes an "if-then" plan for facing this potential roadblock. For example,:

If I think, 'I'm never in the mood to do fun things,' then one small thing I can do to take positive action is [free-response].

To further increase internalization of the teen's chosen message, they are then asked to write a free-response describing what they would say to help a teen experiencing a similar struggle:

Imagine another kid your age, 'Alex,' has the same roadblock thought you just chose. Alex has been feeling really down lately and isn't sure if they can take positive action. Based on what you've learned today about the brain and taking positive action, what would you tell Alex to let them know that they can stand up to their roadblock thought and reverse their negative mood spiral?

Testimonials and evidence from valued others

Testimonials, or personal narratives from others, engage participating teens and increase the salience of the intervention content for the participating teen [60]. Evidence in the form of testimonials from peers and from perceived "experts" are particularly persuasive for teens [61]. The ABC Project presents testimonials about the power of behavioral activation both from hypothetical peers and from research experts. For example, the ABC Project presents a narrative from teen "Kat":

I've played volleyball since I was 8 years old. It's always been my favorite thing. Last year, I decided to try out for my

school's varsity team. My best friend made it, but I got cut … After that, things got tough. I just wanted to hide. At first I wasn't sure how to start feeling like myself again. The only thing I could think of was, I don't know… doing stuff that reminded me of me … I started focusing more on my photography. It was nice, because it was just for me, and it felt good no matter how it ended up. I also kept hanging out with my best friend … After a while I started feeling more like me again. I'm not going to pretend it happened all at once. But doing stuff I liked, even when I didn't totally feel like it, made things easier.

Shamiri-Digital

The Shamiri (means thrive in Swahili) program was initially developed as a group intervention for adolescents experiencing anxiety and depression [62]. It consists of 4 h-long sessions covering growth mindset, gratitude, and value affirmation to be delivered over 4 weeks. These intervention modalities were selected because they were brief, precise, evidence-based, and non-stigmatizing. The Shamiri intervention was found to be effective in reducing adolescent depression and anxiety when delivered by lay providers [62,63] with effects lasting at least 7 months [63]. Shamiri-Digital (https://thrive-online.shamiri.institute/) is the digital single-session adaptation of the full Shamiri intervention. It consists of the same three modules on growth, gratitude, and value affirmation, and it is designed to last for 60 min. Shamiri-Digital has been shown to be effective in reducing depressive symptoms at a 2-week follow-up [43]. Shamiri-Digital has been designed following the B.E.S.T. principles.

Brain science to normalize concepts in the program

The *growth mindset* module emphasizes the fact that it is possible for us to grow in different areas of our life like relationships, math, generosity, etc. It also highlights how our brain changes as we grow in different areas:

Imagine you go to the gym and exercise. After a while, your muscles begin to grow and become stronger. When you stop exercising, the muscles stop growing and might become smaller.

The brain works in the same way. Just like a muscle, your brain gets stronger the more you use it. This happens because our brain cells grow and make many more small connections when we learn. The more you challenge your mind, the more the brain cells grow. Things that you found hard, like algebra or chemistry, start becoming easier.

The gratitude and the values affirmation modules deviate slightly in that they use science, but not brain science, to add credibility to the concepts. For example, the module on gratitude says:

> Scientists say that being grateful makes a person feel happier, more successful, and have better relationships with their friends and family. If we try and be more grateful, we will be able to deal with challenges in our lives.

And the module on values affirmation says:

> Science has shown that remembering our virtues can make us happier and help us make better choices. Research shows that people who think about their virtues are healthier than people who do not think about their virtues. Thinking about our virtues can also improve our energy levels, compassion for others, self-esteem, and our ability to work and study.

Empower youths to a "helper" or "expert" role

Before the modules start, Shamiri-Digital shows a message to the users to emphasize their role in helping improve the intervention for other students. The relevant parts are:

> Your answers will help us understand things that students like you go through.

> We will ask for your advice and suggestions so that we can be able to improve this program for other students in the future.

Saying-is-believing exercises to solidify learning

All three modules include exercises to help adolescents practice what they have learned in the modules. The growth module asks the participants to think of a time they faced a challenge, how they used effort to overcome the challenge, and how they grew in the process. In the gratitude module, the participants were asked to think of three things they were grateful for and why that good thing is important to them. In the virtue affirmation module, the participants were asked to select three virtues out of a list. Following that, the participants are prompted to write one virtue that is very important to them and are asked to detail why it matters to them.

Testimonials and evidence from valued others. A testimonial was provided in the growth mindset module, but not in the other two modules. The testimonial in the growth module narrated how a school student made a conscious effort to improve her relationship with her sister:

> My Growth Story – Learning to Communicate.

> Our families are a major part of who we are. Everyone hopes to have strong relationships with their parents, aunts, uncles, and siblings. But from a young age, my sister and I never got along. We always fought and yelled at each other. It was difficult to be in the same room because we were very different and didn't listen to each other.

> I felt very sad that my sister and I could not have a strong relationship, go out and do things together, or have interesting conversations. Finally, when I entered high school, I realized that my problems with my sister would not change on their own. They would only change if I made an effort to change my behavior.

> From that moment on, I made an effort to be more compassionate, kind, and became less angry. I listened to her more, and paid attention to what she had to say. Slowly, we grew closer. I am now proud to say that my sister and I are closer than I ever thought we could be.

Dissemination and Implementation of Digital Single-Session Interventions

Co-design and coproduction with people/communities in low- and middle-income countries

Treatment approaches and guidelines used in LMICs are mostly based on research in HICs [18]. To increase the acceptability of SSIs in LMICs, it is necessary to incorporate feedback from communities in LMICs. Wasil and colleagues [52] describe the process of developing an SSI for adolescents in India. The first step was to find brief intervention components that have been validated empirically. They narrowed down on intervention components based on growth mindset, gratitude, and behavioral activation. Then they discussed the cultural appropriateness, perceived efficacy, and perceived relevance of the identified interventions with local researchers and school officials. The initial intervention was then developed using the structure followed by previous SSIs [21]. The initial intervention draft was then reviewed in two focus group studies with teachers and students. The feedback received in the focus groups were used to edit and finalize the SSI. For example, case vignettes were made more relatable by including more common concerns and were moved to the beginning of the interventions to increase engagement. This study provides a template for developing or adapting SSIs for LMICs.

Examination of barriers to implementation and acceptability of digital self-help tools by setting

Digital SSIs have been shown to be effective when delivered in school settings [34,43]. In LMICs, however, the resource constraints at the school could limit the accessibility of the SSIs. Osborn and colleagues [43] reported that they could only deliver treatment to 18 students at a time because the school had only 18 Internet-connected computers. A study conducted in rural low-income high schools in Southeastern US, in contrast, did not report this limitation [34]. Another survey conducted on Jamaican adolescents reported that stigma, embarrassment, and low mental health literacy were stronger barriers to help-seeking and digital mental health uptake than were access to smartphones or the Internet [64]. Overall, digital SSIs have the potential to overcome structural barriers that limit access to mental health interventions for the youth in LMICs and low-resource settings in HICs. However, the reach of digital SSIs is moderated by smartphone and Internet penetration in the country. Globally, national policies that prioritize infrastructure to provide fast, affordable Internet access to everyone would add an additional tool to combat youth mental health crisis.

Dissemination of digital single-session interventions through the existing frameworks and social media

The flexibility offered by digital SSIs makes them suitable for dissemination in diverse settings ranging from classrooms [34] to social media [50]. Social media penetration varies widely by country, with more than 80% of the population in North America and Western European countries using the Internet, versus 10% or less in Eastern and Middle Africa [65]. Throughout the globe, the percentage of people accessing the Internet is increasing consistently. With the increasing penetration of smartphones and Internet accessibility in LMICs, the penetration of social media, and the potential reach of digital SSIs is only going to increase over time. Digital SSIs are increasingly becoming a scalable, low-cost treatment option in LMICs and low-resource settings [66].

SUMMARY

This article summarizes the prevalence of and treatment gap in mental health disorders in children and adolescents and highlights how digital SSIs can serve as a potential scalable treatment approach. The article also highlights the scenario in LMICs where the need for accessible interventions is more pressing. Digital SSIs provide an effective and scalable treatment approach that can be delivered as a standalone treatment to individuals who would otherwise receive no treatment. The flexibility offered by digital SSIs also makes them suitable for seamless integration within the traditional

primary care and mental health care frameworks and can be used in conjunction with other long-term treatments for individuals with chronic disorders. Digital SSIs would not be a panacea for the mental health crisis, but with the increasing penetration of smartphones and Internet even in LMICs, digital SSIs are a promising treatment approach that can reduce the treatment gap.

CLINICS CARE POINTS

- Both digital and therapist-delivered Single-Session Interventions may be offered youth on lengthy waiting lists for treatment in order to reduce wait time and prevent symptoms from worsening before longer-term treatment can begin.

- Single-Session Interventions may be useful to offer in treatment settings where multi-session approaches are less feasible, such as schools, primary care clinics, and emergency settings.

- Single-Session Interventions may be sufficient to meet some youths' clinical needs, but they are not meant to replace other forms of treatment; rather, they may bridge gaps in systems of care that traditional, multi-session therapies cannot fill.

REFERENCES

[1] WHO. Child and adolescent mental and brain health. Accessed 2 December 2022. Available at: https://www.who.int/activities/improving-the-mental-and-brain-health-of-children-and-adolescents.

[2] Gillies D, Christou MA, Dixon AC, et al. Prevalence and characteristics of self-harm in adolescents: meta-analyses of community-based studies 1990–2015. J Am Acad Child Adolesc Psychiatry 2018;57(10):733–41.

[3] Bitsko RH, Claussen AH, Lichstein J, et al. Mental health surveillance among children — United States, 2013–2019. MMWR Suppl 2022;71(2):1–42.

[4] Shorey S, Ng ED, Wong CHJ. Global prevalence of depression and elevated depressive symptoms among adolescents: A systematic review and meta-analysis. Br J Clin Psychol 2022;61(2):287–305.

[5] Douglas J, Scott J. A systematic review of gender-specific rates of unipolar and bipolar disorders in community studies of pre-pubertal children. Bipolar Disord 2014;16(1):5–15.

[6] Biswas T, Scott JG, Munir K, et al. Global variation in the prevalence of suicidal ideation, anxiety and their correlates among adolescents: a population based study of 82 countries. eClinicalMedicine 2020;24:100395.

[7] Racine N, McArthur BA, Cooke JE, et al. Global prevalence of depressive and anxiety symptoms in children

and adolescents during COVID-19: a meta-analysis. JAMA Pediatr 2021;175(11):1142.

[8] Mei C, Fitzsimons J, Allen N, et al. Global research priorities for youth mental health. Early Interv Psychiatry 2020;14(1):3–13.

[9] Sawyer MG, Reece CE, Sawyer AC, et al. Adequacy of treatment for child and adolescent mental disorders in Australia: A national study. Aust N Z J Psychiatry 2019; 53(4):326–35.

[10] Anderson JK, Howarth E, Vainre M, et al. A scoping literature review of service-level barriers for access and engagement with mental health services for children and young people. Child Youth Serv Rev 2017;77: 164–76.

[11] Schnyder N, Sawyer MG, Lawrence D, et al. Barriers to mental health care for Australian children and adolescents in 1998 and 2013–2014. Aust N Z J Psychiatry 2020;54(10):1007–19.

[12] Jensen PS, Goldman E, Offord D, et al. Overlooked and underserved: "action signs" for identifying children with unmet mental health needs. Pediatrics 2011;128(5): 970–9.

[13] Breland DJ, McCarty CA, Zhou C, et al. Determinants of mental health service use among depressed adolescents. Gen Hosp Psychiatry 2014;36(3):296–301.

[14] Wang C, Barlis J, Do KA, et al. Barriers to mental health help seeking at school for Asian– and Latinx–American adolescents. School Ment Health 2020;12(1):182–94.

[15] Planey AM, Smith SM, Moore S, et al. Barriers and facilitators to mental health help-seeking among African American youth and their families: a systematic review study. Child Youth Serv Rev 2019;101: 190–200.

[16] Clausen CE, Skokauskas N. Child and Adolescent Mental Health: How can we help improve access to care? J Indian Assoc Child Adolesc Ment Health 2018;14(1): 10–8.

[17] Docherty M, Shaw K, Goulding L, et al. Evidence-based guideline implementation in low and middle income countries: lessons for mental health care. Int J Ment Health Syst 2017;11(1):8.

[18] Patel V, Kieling C, Maulik PK, et al. Improving access to care for children with mental disorders: a global perspective. Arch Dis Child 2013;98(5):323–7.

[19] Kieling C, Baker-Henningham H, Belfer M, et al. Child and adolescent mental health worldwide: evidence for action. Lancet 2011;378(9801):1515–25.

[20] Schleider JL, Dobias ML, Sung JY, et al. Future directions in single-session youth mental health interventions. J Clin Child Adolesc Psychol 2020;49(2):264–78.

[21] Schleider JL, Weisz JR. Little treatments, promising effects? Meta-analysis of single-session interventions for youth psychiatric problems. J Am Acad Child Adolesc Psychiatry 2017;56(2):107–15.

[22] Dobias ML, Schleider JL, Jans L, et al. An online, single-session intervention for adolescent self-injurious

thoughts and behaviors: results from a randomized trial. Behav Res Ther 2021;147:103983.

[23] Schleider JL, Mullarkey MC, Fox KR, et al. A randomized trial of online single-session interventions for adolescent depression during COVID-19. Nat Hum Behav 2022; 6(2):258–68.

[24] Schleider JL, Dobias M, Sung J, et al. Acceptability and utility of an open-access, online single-session intervention platform for adolescent mental health. JMIR Ment Health 2020;7(6):e20513.

[25] Harpaz-Rotem I, Leslie D, Rosenheck RA. Treatment retention among children entering a new episode of mental health care. Psychiatr Serv 2004;55(9): 1022–8.

[26] Hoyt MF, Bobele M, Slive A, et al. Single-session/one-at-a-time walk-in therapy. In: Hoyt MF, Bobele M, Slive A, editors. et al., Single-session therapy by walk-in or appointment. 1st edition. New York: Routledge; 2018. p. 3–24.

[27] Wright B, Tindall L, Scott AJ, et al. One session treatment (OST) is equivalent to multi-session cognitive behavioral therapy (CBT) in children with specific phobias (ASPECT): results from a national non-inferiority randomized controlled trial. J Child Psychol Psychiatry 2022;jcpp.13665. https://doi.org/10.1111/jcpp.13665.

[28] Wang HI, Wright B, Tindall L, et al. Cost and effectiveness of one session treatment (OST) for children and young people with specific phobias compared to multi-session cognitive behavioural therapy (CBT): results from a randomised controlled trial. BMC Psychiatry 2022;22(1):547.

[29] Diedrichs PC, Atkinson MJ, Steer RJ, et al. Effectiveness of a brief school-based body image intervention 'Dove Confident Me: Single Session' when delivered by teachers and researchers: results from a cluster randomised controlled trial. Behav Res Ther 2015;74:94–104.

[30] Mejia A, Calam R, Sanders MR. A pilot randomized controlled trial of a brief parenting intervention in low-resource settings in panama. Prev Sci 2015;16(5): 707–17.

[31] Perkins R. The effectiveness of one session of therapy using a single-session therapy approach for children and adolescents with mental health problems. Psychol Psychother Theory Res Pract 2006;79(2):215–27.

[32] Yeager DS, Bryan CJ, Gross JJ, et al. A synergistic mindsets intervention protects adolescents from stress. Nature 2022;607(7919):512–20.

[33] Feldman DB, Dreher DE. Can hope be changed in 90 minutes? Testing the efficacy of a single-session goal-pursuit intervention for college students. J Happiness Stud 2012; 13(4):745–59.

[34] Schleider JL, Burnette JL, Widman L, et al. Randomized trial of a single-session growth mind-set intervention for rural adolescents' internalizing and externalizing problems. J Clin Child Adolesc Psychol 2020;49(5): 660–72.

[35] Schleider J, Weisz J. A single-session growth mindset intervention for adolescent anxiety and depression: 9-month outcomes of a randomized trial. J Child Psychol Psychiatry 2018;59(2):160–70.

[36] Calvete E, Fernández-Gonzalez L, Orue I, et al. The effect of an intervention teaching adolescents that people can change on depressive symptoms, cognitive schemas, and hypothalamic-pituitary-adrenal axis hormones. J Abnorm Child Psychol 2019;47(9):1533–46.

[37] Cardamone-Breen MC, Jorm AF, Lawrence KA, et al. A single-session, web-based parenting intervention to prevent adolescent depression and anxiety disorders: randomized controlled trial. J Med Internet Res 2018;20(4): e148.

[38] Venturo-Conerly KE. Single-session interventions for adolescent anxiety and depression symptoms in Kenya: a cluster-randomized controlled trial. Behav Res Ther 2022;9. https://doi.org/10.1016/j.brat.2022.104040.

[39] Cartwright-Hatton S, Ewing D, Dash S, et al. Preventing family transmission of anxiety: feasibility RCT of a brief intervention for parents. Br J Clin Psychol 2018;57(3): 351–66.

[40] White C, Shanley DC, Zimmer-Gembeck MJ, et al. Outcomes of in situ training for disclosure as a standalone and a booster to a child protective behaviors education program. Child Maltreat 2019;24(2):193–202.

[41] Aggarwal S, Patton G. Engaging families in the management of adolescent self-harm. Evid Based Ment Health 2018;21(1):16–22.

[42] McDanal R, Rubin A, Fox KR, et al. Associations of LGBTQ+ identities with acceptability and efficacy of online single-session youth mental health interventions. Behav Ther 2022;53(2):376–91.

[43] Osborn TL, Rodriguez M, Wasil AR, et al. Single-session digital intervention for adolescent depression, anxiety, and well-being: Outcomes of a randomized controlled trial with Kenyan adolescents. J Consult Clin Psychol 2020;88(7);657–68.

[44] Pretorius C, Chambers D, Cowan B, et al. Young people seeking help online for mental health: cross-sectional survey study. JMIR Ment Health 2019;6(8): e13524.

[45] Wetterlin FM, Mar MY, Neilson EK, et al. eMental health experiences and expectations: a survey of youths' web-based resource preferences in Canada. J Med Internet Res 2014;16(12):e293.

[46] Pretorius C, Chambers D, Coyle D. Young people's online help-seeking and mental health difficulties: systematic narrative review. J Med Internet Res 2019;21(11): e13873.

[47] Williams KA, Chapman MV. Comparing health and mental health needs, service use, and barriers to services among sexual minority youths and their peers. Health Soc Work 2011;36(3):197–206.

[48] Acevedo-Polakovich ID, Bell B, Gamache P, et al. Service accessibility for lesbian, gay, bisexual, transgender, and questioning youth. Youth Soc 2013;45(1):75–97.

[49] Schleider JL. The fundamental need for lived experience perspectives in developing and evaluating psychotherapies. J Consult Clin Psychol 2023;91(3):119–21.

[50] Dobias ML, Morris RR, Schleider JL. Single-session interventions embedded within tumblr: acceptability, feasibility, and utility study. JMIR Form Res 2022;6(7): e39004.

[51] Ching BC, Bennett SD, Morant N, et al. Growth mindset in young people awaiting treatment in a paediatric mental health service: A mixed methods pilot of a digital single-session intervention. Clin Child Psychol Psychiatry 2022. https://doi.org/10.1177/13591045221105193 135910452211051.

[52] Wasil AR, Park SJ, Gillespie S, et al. Harnessing single-session interventions to improve adolescent mental health and well-being in India: Development, adaptation, and pilot testing of online single-session interventions in Indian secondary schools. Asian J Psychiatry 2020;50:101980.

[53] Mullarkey M, Dobias M, Sung J, et al. Web-based single session intervention for perceived control over anxiety during COVID-19: randomized controlled trial. JMIR Ment Health 2022;9(4):e33473.

[54] Lewin GW. Constructs in field theory. In: Cartwright D, editor. Resolving social conflicts and field theory in social science. New York, NY: Harper and Brothers; 1944. p. 191–9.

[55] Snyder CR, Sympson SC, Ybasco FC, et al. State hope scale. Published online September 12, 2011. https://doi.org/10.1037/t01180-000

[56] Jacobson NS, Dobson KS, Truax PA, et al. A component analysis of cognitive-behavioral treatment for depression. J Consult Clin Psychol 1996;64(2):295–304.

[57] Samdal O, Rowling L. Implementation strategies to promote and sustain health and learning in school. In: Simovska V, Mannix McNamara P, editors. Schools for health and Sustainability. Dordrecht: Springer Netherlands; 2015. p. 233–52. https://doi.org/10.1007/978-94-017-9171-7_11.

[58] Aronson E. The power of self-persuasion. Am Psychol 1999;54(11):875–84.

[59] Yeager DS, Walton GM. Social-psychological interventions in education: they're not magic. Rev Educ Res 2011;81(2):267–301.

[60] Quintero Johnson JM, Yilmaz G, Najarian K. Optimizing the presentation of mental health information in social media: the effects of health testimonials and platform on source perceptions, message processing, and health outcomes. Health Commun 2017;32(9):1121–32.

[61] Borah P, Xiao X. The importance of 'likes': the interplay of message framing, source, and social endorsement on credibility perceptions of health information on facebook. J Health Commun 2018;23(4):399–411.

[62] Osborn TL, Wasil AR, Venturo-Conerly KE, et al. Group intervention for adolescent anxiety and depression: outcomes of a randomized trial with adolescents in kenya. Behav Ther 2020;51(4):601–15.

[63] Osborn TL, Venturo-Conerly KE, Arango GS, et al. Effect of shamiri layperson-provided intervention vs study skills control intervention for depression and anxiety symptoms in adolescents in kenya: a randomized clinical trial. JAMA Psychiatr 2021;78(8):829.

[64] Maloney CA, Abel WD, McLeod HJ. Jamaican adolescents' receptiveness to digital mental health services: a cross-sectional survey from rural and urban communities. Internet Interv 2020;21:100325.

[65] Social media: worldwide penetration rate 2022. Statista. Accessed 3 January, 2023. Available at: https://www.statista.com/statistics/269615/social-network-penetration-by-region/.

[66] Wasil AR, Kacmarek CN, Osborn TL, et al. Economic evaluation of an online single-session intervention for depression in Kenyan adolescents. J Consult Clin Psychol 2021;89(8):657–67.

Advances in Psychiatry and Behavioral Health 3 (2023) 139–147

ADVANCES IN PSYCHIATRY AND BEHAVIORAL HEALTH

Temperament, Parenting, and Child Anxiety

Elizabeth M. Aaron, MA, Nicole M. Baumgartner, MA, Elizabeth J. Kiel, PhD*

Department of Psychology, Miami University, 90 North Patterson Avenue, Oxford, OH 45056, USA

KEYWORDS

• Temperament • Behavioral inhibition • Parenting • Child • Parent–child • Anxiety • Development

KEY POINTS

- Inhibited temperament is a risk factor for child anxiety. Inhibited temperament and anxiety share biological and behavioral correlates, and environmental and cultural contexts impact the risk pathway.
- There are anxiety-promoting (eg, overcontrolling) and anxiety-dampening (eg, autonomy-encouragement) parenting behaviors. Parenting behaviors that promote or dampen anxiety may differ across various caregivers and identities.
- Child inhibited temperament and anxiogenic parenting interact with and bidirectionally relate to one another in the pathway to child anxiety, which is contextualized by culture.

INTRODUCTION

Theories of anxiety development posit that biological, genetic, and environmental factors all play roles in the trajectory to anxiety outcomes [1,2]. Temperament, which is theorized to be at least partly genetic and biologically-based, represents predispositions to respond to the environment with various patterns of reactivity and regulation [3]. Parenting is a primary means by which the environment affects children, particularly during early developmental periods. Thus, considering the roles of temperament and parenting has been a major focus for theories and empirical studies seeking to explain how and under what circumstances anxiety develops. As such, this chapter focuses on advances in the field's understanding of child temperament and parenting behaviors as key factors examined within the developmental pathway toward anxiety. The cultural and socio-temporal surroundings of research theories and empirical findings are discussed to contextualize the current knowledge base and stimulate areas of future research.

TEMPERAMENT

There are multiple dimensions of temperament that have been linked to child anxiety development, including negative affectivity, effortful control, and inhibited temperament [4,5]. Inhibited temperament, also known as behavioral inhibition or fearful temperament, is the most widely researched dimension within the study of child anxiety, and therefore this chapter will focus on this temperamental dimension.

Behavioral Correlates

Inhibited temperament is defined by withdrawal and shyness when in new environments or when presented with novel stimuli [6,7]. Children with high inhibited temperament are reactive to unknown stimuli, moving away from unfamiliar toys or strangers and moving closer to caregivers in the presence of these stimuli. Children with high inhibited temperament tend to have attentional and cognitive biases toward threat, demonstrating difficulty with shifting their attention away from threat cues and interpreting ambiguous situations as threatening [8].

---

*Corresponding author, *E-mail address:* kielluej@miamioh.edu

https://doi.org/10.1016/j.ypsc.2023.03.017
2667-3827/23/

The prevalence of high inhibited temperament may differ across cultures. For example, one study found that Mexican-American immigrants displayed more shyness than Mexican-Americans born in the United States [9], and early research found that higher inhibited behaviors were displayed by Chinese children as compared to Canadian children [10]. Differences in rates of high inhibited temperament may be due to the social desirability of inhibition within these cultural contexts [11]. However, more recent research indicates that the social desirability of shyness may be decreasing in urbanized areas of China [11], which suggests that further research is needed.

Recent research indicates that the context in which inhibited temperament is observed impacts its correlates. For instance, the related construct of dysregulated fear assesses children's high levels of inhibition and fear in low-threat contexts, in particular [12]. Dysregulated fear was found to uniquely predict adolescent social anxiety symptoms [13]. Further, inhibited temperament shown in a social context relates differently to anxiety outcomes than inhibited temperament shown in a non-social context [14,15]. In a sample of primarily White Americans, social inhibited temperament related to separation anxiety and social anxiety, whereas non-social inhibited temperament was associated with specific phobia [14]. Importantly, the context in which inhibited temperament is assessed may also impact correlates differently across cultural contexts. In a Native American sample, retrospective reports of nonsocial behavioral inhibition were specifically associated with later social anxiety development in adolescence [16], indicating potentially different relations between social versus nonsocial behavioral inhibition and anxiety outcomes in White and Native American populations.

Although nuances exist, inhibited temperament and its related constructs (eg, dysregulated fear, social, and nonsocial behavioral inhibition) are linked to child anxiety development across cultural contexts, including in Western, Eastern European, and African regions [17,18] and in diverse racial and ethnic groups in the United States, including Native American, Chinese American, and Hispanic American groups.[16,19–21] High child inhibited temperament is also one of the strongest predictors of social anxiety disorder, in particular [22]. Inhibited temperament and anxiety share behavioral correlates such as social withdrawal and attentional biases to threat, indicating that children with high inhibited temperament have a behavioral risk for anxiety development [23]. Additionally, inhibited temperament and anxiety share notable biological and psychophysiological correlates that further strengthen anxiety risk for inhibited children.

Biological Correlates

Like other temperament constructs, inhibited temperament is theorized to be at least partly biologically based [3]. Kagan [24] theorized that the amygdala, a part of the brain that detects emotional valence and environmental threat, has a low threshold for arousal, or could be considered overactive, in inhibited children. This relation was later born out with adults who had previously been classified as behaviorally inhibited as toddlers [25]. Given the amygdala's connection to both cortical and subcortical structures, amygdala reactivity has downstream effects on biological outputs commonly associated with inhibited temperament, including cortisol reactivity, high and stable heart rate, and neural indices of withdrawal and dysregulated responses to fear and novelty [26,27].

Advances in the knowledge base have provided additional evidence for the biological bases of inhibited behavior and its link to anxiety. For example, children with extreme inhibition show sustained elevation of cortisol, a stress hormone released downstream from the amygdala's activation of the hypothalamic-pituitary-adrenal system [28–30]. Additionally, these children show higher heart rate variability [31], an index of parasympathetic control over fight-or-flight responses. These elevations in cortisol and heart rate variability reveal the sustained reactivity shown by children with extreme inhibition as compared with the recovery and regulation shown by less inhibited children. At the neural level, children with early emerging shyness, conceptually similar to inhibited temperament, show greater relative right-frontal electroencephalogram (EEG) asymmetry, a pattern characterizing tendencies toward withdrawal, compared with children who were not shy or developed shyness later in childhood [32]. Additionally, dysregulated fear has been shown to predict coupling across the delta and beta EEG frequency bands in a manner indicative of neural over-control of fearfulness in low-threat contexts [33]. Neural indices of threat and novelty detection, measured as event-related potentials, can be observed from EEG when children complete tasks involving attention bias toward novel or threatening faces, oddball detection, and conflict and error monitoring [34]. Thus, inhibited temperament has been linked to patterns of reactivity and regulation across several systems.

Biologically-based reactivity and regulation function as moderators of the predictive link between inhibited temperament and anxiety risk. Inhibited temperament has been most strongly linked to anxiety when children show maladaptive patterns of heart rate variability, either by itself [31] or in the context of high negative emotionality [35]. Thus, physiological dysregulation may determine when behavioral measures of inhibited temperament continue to follow a trajectory toward risk. Recent advances have uncovered additional nuance. Ugarte and colleagues [36], for example, found a curvilinear association between respiratory sinus arrhythmia (RSA), a metric of heart rate variability, and internalizing problems including anxiety, wherein both low and high RSA related to maladjustment. Thus, biology's role in inhibited temperament and its risk for anxiety is complex, with much knowledge yet to uncover. Of course, children's temperamental predispositions do not exist in a vacuum, and thus the parenting environment is essential to consider.

PARENTING

When studying the role of parenting in relation to increased anxiety risk, there are a myriad of parenting behaviors to consider, as many different attitudes, perceptions, and contexts determine how a parent may engage with their child (Fig. 1).

Broadly, it is beneficial to examine behaviors that promote and behaviors that dampen or discourage further anxiety development. Behaviors that are often associated with promoting anxiety development include harsh expressions of anger, emotional withdrawal, rejection, overcontrol, and intrusiveness [37,38]. An anxiety-promoting behavior that is frequently discussed in the literature is that of overprotection, in which parents shield their children from new experiences or potential risk, denying them the opportunity to learn to tolerate uncertainty and cope with novelty. There is a strong positive association between parental overprotection and child anxiety development [39]. Conversely, behaviors that are often associated with dampening further anxiety development include sensitivity, encouragement to engage or approach, warmth, and nurturance [38]. An anxiety-dampening behavior frequently highlighted in the anxiety literature is encouragement of independence, or the encouragement of the child to try new things and take appropriate risks, modeling to the child that the environment is safe. Parents higher in encouragement of independence are less likely to have anxious children [40].

The parenting behaviors that are most relevant to child anxiety development may be dependent on the child's age, as well. For example, in the first few months of a child's life, parental sensitivity in predominantly White, Western families may be especially important with regard to the infant's ability to regulate their emotions, as parents who engage in high levels of sensitivity have infants who are better able to self-regulate [38]. However, as children age, the role of sensitivity is not as clear, and does not seem to have as profound an impact on the child's self-regulation capabilities [38]. Conversely, parental overcontrol has been shown to predict anxiety outcomes from infancy through adolescence, demonstrating more consistent relations across child development [37].

Parenting Among Diverse Caregivers

Although the literature on parenting, temperament, and anxiety development is well-established, it has largely

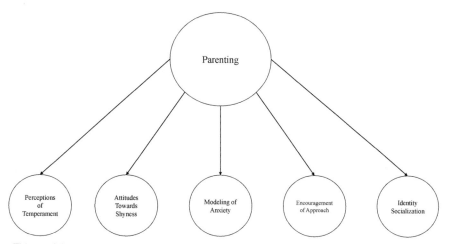

FIG. 1 This model contains a non-exhaustive list of factors that are included in the study parenting. For sake of clarity, only factors that are explicitly discussed in the chapter are depicted.

focused on mothers, with less emphasis on other caregivers. Though a call was put forth in 1975 for more research on caregivers other than mothers [41], few studies have answered this call.

Theory would suggest that it is imperative to study caregivers other than mothers. Although mothers and fathers, for example, likely engage in many similar behaviors, recent literature suggests that each caregiver has an impact on the child that is unique from that of the other parent [42]. In White, Western families, the mother is often considered a nurturing figure for the child, whereas the father's role may largely encompass encouraging the child to explore the world around them [43]. Fathers who model approach toward novelty, trying new things, or meeting new people may teach their children tolerance of uncertainty, decreasing their risk for anxiety. One setting in which fathers can encourage tolerance of uncertainty is the play environment. Fathers often engage in rough-and-tumble play, displaying behaviors such as play-wrestling which teach children to take appropriate risks and to overcome limits [43]. Fathers who do not engage in this play, or who place strict limits on play, may be unintentionally promoting further inhibition, increasing anxiety risk. Though fathers have a crucial role in temperament and anxiety development, few empirical studies include fathers.

Although the field has shown some advancement in studying caregiving more broadly, still only 15% of studies on parenting and anxiety include a caregiver that is not a mother, and the majority of the ones that do focus on fathers [38]. Thus, the literature largely neglects alternative family structures and other caregivers. Moving forward, the literature should broaden its scope so as to more accurately capture the role of all caregivers in anxiety development.

Parenting in underrepresented cultures and identities

The parent–child temperament and anxiety literature is also limited in that most studies are comprised of White, upper-middle class parents in heterosexual relationships. The dynamics of lesbian, gay, bisexual, transgender, queer, and additional gender and sexual orientation identity (LGBTQ+) families, families of color, families of low SES, and families in developing countries may function differently in relation to child anxiety than those in traditionally -studied WEIRD (Western, Educated, Industrialized, Rich, Democratic) populations, pointing to the importance of representing them in research.

Although parents in heterosexual, gay, and lesbian relationships have been found to similarly distribute childcare tasks [44], recent research reveals some potential differences among individual parents. Gay fathers, for example, were found to display higher warmth, view inhibition less negatively, and spend more time, on average, with their children than heterosexual fathers [45].

Moreover, recent literature continues to highlight that the experience of oppression impacts parenting strategies for minoritized groups. In Black families, specifically, discussions regarding race and discrimination have been identified as key protective factors for children, leading to a lower likelihood of internalizing racism, thus improving socioemotional outcomes [46]. Parental behaviors that encourage pride in identity may be especially important in reducing anxiety risk of Black children, yet few studies on parenting and child anxiety development include explicit measures of conversations about discrimination. Additionally, families oppressed based on SES may parent differently due to limited resources and other environmental factors. Children in families of low SES may have a higher anxiety risk due to living in unsafe neighborhoods, not having as much time to spend at home, and experiencing stress that limits their own regulatory abilities [47,48]. Strength-focused research may identify unique aspects of resilience in families of low SES. As such, studies should consider how experiences of oppression impact parenting strategies.

The parent–child dynamic is impacted by cultural values and life experiences, yet the parenting literature largely focuses on the same privileged populations. Future studies need to include underrepresented populations, and give particular attention to the ways in which experiences of oppression interact with parenting to predict anxiety development. For example, families with undocumented immigrant parents face a series of unique stressors, including persistent fears of separation and difficult conversations around documentation status, that are not reflected in the current literature [49]. As such, researchers should take caution in overgeneralizing their results to all populations. Cultural context and life experiences must also be considered when examining the complex relations between temperament and parenting in the pathway to child anxiety.

TEMPERAMENT AND PARENTING

Theory and research indicate that children and parents interact with one another in a dynamic and reciprocal manner, with various factors influencing how they respond to one another and engage with their environments [2,50]. Substantial research shows a link between child temperament and parenting behavior [5,7,17], and one factor that requires consideration in these relations is parental perceptions of child temperament [51].

Parental Perceptions of Temperament

Parental perceptions of child temperament likely impact how caregivers parent their children. More positive perceptions of inhibited temperament may lead to more accepting parenting behaviors and more negative perceptions may lead to more controlling parenting behaviors [11]. When parents perceive their children's inhibition as socially inappropriate, they may engage in overcontrolling behaviors in an attempt to reduce these displays of inhibition.

Importantly, perceptions of child inhibited temperament and shyness are different across cultural contexts [11]. For example, child shyness may be less valued, and thus perceived more negatively, by American families [51] whereas child shyness may be more valued, and thus more accepted by parents, in China and Korea [10,52]. These cultural differences in perceptions of shyness may be due to cultural values of sociability and independence in American contexts and cultural values of collectivism, interdependence, and modesty in Chinese and Korean contexts [11]. However, there are notable recent advances in the literature that indicate shifts in perceptions of shyness in urban China, which has experienced more Western influence, with increasing negative parental attitudes toward shy children and worse outcomes for these children as compared with previous findings in this population [11]. These findings reveal the complexity of culture and its influence on the parent–child relationship. This complexity is also shown in research examining the relations among temperament, parenting, and child anxiety, which includes correlations, main effects, moderations, and mediations within various cultural contexts (Fig. 2).

Concurrent Relations

There are concurrent relations between child temperament and parenting behavior across cultural contexts [5,53,54]. Child negative affect and low sociability (ie, inhibition) positively relate to authoritarianism (ie, strict parenting with low warmth) in Indian, American, and Chinese contexts [53,54]. That is, when children display high levels of distress and inhibition, their parents are more likely to engage in critical parenting across Western and Eastern contexts. Additionally, overcontrolling parenting positively relates to child inhibition in Western and Eastern contexts [7,17]. When children are withdrawn, their parents may be more likely to engage in parenting behaviors that limit child autonomy.

Theory and research have examined more complex models building on these concurrent relations. A recent review of child anxiety development posited a conceptual model in which anxiogenic parenting serves both a moderating and mediating role in the relation between child inhibited temperament and child anxiety [55]. Research in Western and Eastern contexts provides empirical evidence supporting this developmental model.

Moderations

Some theories suggest that environmental factors provide the context within which predisposing factors lead to anxiety [1,55]. In line with these theories, research has investigated the interaction between child inhibited temperament and parenting behavior in the prediction of child anxiety and anxiety-related outcomes. Some literature has assessed this interaction concurrently, with early research finding that high inhibition related to greater social reticence solely within the context of high maternal intrusiveness [5]. Recent literature has examined this interaction longitudinally, strengthening the interpretation of directional effects. Several studies have found that parenting behaviors such as overinvolvement, excessive support, and encouragement to approach novelty moderate the prospective relation between child inhibited temperament and child anxiety symptoms in Western contexts [40,56–58]. For example, Hudson and colleagues [56] found that for inhibited children, anxiety symptoms decreased more slowly from age 4 to 12 years within the context of high parental involvement compared with low parental involvement.

Emerging literature in Eastern contexts indicates that parenting may also moderate the relation between inhibited temperament and anxiety within these cultures [18]. For example, Turkish children's high inhibition predicted greater child anxiety within the context of low, but not high, levels of maternal warmth [17]. Further, high child inhibited temperament had a marginally stronger positive relation with anxiety in the context of high parental overprotection in South Africa [18]. Lastly, in Chinese American families, maternal encouragement of modesty and maternal praise served as adaptive parenting contexts, weakening the positive relation between child shyness and anxious behavior [19,20].

Parental encouragement is another adaptive contextual factor, with the goal of this encouragement differing across cultural contexts (ie, encouragement

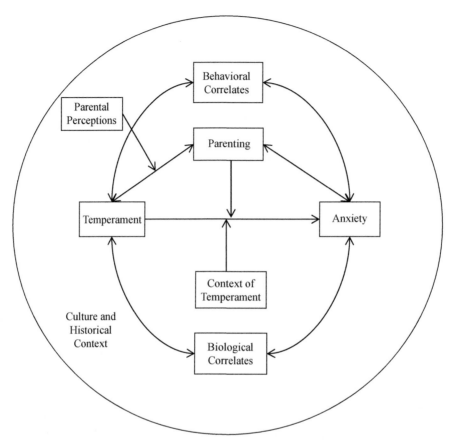

FIG. 2 This conceptual model depicts the relations between temperament, parenting, anxiety, and their correlates as reviewed in this chapter. The model builds off of models developed by Liu and Pérez-Edgar and Vélez-Agosto et al. (*Modified from* Liu P, Pérez-Edgar KE. Developmental pathways from early behavioral inhibition to later anxiety: an integrative review of developmental psychopathology research and translational implications. Adolesc Res Rev. 2019;4(1):45-58; and Vélez-Agosto NM, Soto-Crespo JG, Vizcarrondo-Oppenheimer M, Vega-Molina S, García Coll C. Bronfenbrenner's bioecological theory revision: moving culture from the macro into the micro. Perspect Psychol Sci. 2017;12(5):900-910.)

to approach novelty, encouragement to be modest). The moderate evidence for an interaction between parenting and child inhibited temperament in the prediction of child anxiety is important to consider in tandem with evidence that parenting and temperament also have bidirectional and mechanistic relations.

Bidirectional and Mechanistic Relations

Research on temperament, parenting, and anxiety has primarily focused on parent-driven effects, such as over-involved parenting predicting increases in child inhibited temperament and anxiety [59]. However, child-driven effects are critical to parenting behaviors, as well, with child inhibition predicting parental over-protection [39]. Further, child temperamental risk for

anxiety and anxious symptoms predict, and are predicted by, parenting behavior over time [13,49]. This empirical evidence for bidirectional effects supports theory positing an anxious-coercive cycle [2]. It is theorized that child inhibited temperament and overcontrolling parenting serve to reinforce each other within this cycle. First, child withdrawal pulls for parental overcontrol to help manage the situation. Then, when parents engage in high overcontrol, they give their children little autonomy, which may lead children to believe that they have little control over their surroundings [60]. This low self-efficacy increases child inhibition, thus continuing the cycle. This theory supports both parent-driven and child-driven effects, and, more specifically, bidirectional effects. Additionally, this theory suggests that parenting behavior may serve as the mechanistic link between child temperament and child anxiety and internalizing problems, which has been examined recently in the field [61–63]. For example, child dysregulated fear positively predicts child separation anxiety through maternal intrusive parenting behavior [63]. There are few studies in Southern and Eastern regions and with racially and ethnically diverse samples that have assessed the bidirectional and mechanistic relations between anxiety-relevant temperament and parenting dimensions. This is an important future avenue of research, particularly in recognizing how cultural perceptions may impact these bidirectional relations.

In summary, child temperament not only predicts anxiogenic parenting behaviors, but interacts with these behaviors in the trajectory to anxiety outcomes. Further, research suggests that parenting also predicts child temperament and child anxiety, yielding bidirectional relations over time. Lastly, culture provides a nuanced context that impacts these complex relations.

DISCUSSION

There is strong theoretical and empirical evidence supporting a developmental pathway to child anxiety that is marked by complex relations between child temperament and parenting behavior. Importantly, this pathway occurs within a nuanced cultural context. The latest research in the field has added to our understanding of these relations, and also points toward important future directions. Recent advances in the temperament literature highlight the dynamic interplay of biological and behavioral correlates of inhibited temperament. Future research would benefit from continuing to investigate these correlates in tandem, particularly building on recent findings regarding the importance of the context in which inhibited temperament is demonstrated and the presence of curvilinear relations [13,15,36].

Further research on the relations among child temperament, parenting, and child anxiety in samples that represent diverse races, ethnicities, socioeconomic statuses, gender identities, sexual orientations, and family structures is needed. There is little to no research on these relations in Latinx and Black American families, and little research outside of the Western context. Additionally, more longitudinal research is needed to parse apart the directionality of these relations across main effect, moderation, and mediation analyses. Few studies have assessed these variables over time, and therefore our understanding of directionality is limited.

SUMMARY

Temperament and parenting continue to be major foci of theory and empirical studies of anxiety risk and development. Children come into the world with varying levels of temperamentally-based dispositions to respond to novelty, uncertainty, and challenge with vigilance, withdrawal, and avoidance. They also receive and influence parenting practices within mutually influential caregiving relationships that act as conduits of culturally-based values. Contemporary theory and empirical studies have been able to provide a more nuanced understanding of these complex, dynamic patterns. Future directions include a simultaneous focus on becoming increasingly fine-grained in understanding the profiles and mechanisms of parent–child interactions, as well as adjusting the lens to appreciate how culture and societal change contextualize them.

CLINICS CARE POINTS

- Inhibited temperament can predispose children toward the development of anxiety. Early intervention targeting the families of toddlers and preschoolers showing extreme wariness, avoidance, and withdrawal may prevent the development of anxiety symptoms and problems.
- Parenting behaviors that promote anxiety by reinforcing avoidance, increasing negative emotion, or undermining independence may be targeted in parent-focused interventions for child anxiety. However, it should be acknowledged that avoidance and dependence may be elicited by anxiety-prone children, so parent-focused interventions should provide adequate empathy and support to caregivers.
- Temperament and parenting relate to anxiety differently across family identities and cultures, depending on the values and goals surrounding both anxiety and typical development. Interventions must be sensitive to the cultural context of the child and family.

FUNDING

Elizabeth Kiel was funded by R01 MH113669 from the National Institute for Mental Health during the writing of this article.

DISCLOSURE

The authors have nothing to disclose.

REFERENCES

[1] Barlow DH. Unraveling the mysteries of anxiety and its disorders from the perspective of emotion theory. Am Psychol 2000;55(11):1247–63.

[2] Dadds MR, Roth JH. Family processes in the development of anxiety problems. In: Vasey MW, Dadds MR, editors. The developmental psychopathology of anxiety. Oxford University Press; 2001. p. 278–303. https://doi.org/10.1093/med:psych/9780195123630.003.0013.

[3] Shiner RL, Buss KA, McClowry SG, et al. What is temperament now? Assessing progress in temperament research on the twenty-fifth anniversary of Goldsmith et al. (1987). Child Dev Perspect 2012;6(4):436–44.

[4] Lonigan CJ, Vasey MW. Negative affectivity, effortful control, and attention to threat-relevant stimuli. J Abnorm Child Psychol 2008;37(3):387–99.

[5] Rubin KH, Burgess KB, Hastings PD. Stability and social-behavioral consequences of toddlers' inhibited temperament and parenting behaviors. Child Dev 2002;73(2):483–95.

[6] Kagan J, Reznick JS, Clarke C, et al. Behavioral inhibition to the unfamiliar. Child Dev 1984;55(6):2212–25.

[7] Kiel EJ, Buss KA. Prospective relations among fearful temperament, protective parenting, and social withdrawal: the role of maternal accuracy in a moderated mediation framework. J Abnorm Child Psychol 2011;39(7):953–66.

[8] Fox NA, Henderson HA, Marshall PJ, et al. Behavioral inhibition: linking biology and behavior within a developmental framework. Annu Rev Psychol 2005;56:235–62.

[9] Polo AJ, López SR. Culture, context, and the internalizing distress of Mexican American youth. J Clin Child Adolesc Psychol 2009;38(2):273–85.

[10] Chen X, Hastings PD, Rubin KH, et al. Child-rearing attitudes and behavioral inhibition in Chinese and Canadian toddlers: a cross-cultural study. Dev Psychol 1998;34(4):677–86.

[11] Chen X. Culture and shyness in childhood and adolescence. New Ideas Psychol 2019;53:58–66.

[12] Buss KA. Which fearful toddlers should we worry about? Context, fear regulation, and anxiety risk. Dev Psychol 2011;47(3):804–19.

[13] Buss KA, Cho S, Morales S, et al. Toddler dysregulated fear predicts continued risk for social anxiety symptoms in early adolescence. Dev Psychopathol 2021;33(1):252–63.

[14] Dyson MW, Klein DN, Olino TM, et al. Social and non-social behavioral inhibition in preschool-age children: differential associations with parent-reports of temperament and anxiety. Child Psychiatry Hum Dev 2011;42(4):390–405.

[15] Hofer PD, Wahl K, Meyer AH, et al. The role of behavioral inhibition, perceived parental rearing, and adverse life events in adolescents and young adults with incident obsessive-compulsive disorder. J Obsessive Compuls Relat Disord 2018;19:116–23.

[16] West AE, Newman DL. Childhood behavioral inhibition and the experience of social anxiety in American Indian adolescents. Cultur Divers Ethnic Minor Psychol 2007;13(3):197–206.

[17] Bahtiyar-Saygan B, Berument SK. The role of temperament and parenting on anxiety problems among toddlers: moderating role of parenting and mediating role of attachment. Infant Ment Health J 2022;43(4):533–45.

[18] Howard M, Muris P, Loxton H, et al. Anxiety-proneness, anxiety symptoms, and the role of parental overprotection in young South African children. J Child Fam Stud 2017;26(1):262–70.

[19] Balkaya M, Cheah CSL, Yu J, et al. Maternal encouragement of modest behavior, temperamental shyness, and anxious withdrawal linkages to Chinese American children's social adjustment: a moderated mediation analysis. Soc Dev 2018;27(4):876–90.

[20] Gao D, Hart CH, Cheah CSL, et al. Chinese American children's temperamental shyness and responses to peer victimization as moderated by maternal praise. J Fam Psychol 2021;35(5):680–90.

[21] Gudino OG, Lau AS. Parental cultural orientation, shyness, and anxiety in Hispanic children: an exploratory study. J Appl Dev Psychol 2010;31(3):202–10.

[22] Clauss JA, Blackford JU. Behavioral inhibition and risk for developing social anxiety disorder: a meta-analytic study. J Am Acad Child Adolesc Psychiatry 2012;51(10):1066–75.e1.

[23] Pérez-Edgar KE, Guyer AE. Behavioral inhibition: temperament or prodrome? Curr Behav Neurosci Rep 2014;1(3):182–90.

[24] Kagan J. Early predictors of the two types. Galen's Prophecy: Temperament in Human Nature. Routledge 1994;170–207.

[25] Schwartz CE, Wright CI, Shin LM, et al. Inhibited and uninhibited infants "grown up": adult amygdalar response to novelty. Science 2003;300(5627):1952–3.

[26] Reznick JS, Kagan J, Snidman N, et al. Inhibited and uninhibited children: a follow-up study. Child Dev 1986;57(3):660–80.

[27] McManis MH, Kagan J, Snidman NC, et al. EEG asymmetry, power, and temperament in children. Dev Psychobiol 2002;41(2):169–77.

[28] Buss KA, Davidson RJ, Kalin NH, et al. Context-specific freezing and associated physiological reactivity as a dysregulated fear response. Dev Psychol 2004;40(4):583–94.

[29] Davis EL, Buss KA. Moderators of the relation between shyness and behavior with peers: cortisol dysregulation and maternal emotion socialization. Soc Dev 2012;21(4):801–20.

[30] Tarullo AR, Mliner S, Gunnar MR. Inhibition and exuberance in preschool classrooms: associations with peer social experiences and changes in cortisol across the preschool year. Dev Psychol 2011;47(5):1374–88.

[31] Buss KA, Davis EL, Ram N, et al. Dysregulated fear, social inhibition, and respiratory sinus arrhythmia: a replication and extension. Child Dev 2018;89(3):e214–28.

[32] Poole KL, Schmidt LA. Early- and later-developing shyness in children: an investigation of biological and behavioral correlates. Dev Psychobiol 2020;62(5):644–56.

[33] Phelps RA, Brooker RJ, Buss KA. Toddlers' dysregulated fear predicts delta–beta coupling during preschool. Dev Cogn Neurosci 2016;17:28–34.

[34] Fox NA, Buzzell GA, Morales S, et al. Understanding the emergence of social anxiety in children with behavioral inhibition. Biol Psychiatry 2021;89(7):681–9.

[35] Smith KA, Hastings PD, Henderson HA, et al. Multidimensional emotion regulation moderates the relation between behavioral inhibition at age 2 and social reticence with unfamiliar peers at age 4. J Abnorm Child Psychol 2019;47(7):1239–51.

[36] Ugarte E, Liu S, Hastings PD. Parasympathetic activity, emotion socialization, and internalizing and externalizing problems in children: longitudinal associations between and within families. Dev Psychol 2021;57(9): 1525–39.

[37] Ryan SM, Ollendick TH. The interaction between child behavioral inhibition and parenting behaviors: effects on internalizing and externalizing symptomology. Clin Child Fam Psychol Rev 2018;21(3):320–39.

[38] Samdan G, Kiel N, Petermann F, et al. The relationship between parental behavior and infant regulation: a systematic review. Dev Rev 2020;57:1–31.

[39] Edwards SL, Rapee RM, Kennedy S. Prediction of anxiety symptoms in preschool-aged children: examination of maternal and paternal perspectives. J Child Psychol Psychiatry 2010;51(3):313–21.

[40] McLeod BD, Wood JJ, Weisz JR. Examining the association between parenting and childhood anxiety: a meta-analysis. Clin Psychol Rev 2007;27(2):155–72.

[41] Volling BL, Stevenson MM, Safyer P, et al. In search of the father-infant activation relationship: a person-centered approach. Monogr Soc Res Child Dev 2019;84(1):50–63.

[42] Cabrera NJ, Volling BL. Moving research on fathering and children's development forward: priorities and recommendations for the future. Monogr Soc Res Child Dev 2019;84(1):107–17.

[43] Paquette D. Theorizing the father-child relationship: mechanisms and developmental outcomes. Hum Dev 2004;47(4):193–219.

[44] Farr RH, Bruun ST, Patterson CJ. Longitudinal associations between coparenting and child adjustment among lesbian, gay, and heterosexual adoptive parent families. Dev Psychol 2019;55(12):2547–60.

[45] Neresheimer CD, Daum MM. Parenting styles of gay fathers. J GLBT Fam Stud 2021;17(2):102–17.

[46] Murry VM, Cooper SM, Burnett M, et al. Rural African Americans' family relationships and well-being. In: Glick JE, McHale SM, King V, editors. Rural families and communities in the United States: facing challenges and leveraging opportunities. Springer; 2020. p. 169–200. https://doi.org/10.1007/978-3-030-37689-5_7.

[47] Strickhouser JE, Sutin AR. Family and neighborhood socioeconomic status and temperament development from childhood to adolescence. J Pers 2020;88(3):515–29.

[48] Padilla CM, Hines CT, Ryan RM. Infant temperament, parenting and behavior problems: variation by parental education and income. J Appl Dev Psychol 2020;70: 1–10.

[49] Berger Cardoso J, Scott JL, Faulkner M, et al. Parenting in the Context of Deportation Risk. J Marriage Fam 2018; 80(2):301–16.

[50] Gouze KR, Hopkins J, Bryant FB, et al. Parenting and anxiety: bi-directional relations in young children. J Abnorm Child Psychol 2017;45(6):1169–80.

[51] Rubin KH, Coplan RJ, Bowker JC. Social withdrawal in childhood. Annu Rev Psychol 2009;60:141–71.

[52] Kim J, Rapee RM, Ja Oh K, et al. Retrospective report of social withdrawal during adolescence and current maladjustment in young adulthood: cross-cultural comparisons between Australian and South Korean students. J Adolesc 2008;31(5):543–63.

[53] Porter CL, Hart CH, Yang C, et al. A comparative study of child temperament and parenting in Beijing, China and the western United States. Int J Behav Dev 2005;29(6):541–51.

[54] Sahithya BR, Manohari SM, Vijaya R. Parenting styles and its impact on children – a cross cultural review with a focus on India. Ment Health Relig Cult 2019;22(4):357–83.

[55] Liu P, Pérez-Edgar KE. Developmental pathways from early behavioral inhibition to later anxiety: an integrative review of developmental psychopathology research and translational implications. Adolesc Res Rev 2019;4(1):45–58.

[56] Hudson JL, Murayama K, Meteyard L, et al. Early childhood predictors of anxiety in early adolescence. J Abnorm Child Psychol 2019;47(7):1121–33.

[57] Kiel EJ, Premo JE, Buss KA. Maternal encouragement to approach novelty: a curvilinear relation to change in anxiety for inhibited toddlers. J Abnorm Child Psychol 2016;44(3):433–44.

[58] Lewis-Morrarty E, Degnan KA, Chronis-Tuscano A, et al. Maternal over-control moderates the association between early childhood behavioral inhibition and adolescent social anxiety symptoms. J Abnorm Child Psychol 2012;40(8):1363–73.

[59] Bayer JK, Morgan A, Prendergast LA, et al. Predicting temperamentally inhibited young children's clinical-level anxiety and internalizing problems from parenting and parent wellbeing: a population study. J Abnorm Child Psychol 2019;47(7):1165–81.

[60] Chorpita BF, Barlow DH. The development of anxiety: the role of control in the early environment. Psychol Bull 1998;124(1):3–21.

[61] Ezpeleta L, Penelo E, de la Osa N, et al. Irritability and parenting practices as mediational variables between temperament and affective, anxiety, and oppositional defiant problems. Aggress Behav 2019;45(5):550–60.

[62] Liu P, Kryski KR, Smith HJ, et al. Transactional relations between early child temperament, structured parenting, and child outcomes: a three-wave longitudinal study. Dev Psychopathol 2020;32(3):923–33.

[63] Maag B, Phelps RA, Kiel EJ. Do maternal parenting behaviors indirectly link toddler dysregulated fear and child anxiety symptoms? Child Psychiatry Hum Dev 2021; 52(2):225–35.

Advances in Psychiatry and Behavioral Health 3 (2023) 149–157

ADVANCES IN PSYCHIATRY AND BEHAVIORAL HEALTH

Perfect Storms and Double-Edged Swords: Recent Advances in Research on Adolescent Social Media Use and Mental Health

Sophia Choukas-Bradley, PhD*, Zelal Kilic, BA, Claire D. Stout, BA, Savannah R. Roberts, MA

Department of Psychology, University of Pittsburgh, 210 South Bouquet Street, 3137 Sennott Square (Main Office, 3rd Floor), Pittsburgh, PA 15260, USA

KEYWORDS

- Social media • Adolescence • Mental health • Depression • Suicide • Body image • Disordered eating
- Sexual and gender minority youth

KEY POINTS

- Adolescence is a developmental period characterized by identity exploration, increased importance of peers, and heightened vulnerability to mental health concerns.
- The features of social media, combined with adolescent developmental features, may create a "perfect storm" for maximally influencing adolescents' body image and mental health.
- Yet social media may also serve as a "double-edged sword," conferring both benefits and risks for adolescents' mental health.
- Recent advances have moved beyond a focus on screen-time, toward a nuanced understanding of the specific social media experiences that affect mental health in positive and negative ways.
- We provide an overview of some of the key advances, highlighting what we do and do not know about how social media use affects—and is affected by—adolescent mental health.

INTRODUCTION

Over roughly the past decade, adolescents' mental health concerns have increased, sparking important debates about the role of social media [1–3]. Adolescents' experiences with social media are diverse and nuanced, with a wide range of possible implications for mental health. Recently, researchers have called for a shift away from focusing on screen-time, and toward identification of the specific social media experiences that may promote or hinder positive mental health and development [4–7]. In this article, we first address key

features of adolescence as a developmental period, followed by a discussion of the ways that social media may affect adolescents' body image concerns, disordered eating, depression, and suicidality. We provide examples of recent advances toward a more nuanced understanding of how social media affects adolescents' mental health, with a primary focus on US youth. We address how social media may provide the "perfect storm" for exacerbating some adolescents' mental health risks—but we also acknowledge that, for many youth, social media likely serves as a "double-edged

---

*Corresponding author, *E-mail address:* scb.1@pitt.edu

https://doi.org/10.1016/j.ypsc.2023.03.007
2667-3827/23/

sword," with a complex set of possible risks and benefits.

KEY DEVELOPMENTAL FEATURES OF ADOLESCENCE: IDENTITY DEVELOPMENT, PEER RELATIONSHIPS, AND VULNERABILITY FOR MENTAL HEALTH CONCERNS

Adolescence is a developmental period marked by tremendous growth and change. The dramatic hormonal, neural, somatic, and social-cognitive changes of this period contribute to a paradox, in which adolescents are highly egocentric, while also highly attuned to their peers [8–10]. Furthermore, adolescence is a period characterized by identity exploration and development [4]. Amid these developmental changes, adolescents are vulnerable to a broad range of mental health concerns.

Depression is one of the most common mental disorders diagnosed in young people in the United States, with higher rates in adolescence compared with childhood [11]. Furthermore, suicide is a major public health concern and a leading cause of death for adolescents and emerging adults in the United States and worldwide [12]. In the past 2 decades, rates of depression and suicidal ideation, planning, attempts, and deaths among youth have increased sharply [13,14]. Body image concerns and disordered eating are also prevalent during adolescence and emerging adulthood [15].

Adolescents' identities affect their mental health experiences. Research consistently indicates that adolescent girls, relative to boys, are at heightened risk for depression, suicidality, body image concerns, and disordered eating [15–17]. Sexual and gender minority (SGM) adolescents are also at heightened risk for a range of mental health concerns and suicidality, compared with their heterosexual, cisgender peers [18–21]—disparities likely explained by minority stress processes [22–25]. Recent study also suggests high and increasing rates of suicidality among youth of color, as well as girls and LGBTQ+ youth [26,27], demonstrating the imperative need to focus attention on marginalized adolescents who have been historically underrepresented in suicide research [28]. Researchers in the field of body image and disordered eating have also recently noted the need for a clearer focus on the experiences of people of color [29,30]. Recent study from our team found associations between Black adolescents' satisfaction with culturally relevant body image areas (skin tone, hair, face) and several indicators of well-being (higher appearance esteem, lower self-objectification, lower depressive symptoms) [31].

HOW DOES SOCIAL MEDIA USE AFFECT ADOLESCENT MENTAL HEALTH?

Recently, Valkenburg and colleagues [32] completed an umbrella review of 25 earlier reviews, concluding that the associations between adolescents' social media use and mental health are inconsistent and complex. We aim to address this complexity in Fig. 1, which shows examples of how specific features of adolescent development may intersect with social media experiences to affect mental health. This framing is consistent with recent review articles and commentaries highlighting the need to move beyond a focus on screen-time and toward a nuanced understanding of specific experiences with social media [4–7]. Furthermore, in keeping with the idea of social media as a double-edged sword, we highlight how specific social media experiences may either positively or negatively affect adolescents' mental health. For example, for youth with marginalized identities, social media may confer benefits related to community and support (perhaps buffering against depressive symptoms) while also increasing the exposure to discrimination and hate speech (perhaps increasing risk for mental health concerns). In the following sections, we provide examples of recent scientific advances regarding how social media may positively and negatively affect mental health.

Social Media Use and Adolescents' Body Image and Disordered Eating

Our research team recently published a theoretical framework for how social media may affect adolescent girls' body image and, in turn, their depressive symptoms and disordered eating [33]. Specifically, we proposed that social media may provide the "perfect storm" for exacerbating girls' body image concerns, by increasing their focus on (1) the physical appearance of peers, social media influencers, and celebrities and (2) their own physical appearance [33]. This article built on our previous work regarding how the specific features of social media (eg, quantifiability, visual nature, 24/7 availability, and publicness) may transform interpersonal experiences [34,35]. We focused this earlier theoretical framework and review on adolescent girls, given their elevated rates of body image concerns and disordered eating, as well as unique gendered sociocultural pressures related to physical appearance, such as the objectification of women and internalization of specific body ideals [36,37]. However, recent empirical work (including from our team) has also documented significant associations between boys' appearance-related social media experiences and body image and

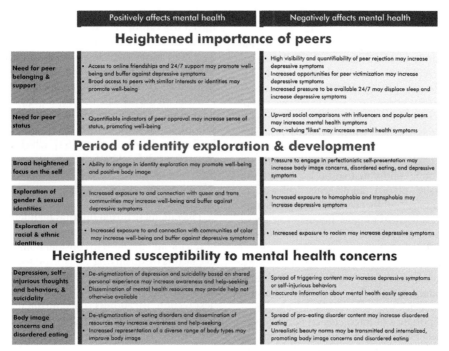

Positively affects mental health	Negatively affects mental health

Heightened importance of peers

	Positively affects mental health	Negatively affects mental health
Need for peer belonging & support	• Access to online friendships and 24/7 support may promote well-being and buffer against depressive symptoms • Broad access to peers with similar interests or identities may promote well-being	• High visibility and quantifiability of peer rejection may increase depressive symptoms • Increased opportunities for peer victimization may increase depressive symptoms • Increased pressure to be available 24/7 may displace sleep and increase depressive symptoms
Need for peer status	• Quantifiable indicators of peer approval may increase sense of status, promoting well-being	• Upward social comparisons with influencers and popular peers may increase mental health symptoms • Over-valuing "likes" may increase mental health symptoms

Period of identity exploration & development

Broad heightened focus on the self	• Ability to engage in identity exploration may promote well-being and positive body image	• Pressure to engage in perfectionistic self-presentation may increase body image concerns, disordered eating, and depressive symptoms
Exploration of gender & sexual identities	• Increased exposure to and connection with queer and trans communities may increase well-being and buffer against depressive symptoms	• Increased exposure to homophobia and transphobia may increase depressive symptoms
Exploration of racial & ethnic identities	• Increased exposure to and connection with communities of color may increase well-being and buffer against depressive symptoms	• Increased exposure to racism may increase depressive symptoms

Heightened susceptibility to mental health concerns

Depression, self-injurious thoughts and behaviors, & suicidality	• De-stigmatization of depression and suicidality based on shared personal experience may increase awareness and help-seeking • Dissemination of mental health resources may provide help not otherwise available	• Spread of triggering content may increase depressive symptoms or self-injurious behaviors • Inaccurate information about mental health easily spreads
Body image concerns and disordered eating	• De-stigmatization of eating disorders and dissemination of resources may increase awareness and help-seeking • Increased representation of a diverse range of body types may improve body image	• Spread of pro-eating disorder content may increase disordered eating • Unrealistic beauty norms may be transmitted and internalized, promoting body image concerns and disordered eating

FIG. 1 Examples of how features of adolescent development may intersect with positive and negative social media experiences to affect mental health.

mental health concerns [8,38]. Our team has also found high levels of body image concerns and disordered eating among gender minority youth [21,39] but to our knowledge, no published research has yet examined social media-specific appearance concerns among gender minority youth.

Adolescents are often exposed to social media content that is associated with body image disturbances and disordered eating. *Thinspiration* and *fitspiration* refer to content that encourages weight-loss and muscle-building, respectively, and is especially sought out by adolescent girls with preexisting body image concerns [40]. Furthermore, *pro-ana* and *pro-mia* content refers to online material designed to encourage eating disorders and dissuade recovery. Adolescent girls are the largest followers of pro-eating disorder content [41], and even without users' intentionally seeking it out, social media algorithms may funnel adolescent girls to this content [42]. Consistent with the double-edged sword theme, "body-positive content" has arisen as an alternative, portraying a more diverse range of body sizes and appearances as attractive. However, body-positive media has been critiqued for reinforcing the importance of attractiveness for self-worth [43].

Ultimately, it seems that images without human figures, or those that are nonappearance focused, may be most helpful for promoting positive body image [44].

One line of research in our laboratory focuses on appearance-related social media consciousness (ASMC), defined as preoccupation with one's attractiveness to a social media audience [8]. Consistent with the overarching goal of understanding specific social media experiences with mental health implications, we have found ASMC to predict US adolescents' disordered eating and depressive symptoms, above and beyond overall time spent on social media [8,38]. Moreover, we have developed and validated a scale, the ASMC scale, freely available and validated for use with adolescents and emerging adults [8,45]. Other recent research shows that specific behaviors on social media are linked to disordered eating, such as selfie-posting, photo-editing [46–48], and social comparison with others' photos [49]. However, some research has found that *avoidance* of posting selfies is associated with greater disordered eating among adolescent girls and boys [46], highlighting the nuances of appearance-focused social media behaviors and their associations with disordered eating.

Social Media Use and Adolescents' Depressive Symptoms and Suicidality

The role of social media in adolescent depression is one of the most hotly debated areas of psychological research. In one widely discussed and contested article, Twenge and colleagues (2018) identified cross-sectional correlations between screen-time and depressive symptoms in a large epidemiological sample of US adolescents [3]. Other researchers wrote rebuttals [1], with Heffer and colleagues (2019) publishing an "empirical reply," demonstrating in a sample of Canadian early adolescents and young adults that social media use did not longitudinally predict adolescents' subsequent depressive symptoms, and that earlier depressive symptoms *did* predict subsequent higher frequency of social media use among adolescent girls (and not among boys or young adults) [50]. This study reflected one of the first longitudinal studies to challenge previous assumptions about social media *causing* mental health problems—but, importantly, the study relied on a simple measure of screen-time.

Given the importance of interpersonal constructs in understanding suicide [51,52], and that adolescents are especially sensitive to peer influence [53], it is crucial to investigate the qualities of online interpersonal interactions. To date, research has linked various positive and negative social media experiences and behaviors such as social connectedness, social comparison, and online victimization to depression and suicidality [54–56]. Many studies focus on proxies for frequency of social media use (eg, screen time), overall finding significant but small associations between social media use and depressive symptoms [57]. However, a recent meta-analysis examining the role of social media in self-injurious thoughts and behaviors found no association between frequency of social media use and suicide, highlighting the need to qualify teens' experiences on social media [58].

Among suicidal teens, less time spent on social media has been associated with *increased* suicidal ideation longitudinally, suggesting that social engagement on social media may buffer against suicidality by increasing feelings of social belonging and reducing social withdrawal [59]. Furthermore, online-only friendships have been shown to attenuate the risk for suicide, especially in teens who experience high friendship stress in their daily lives, suggesting that online social support may be a protective factor against suicide [60]. In particular, marginalized youth at high risk for suicide, who may lack access to consistent social support, could benefit from online friendships and social networks [61,62].

Although these recent findings highlight how social media use can be beneficial, a large body of literature points to negative online interactions such as cyberbullying and social exclusion leading to increased depressive symptoms and increased risk for suicidality [63]. In addition to negative online experiences, higher levels of social media use can also impact teens' well-being by interfering with in-person social interactions [64], causing sleep disturbances [65] and inducing high levels of social comparison [54], which can in turn increase the risk for depressive symptoms and suicidality [66]. Furthermore, as discussed above, appearance-related social media concerns have been linked to depressive symptoms [33].

Overall, these mixed findings highlight the complexities of investigating online interactions in the context of suicide and the need to consider both risk and protective factors by qualifying teens' experiences. The picture becomes more complex when considering the experiences of youth with marginalized identities. In the next section, we address social media use among SGM adolescents' mental health, as an example of these complexities.

Social Media Use and Sexual and Gender Minority Adolescents' Mental Health

SGM youth may spend more time online than their heterosexual, cisgender peers [67], and they may use social media to meet unique needs. For example, sexual minority adolescents are more likely than their heterosexual peers to join an online group to feel less alone [61]. For SGM youth, social media may provide a space for connection with other SGM people, identity exploration, validation, self-expression, and support [68–75]. In fact, using social media for sexual identity development may be associated with positive mental health outcomes for SGM youth, namely lower levels of reported paranoia [76], and SGM-specific social support online may improve identity acceptance [62].

Participating in the SGM community online may feel safer and more supportive than participating offline [73]. For transgender youth of color, social media may be particularly useful to explore the connection between their racial/ethnic identities and gender identities [77]. Social media also provides the space for adolescents to access SGM-related information such as terminology, sex education, and gender-affirming care [68,69,72,74,75]. For rural and nonmetropolitan youth who have less access to SGM resources, social media may provide a particularly useful context for connection and education [74,78–80].

Unfortunately, social media may also provide a space for transphobic and homophobic sentiments, as well as harassment and victimization [69,75]. Although some youth cope adaptively with negative comments online, such as minimizing exposure to content or reaching out to peers for support, others engage in maladaptive ways, including self-harming behaviors [81]. Sexual minority youth may also be more likely to view self-harming videos than their heterosexual peers [61]. Cyberbullying seems to be prevalent for SGM youth, and experiencing cyberbullying is associated with suicidal ideation and attempts, depression, and poor self-esteem [82]. Sexual minority youth are more likely than their heterosexual peers to have online friends, and also to think these friends provide better emotional support than their offline friends [83]. However, online social support does not seem to reduce the odds of online or in-person bully victimization for SGM youth, whereas in-person peer social support may provide this protective effect [83]. Moreover, SGM youth can experience more negative experiences on social media than their heterosexual, cisgender peers, and these experiences may culminate in symptoms of depression [84].

FUTURE DIRECTIONS, FINAL REFLECTIONS, AND CONCLUSIONS

Recent advances suggest that social media use affects—and is affected by—adolescent mental health in complex ways. Early work focused on screen-time and concluded that social media is deleterious for teens' mental health [3]. Advances in our methods and conceptualizations have led us to a more nuanced place as a field: recognizing that social media offers risks and opportunities that are as diverse as the adolescents experiencing them, with complex implications for mental health.

Consistent with bidirectional and transactional models of media use recently discussed by Valkenburg (2022) [85], preexisting mental health and identity characteristics may shape adolescents' social media experiences, as well as their responses to them. These recent theoretical models of social media use are grounded in earlier theories regarding differential susceptibility to media effects [86] and broader theories regarding differential susceptibility to the environment [87]. Recently, scholars interested in links between social media use and mental health have begun to use person-centered analyses to examine within-person effects. For example, Valkenburg and colleagues have conducted experience sampling studies, with tens of thousands of data points, to understand person-specific effects on a broad range of outcomes [88–90]. Such analyses can shed light on individual differences, rather than focusing on average effects. However, like most research advances, this new approach is not without critiques [91].

The questions of how, when, why, and for whom social media affects mental health are far from being resolved. Moreover, given the rapid evolution of digital technologies and adolescents' ways of using them [92], combined with dramatic shifts in the US adolescent population [93], it is difficult to predict what key questions will emerge in future years. However, one thing is clear: as social media technologies advance and become more complicated, so must our methods and conceptualizations. It is imperative to continue moving beyond a static debate about screen time and toward a nuanced consideration of the content of adolescents' social media use, the functions of specific uses based on developmental and interpersonal needs, and the implications for well-being across development.

CLINICS CARE POINTS

- When working with adolescent patients experiencing mental health concerns, providers should assess for specific uses of social media, rather than simply overall time spent on social media.
- For adolescent patients presenting with body image concerns and disordered eating, look for social media behaviors that may increase risk (e.g., excessive selfie-editing and posting, social comparisons with idealized images, exposure to pro-eating disorder content), and encourage a focus on content not focused on physical appearance.
- For adolescent patients presenting with depressive symptoms, assess for exposure to harmful social media interactions (e.g., social exclusion, cyberbullying) and other social media risk factors (e.g., social comparisons, excessive focus on physical appearance), while encouraging the use of social media for social connection and social support.
- For LGBTQ+ adolescent patients, additionally assess for LGBTQ-specific uses of social media that may provide critical support (e.g., connection with LGBTQ+ communities, affirmation of one's identities), while discouraging engagement with homophobic or transphobic content that may increase distress (e.g., muting specific words or phrases).

DISCLOSURE

The authors have no conflicts of interest to disclose. This article is based upon work supported by the National Science Foundation, United States (NSF) Graduate Research Fellowship under Grant No. 1940700 awarded to Savannah R. Roberts. Any opinion, findings, and conclusions or recommendations expressed in this material are those of the authors and do not necessarily reflect the views of the NSF.

REFERENCES

[1] Daly M. Social-media use may explain little of the recent rise in depressive symptoms among adolescent girls. Clin Psychol Sci 2018;6(3):295.

[2] Orben A. Teenagers, screens and social media: a narrative review of reviews and key studies. Soc Psychiatry Psychiatr Epidemiol 2020;55(4):407–14.

[3] Twenge JM, Joiner TE, Rogers ML, et al. Increases in depressive symptoms, suicide-related outcomes, and suicide rates among U.S. adolescents after 2010 and links to increased new media screen time. Clin Psychol Sci 2018; 6(1):3–17.

[4] Granic I, Morita H, Scholten H. Young people's digital interactions from a narrative identity perspective: implications for mental health and wellbeing. Psychol Inq 2020;31(3):258–70.

[5] Hamilton JL, Nesi J, Choukas-Bradley S. Reexamining social media and socioemotional well-being among adolescents through the lens of the COVID-19 pandemic: a theoretical review and directions for future research. Perspect Psychol Sci 2022;17(3):662–79.

[6] Odgers CL, Jensen MR. Annual Research Review: Adolescent mental health in the digital age: facts, fears, and future directions. J Child Psychol Psychiatry 2020; 61(3):336–48.

[7] Prinstein MJ, Nesi J, Telzer EH. Commentary: an updated agenda for the study of digital media use and adolescent development – future directions following Odgers & Jensen (2020). J Child Psychol Psychiatry 2020;61(3):349–52.

[8] Choukas-Bradley S, Nesi J, Widman L, et al. The Appearance-Related Social Media Consciousness Scale: development and validation with adolescents. Body Image 2020;33:164–74.

[9] Dahl RE, Allen NB, Wilbrecht L, et al. Importance of investing in adolescence from a developmental science perspective. Nature 2018;554(7693):441–50.

[10] Markey CN. Invited Commentary: Why body image is important to adolescent development. J Youth Adolesc 2010;39(12):1387–91.

[11] Bitsko RH, Claussen AH, Lichstein J, et al. Mental health surveillance among children — United States, 2013–2019. MMWR Suppl 2022;71(2):1–42.

[12] Glenn CR, Kleiman EM, Kellerman J, et al. Annual research review: a meta-analytic review of worldwide suicide rates in adolescents. J Child Psychol Psychiatry 2020;61(3):294–308.

[13] Burstein B, Agostino H, Greenfield B. Suicidal attempts and ideation among children and adolescents in US emergency departments, 2007-2015. JAMA Pediatr 2019;173(6):598.

[14] Twenge JM, Cooper AB, Joiner TE, et al. Age, period, and cohort trends in mood disorder indicators and suicide-related outcomes in a nationally representative dataset, 2005–2017. J Abnorm Psychol 2019;128(3):185–99.

[15] Larson N, Loth KA, Eisenberg ME, et al. Body dissatisfaction and disordered eating are prevalent problems among U.S. young people from diverse socioeconomic backgrounds: findings from the EAT 2010–2018 study. Eat Behav 2021;42:101535.

[16] Breslau J, Gilman SE, Stein BD, et al. Sex differences in recent first-onset depression in an epidemiological sample of adolescents. Transl Psychiatry 2017;7(5):e1139.

[17] Kann L, Kinchen S, Shanklin SL, et al. Youth risk behavior surveillance–United States, 2013. MMWR Suppl 2014;63(4):1–168.

[18] Guz S, Kattari SK, Atteberry-Ash B, et al. Depression and suicide risk at the cross-section of sexual orientation and gender identity for youth. J Adolesc Health 2021;68(2): 317–23.

[19] James SE, Herman JL, Rankin S, et al. The report of the 2015 U.S. Transgender Survey. Washington, DC: National Center for Transgender Equality; 2016.

[20] Park IY, Speer R, Whitfield DL, et al. Predictors of bullying, depression, and suicide attempts among youth: the intersection of race/ethnicity by gender identity. Child Youth Serv Rev 2022;139:106536.

[21] Roberts SR, Salk RH, Thoma BC, et al. Disparities in disordered eating between gender minority and cisgender adolescents. Int J Eat Disord 2021;54(7): 1135–46.

[22] Burton CM, Marshal MP, Chisolm DJ, et al. Sexual minority-related victimization as a mediator of mental health disparities in sexual minority youth: a longitudinal analysis. J Youth Adolesc 2013;42(3):394–402.

[23] Chodzen G, Hidalgo MA, Chen D, et al. Minority stress factors associated with depression and anxiety among transgender and gender-nonconforming youth. J Adolesc Health 2019;64(4):467–71.

[24] Cogan CM, Scholl JA, Lee JY, et al. Potentially traumatic events and the association between gender minority stress and suicide risk in a gender-diverse sample. J Trauma Stress 2021;34(5):977–84.

[25] Fulginiti A, Rhoades H, Mamey MR, et al. Sexual minority stress, mental health symptoms, and suicidality among LGBTQ youth accessing crisis services. J Youth Adolesc 2021;50(5):893–905.

[26] Centers for Disease Control. U.S. teen girls experiencing increased sadness and violence: Press release; 2023. Available at: https://www.cdc.gov/nchhstp/newsroom/2023/increased-sadness-and-violence-press-release.html. Accessed February 27, 2023.

[27] Lindsey MA, Sheftall AH, Xiao Y, et al. Trends of suicidal behaviors among high school students in the United States: 1991–2017. Pediatrics 2019;144(5):e20191187.

[28] Polanco-Roman L, Miranda R. A cycle of exclusion that impedes suicide research among racial and ethnic minority youth. Suicide Life Threat Behav 2022;52(1):171–4.

[29] Burke NL, Schaefer LM, Hazzard VM, et al. Where identities converge: the importance of intersectionality in eating disorders research. Int J Eat Disord 2020;53(10): 1605–9.

[30] Watson LB, Lewis JA, Moody AT. A sociocultural examination of body image among Black women. Body Image 2019;31:280–7.

[31] Ladd BA, Maheux AJ, Roberts SR, et al. Black adolescents' appearance concerns, depressive symptoms, and self-objectification: exploring the roles of gender and ethnic-racial identity commitment. Body Image 2022; 43:314–25.

[32] Valkenburg PM, Meier A, Beyens I. Social media use and its impact on adolescent mental health: an umbrella review of the evidence. Curr Opin Psychol 2022;44:58–68.

[33] Choukas-Bradley S, Roberts SR, Maheux AJ, et al. The perfect storm: a developmental–sociocultural framework for the role of social media in adolescent girls' body image concerns and mental health. Clin Child Fam Psychol Rev 2022;25(4):681–701.

[34] Nesi J, Choukas-Bradley S, Prinstein MJ. Transformation of adolescent peer relations in the social media context: part 1—a theoretical framework and application to dyadic peer relationships. Clin Child Fam Psychol Rev 2018;21(3):267–94.

[35] Nesi J, Choukas-Bradley S, Prinstein MJ. Transformation of adolescent peer relations in the social media context: part 2—application to peer group processes and future directions for research. Clin Child Fam Psychol Rev 2018;21(3):295–319.

[36] Fredrickson BL, Roberts TA. Objectification theory: toward understanding women's lived experiences and mental health risks. Psychol Women Q 1997;21(2): 173–206.

[37] Thompson JK, Heinberg LJ, Altabe M, et al. Exacting beauty: theory, assessment, and treatment of body image disturbance. American Psychological Association; 1999. https://doi.org/10.1037/10312-000.

[38] Maheux AJ, Roberts SR, Nesi J, et al. Longitudinal associations between appearance-related social media consciousness and adolescents' depressive symptoms. J Adolesc 2022;94(2):264–9.

[39] Romito M, Salk RH, Roberts SR, et al. Exploring transgender adolescents' body image concerns and disordered eating: semi-structured interviews with nine gender minority youth. Body Image 2021;37:50–62.

[40] Carrotte ER, Vella AM, Lim MS. Predictors of "liking" three types of health and fitness-related content on social media: a cross-sectional study. J Med Internet Res 2015; 17(8):e205.

[41] Bert F, Gualano MR, Camussi E, et al. Risks and threats of social media websites: Twitter and the proana movement. Cyberpsychology Behav Soc Netw 2016;19(4): 233–8.

[42] Tech transparency project. Pills, cocktails, and anorexia: facebook allows harmful Ads to target teens. Tech Transparency Project; 2021. Available at: https://www.techtransparencyproject.org/articles/pills-cocktails-and-anorexia-facebook-allows-harmful-ads-target-teens. Accessed November 15, 2022.

[43] Cohen R, Newton-John T, Slater A. The case for body positivity on social media: perspectives on current advances and future directions. J Health Psychol 2021; 26(13):2365–73.

[44] Rodgers RF, Paxton SJ, Wertheim EH. #Take idealized bodies out of the picture: a scoping review of social media content aiming to protect and promote positive body image. Body Image 2021;38:10–36.

[45] Maheux AJ, Roberts SR, Nesi J, et al. Psychometric properties and factor structure of the Appearance-Related Social Media Consciousness Scale among emerging adults. Body Image 2022;43:63–74.

[46] Lonergan AR, Bussey K, Fardouly J, et al. Protect me from my selfie: examining the association between photo-based social media behaviors and self-reported eating disorders in adolescence. Int J Eat Disord 2020;53(5): 755–66.

[47] McLean SA, Paxton SJ, Wertheim EH, et al. Photoshopping the selfie: self photo editing and photo investment are associated with body dissatisfaction in adolescent girls. Int J Eat Disord 2015;48(8):1132–40.

[48] Wilksch SM, O'Shea A, Ho P, et al. The relationship between social media use and disordered eating in young adolescents. Int J Eat Disord 2020;53(1):96–106.

[49] Zimmer-Gembeck MJ, Webb HJ, Kerin J, et al. Risk factors and temporal patterns of disordered eating differ in adolescent boys and girls: testing gender specific appearance anxiety models. Dev Psychopathol 2021;33(3):856–67.

[50] Heffer T, Good M, Daly O, et al. The longitudinal association between social-media use and depressive symptoms among adolescents and young adults: an empirical reply to Twenge et al. (2018). Clin Psychol Sci 2019;7(3):462–70.

[51] Chu C, Buchman-Schmitt JM, Stanley IH, et al. The interpersonal theory of suicide: a systematic review and meta-analysis of a decade of cross-national research. Psychol Bull 2017;143(12):1313–45.

[52] Van Orden KA, Witte TK, Cukrowicz KC, et al. The interpersonal theory of suicide. Psychol Rev 2010;117(2): 575–600.

[53] Burnett S, Sebastian C, Cohen Kadosh K, et al. The social brain in adolescence: evidence from functional magnetic resonance imaging and behavioural studies. Neurosci Biobehav Rev 2011;35(8):1654–64.

[54] Nesi J, Prinstein MJ. Using social media for social comparison and feedback-seeking: gender and popularity

moderate associations with depressive symptoms. J Abnorm Child Psychol 2015;43(8):1427–38.

[55] Rodway C, Tham SG, Richards N, et al. Online harms? suicide-related online experience: a UK-wide case series study of young people who die by suicide. Psychol Med 2022;19:1–12.

[56] Weinstein E, Kleiman EM, Franz PJ, et al. Positive and negative uses of social media among adolescents hospitalized for suicidal behavior. J Adolesc 2021;87(1):63–73.

[57] Ivie EJ, Pettitt A, Moses LJ, et al. A meta-analysis of the association between adolescent social media use and depressive symptoms. J Affect Disord 2020;275:165–74.

[58] Nesi J, Burke TA, Bettis AH, et al. Social media use and self-injurious thoughts and behaviors: a systematic review and meta-analysis. Clin Psychol Rev 2021;87:102038.

[59] Hamilton JL, Biernesser C, Moreno MA, et al. Social media use and prospective suicidal thoughts and behaviors among adolescents at high risk for suicide. Suicide Life Threat Behav 2021;51(6):1203–12.

[60] Massing-Schaffer M, Nesi J, Telzer EH, et al. Adolescent peer experiences and prospective suicidal ideation: the protective role of online-only friendships. J Clin Child Adolesc Psychol 2022;51(1):49–60.

[61] Charmaraman L, Hodes R, Richer AM. Young sexual minority adolescent experiences of self-expression and isolation on social media: cross-sectional survey study. JMIR Ment Health 2021;8(9):e26207.

[62] Wagaman MA, Watts KJ, Lamneck V, et al. Managing stressors online and offline: LGBTQ+ youth in the southern United States. Child Youth Serv Rev 2020;110:104799.

[63] Sampasa-Kanyinga H, Roumeliotis P, Xu H. Associations between cyberbullying and school bullying victimization and suicidal ideation, plans and attempts among Canadian schoolchildren. Scott JG. PLoS One 2014;9(7):e102145.

[64] Ang CS, Teo KM, Ong YL, et al. Investigation of a preliminary mixed method of phubbing and social connectedness in adolescents. Addict Health 2019;11(1). https://doi.org/10.22122/ahj.v11i1.539.

[65] Guo L, Luo M, Wang WX, et al. Association between problematic Internet use, sleep disturbance, and suicidal behavior in Chinese adolescents. J Behav Addict 2018;7(4):965–75.

[66] Twenge JM. Increases in depression, self-harm, and suicide among U.S. adolescents after 2012 and links to technology use: possible mechanisms. Psychiatr Res Clin Pract 2020;2(1):19–25.

[67] GLSEN, CiPHR, CCRC. Out online: the experiences of lesbian, gay, bisexual and transgender youth on the internet. New York, NY: GLSEN; 2013.

[68] Bates A, Hobman T, Bell BT. "Let me do what I please with it … don't decide my identity for me": LGBTQ+ youth experiences of social media in narrative identity development. J Adolesc Res 2020;35(1):51–83.

[69] Berger MN, Taba M, Marino JL, et al. Social media's role in support networks among LGBTQ adolescents: a qualitative study. Sex Health 2021;18(5):421.

[70] Craig SL, McInroy L, McCready LT, et al. Media: a catalyst for resilience in lesbian, gay, bisexual, transgender, and queer youth. J LGBT Youth 2015;12(3):254–75.

[71] Craig SL, Eaton AD, McInroy LB, et al. Can social media participation enhance LGBTQ+ youth well-being? Development of the Social Media Benefits Scale. Soc Media Soc 2021;7(1). https://doi.org/10.1177/2056305121988931:205630512198893.

[72] Greensmith C, King B. "Queer as hell media": affirming LGBTQ+ youth identity and building community in Metro Atlanta, Georgia. J LGBT Youth 2022;19(2):180–97.

[73] McInroy LB, McCloskey RJ, Craig SL, et al. LGBTQ+ youths' community engagement and resource seeking online versus offline. J Technol Hum Serv 2019;37(4):315–33.

[74] Paceley MS, Goffnett J, Sanders L, et al. "Sometimes you get married on Facebook": the use of social media among nonmetropolitan sexual and gender minority youth. J Homosex 2022;69(1):41–60.

[75] Selkie E, Adkins V, Masters E, et al. Transgender adolescents' uses of social media for social support. J Adolesc Health 2020;66(3):275–80.

[76] Ceglarek PJD, Ward LM. A tool for help or harm? How associations between social networking use, social support, and mental health differ for sexual minority and heterosexual youth. Comput Hum Behav 2016;65:201–9.

[77] Singh AA. Transgender youth of color and resilience: negotiating oppression and finding support. Sex Roles 2013;68(11–12):690–702.

[78] Escobar-Viera CG, Choukas-Bradley S, Sidani J, et al. Examining social media experiences and attitudes toward technology-based interventions for reducing social isolation among LGBTQ youth living in rural United States: an online qualitative study. Front Digit Health 2022;4:900695.

[79] McInroy LB, Craig SL, Leung VWY. Platforms and patterns for practice: LGBTQ+ youths' use of information and communication technologies. Child Adolesc Soc Work J 2019;36(5):507–20.

[80] Wike TL, Bouchard LM, Kemmerer A, et al. Victimization and resilience: experiences of rural LGBTQ+ youth across multiple contexts. J Interpers Violence 2022;37(19–20):NP18988–9015.

[81] Craig SL, Eaton AD, McInroy LB, et al. Navigating negativity: a grounded theory and integrative mixed methods investigation of how sexual and gender minority youth cope with negative comments online. Psychol Sex 2020;11(3):161–79.

[82] Abreu RL, Kenny MC. Cyberbullying and LGBTQ youth: a systematic literature review and recommendations for prevention and intervention. J Child Adolesc Trauma 2018;11(1):81–97.

[83] Ybarra ML, Mitchell KJ, Palmer NA, et al. Online social support as a buffer against online and offline peer and

sexual victimization among U.S. LGBT and non-LGBT youth. Child Abuse Negl 2015;39:123–36.

[84] Escobar-Viera CG, Shensa A, Sidani J, et al. Association between LGB sexual orientation and depression mediated by negative social media experiences: national survey study of US young adults. JMIR Ment Health 2020; 7(12):e23520.

[85] Valkenburg PM. Theoretical foundations of social media uses and effects. In: Nesi J, Telzer EH, Prinstein MJ, editors. Handbook of adolescent digital media use and mental health. 1st edition. Cambridge, UK: Cambridge University Press; 2022. p. 39–60.

[86] Valkenburg PM, Peter J. The differential susceptibility to media effects model. J Commun 2013;63(2):221–43.

[87] Belsky J, Pluess M. Beyond diathesis stress: differential susceptibility to environmental influences. Psychol Bull 2009;135(6):885–908.

[88] Pouwels JL, Valkenburg PM, Beyens I, et al. Social media use and friendship closeness in adolescents' daily lives:

an experience sampling study. Dev Psychol 2021;57(2): 309–23.

[89] Siebers T, Beyens I, Pouwels JL, et al. Social media and distraction: an experience sampling study among adolescents. Media Psychol 2022;25(3):343–66.

[90] Valkenburg PM, Pouwels JL, Beyens I, et al. Adolescents' social media experiences and their self-esteem: a person-specific susceptibility perspective. Technol Mind Behav 2021;2(2). https://doi.org/10.1037/tmb0000037.

[91] Vuorre M, Johannes N, Przybylski AK. Three objections to a novel paradigm in social media effects research. PsyArXiv 2022. https://doi.org/10.31234/osf.io/dpuya.

[92] Weinstein E, James C. Behind their screens: what teens are facing (and adults are missing). Cambridge, MA: The MIT Press; 2022.

[93] Office of the Assistant Secretary for Health. America's diverse adolescents. U.S. Department of Health & Human Services; Available at: https://opa.hhs.gov/adolescent-health/adolescent-health-facts/americas-diverse-adolescents. Accessed November 15, 2022.

Geriatrics

Advances in Psychiatry and Behavioral Health 3 (2023) 159–175

ADVANCES IN PSYCHIATRY AND BEHAVIORAL HEALTH

The Next Steps in Reducing Risk for Dementia

Diana Matovic, BPysch(Hons), PhD, Malene Ahern, BAppSc(Physiotherapy), PhD,
Viviana M. Wuthrich, BPsych(Hons), MPsych(Clin), PhD*

School of Psychological Sciences, Centre for Emotional Health, Centre for Ageing, Cognition & Wellbeing, Macquarie University, Sydney, New South Wales 2109, Australia

---

KEYWORDS

- Dementia prevention • Dementia risk screening • Dementia risk reduction

KEY POINTS

- Worldwide dementia prevalence is expected to increase from 55 to 139 million people by 2050. Without a cure, reducing risk for dementia is a priority.
- Evidence suggests that reducing lifestyle factors such as cardiovascular risk, social isolation, physical inactivity, and depression may prevent or delay dementia.
- Treatments using pharmacotherapy, cognitive behavioral therapy, mindfulness, and motivational interviewing are effective in reducing these risks.
- There is a large role for psychiatry and psychology in identifying and treating many risk factors for dementia.

INTRODUCTION/BACKGROUND

This review outlines what is currently known about dementia prevention strategies. This includes understanding the prevalence of dementia and the key modifiable lifestyle and environmental risk factors for dementia that have been identified in large systematic reviews. The currently available dementia risk prediction tools and methods for screening risk are discussed. Diagnostic issues and measurement issues are discussed as related to dementia risk screening. Several key clinical trials of dementia risk reduction are described. This is followed by discussion of barriers and facilitators that exist in the translation of dementia risk screening and early intervention at a population level. The unique role of psychiatry and psychology in increasing the current detection and treatment of risks for dementia is described. Theories of

motivation and behavior change are considered, and the important roles of motivational interviewing and behavior change principles are discussed.

Dementia Prevalence and Impact

There are around 55 million people with dementia worldwide [1]. Given the aging population, it is expected that there will be 78 million people with dementia in 2030 and 139 million in 2050 [1]. Alzheimer's disease is the most common form (∼60%–70% cases), and other major forms include vascular dementia, Lewy body dementia, and frontotemporal dementia [1]. Dementia is the seventh leading cause of death among all diseases globally and a major cause of disability and dependence in older adults [1]. The estimated total global societal cost of dementia, including direct medical

---

*Corresponding author, E-mail address:
Twitter: @DrDianaMatovic
Twitter: @maleneahern; Viviana.Wuthrich@mq.edu.au
Twitter: @VivianaWuthrich

https://doi.org/10.1016/j.ypsc.2023.03.019
2667-3827/23/

and societal care costs and informal care, was US$1.3 trillion in 2019, expected to increase to US$2.8 trillion by 2030 [1]. In 2019, informal carers (commonly family members and friends) spent an average of 5 hours per day providing care for people with dementia [1]. People living with dementia also experience substantial negative individual and social impacts, including symptoms of dementia involving memory loss and confusion, impaired decision-making, difficulties with communication, difficulties managing finances [2], and loneliness [3]. Clinical trials for disease-modifying therapies have demonstrated limited efficacy [1], and as such, there has been increasing global attention on the need to reduce the risk of developing dementia or slowing its trajectory [4]. Although age and gender are the two of the largest risk factors, research has focused on those risk factors that are modifiable in an attempt to reduce the prevalence of people living with dementia [5], health care costs, and on caregiver burden.

Overview of Modifiable Lifestyle and Environmental Risk Factors for Dementia

A number of comprehensive systematic reviews have now identified a range of potentially modifiable risk factors for dementia (Table 1). A 2020 Lancet commissioned systematic review identified 12 lifestyle and environmental factors linked to increased risk for dementia [5], adding the risk factors of excessive alcohol consumption, head injury, and air pollution to the nine risks previously identified in the 2017 Lancet commissioned review [6]. Risk factors vary in importance across the life span with the following life stages associated with the specific risk factors of: early-life stage (<45 years, less education), midlife stage (45–65 years; hearing loss, traumatic brain injury, hypertension, excessive alcohol consumption, obesity), and late-life stage (≥65 years; smoking, depression, social isolation, physical inactivity, air pollution, diabetes). Communalities exist between the risk factors (ie, overlap of variance), but even taking these communalities into account it has been estimated that by reducing all 12 lifestyle risks, up to 40% of dementias worldwide could be prevented or delayed [5].

A recent systematic review of meta-analyses [7] categorized factors associated with risk for different types of dementia including any dementia type (any Dementia), Alzheimer's disease, and Vascular Dementia specifically. The following factors were associated with increased risk for all three dementia categories (any dementia, Alzheimer's disease, vascular dementia): low education, diabetes, smoking, depression, midlife obesity, and high homocysteine. The following factors were

specific to one type of dementia: hypertension (vascular dementia only), atrial fibrillation (any dementia only), low social engagement (any dementia only), hearing loss (any dementia), and statin use (Alzheimer's disease and any dementia). Finally, the following were associated with reduced risk for any dementia: physical activity, fish consumption, light alcohol consumption, and antihypertensives. The World Health Organization (WHO) has also published guidelines for risk reduction for cognitive decline and dementia based on a review of the evidence [8]. The risk factors identified by WHO overlap to a large extent with the risks identified in the Lancet Commission review [5] and systematic review of meta-analyses [7]. Some notable differences are that the WHO recommends regular cognitive stimulation, management of dyslipidaemia, and adherence to a Mediterranean diet, and does not include risk related to hearing loss, social engagement, or depression. The similarities and differences in the identified risk factors between these reviews are illustrated in Table 1. The differences in the identified risks between reviews relates to different study inclusion criteria between the reviews, for instance, differences in the inclusion of observational studies and clinical trials [9].

Importantly, there is some evidence that the more risk factors that a person has the greater the increase in the risk for developing dementia. One meta-analysis found a 20% increase in dementia prevalence with the presence of one risk factor, 65% increase with two risk factors, and 121% increase in dementia for three risk factors relative to no risk factors [10]. This indicates a synergistic effect between the risk factors where the joint effect is greater than the sum of the parts.

There are several important limitations associated with these reviews. First, most of the evidence for risk factors has come from studies conducted in high-income countries and so the findings may not be generalizable to middle- and low-income settings [5,7]. This is particularly important as there is some evidence that population prevalence of individual risk factors varies by country and are associated with different risk estimates (eg, the impact of exposure to environmental factors such as air pollution varies widely by country). This is highlighted by the country-specific prevalence estimates of the nine potentially modifiable risk factors identified in the 2017 Lancet Commission review that indicates up to 40% of dementias could be prevented in China, 41% in India, and 56% in Latin America compared with 35% for the nine risk factors worldwide [5,6]. The most geographically representative evidence was found for alcohol, physical activity, diabetes, high midlife body mass index (BMI), and antihypertensives [7].

TABLE 1
Overview of Risk and Protective Factors for Dementia Identified in Reviews

Risk and Protective Factors	Lancet Commission Review [5] (Any Dementia)	Anstey et al [7] (Any Dementia, AD, and Vascular Dementia)	WHO Guidelines [8] (Cognitive Decline and Any Dementia)
Education	Y	Y	?
Diabetes	Y	Y	Y
Smoking	Y	Y	Y
Depression	Y	Y	N
Midlife obesity	Y	Y	Y
Hypertension	Y	Y	Y
Social engagement	Y	Y	N
Hearing loss	Y	Y	N
Physical activity	Y	Y	Y
Alcohol	Y	Y	Y
Air pollution	Y	-	-
Traumatic brain injury	Y	M	?
Homocysteine	-	Y	-
Antihypertensives	Y	Y	Y
Atrial fibrillation	-	Y	-
Fish consumption	-	Y	?
Statin use	?	Y	Y
Mediterranean/healthy diet	M	IE	Y
Cognitive training/engagement	?	IE	Y
Dyslipidaemia	-	-	Y

Abbreviations: -, risk factor was not discussed; ?, the factor was reviewed or discussed, but the recommendation is unclear; AD, Alzheimer's disease; IE, insufficient evidence; M, mixed findings; N, not a risk factor; WHO, World Health Organization; Y, risk factor.

Interactions Between Modifiable Lifestyle Risk Factors and Genetic Risk Factors

Lifestyle and environmental risk factors for dementia also interact with genetic risk factors. The apoE ε4 gene is the most important genetic risk factor for Alzheimer's disease currently identified, explaining approximately half of the genetic risk for Alzheimer's disease [11]. ApoE ε4 had been found to be an independent risk factor for dementia over an average follow-up of 21 years, even after adjustments for sociodemographic, lifestyle, and vascular factors [11]. Further, there is greater dementia and Alzheimer's disease risk among apoE ε4 carriers compared with non-apoE ε4 carriers when modifiable lifestyle risk factors are present at midlife, including physical inactivity, alcohol drinking, smoking, and dietary fat intake [11]. Another study combined genetic risks into a polygenic risk score for dementia to create low, intermediate, or high genetic risk categories and also created a weighted healthy lifestyle score (including no current smoking, regular physical activity, healthy diet, and moderate alcohol consumption) categorized into either favorable, intermediate, or unfavorable lifestyles [12]. An unfavorable lifestyle and high genetic risk score were significantly associated with higher dementia risk among older adults [12]. However, a favorable lifestyle was associated with a lower dementia risk regardless of genetic risk [12], reflecting the importance of dementia risk screening and lifestyle risk reduction interventions for decreasing dementia prevalence. Given the commonality of many of the risk factors that have been identified for dementia, increased screening and assessment of dementia risk may be a helpful public health strategy for identifying and addressing modifiable risks at scale.

CLINICAL ASSESSMENT
Risk Prediction Tools

A number of dementia risk prediction tools have been developed primarily for research use. These tools differ along several important dimensions including the risk/ protective factors measured, life-stage (midlife and/or late-life), inclusion of data from clinical or genetic measures, dementia type (Alzheimer's disease and/or any dementia), use of clinician ratings or self-report, and target screening setting (eg, online, primary care) [13]. Most of the tools are currently designed to quantify risk likelihood using algorithms [4,14] with some of the algorithms requiring clinical data (eg, apoE ϵ4, cerebral MRI, and carotid artery ultrasound) [15,16]. The main risk screening tools that measure lifestyle and environmental factors are the: Cardiovascular Risk Factors, Aging, and Dementia (CAIDE) [17], Lifestyle for Brain Health (LIBRA) [18], Australian National University's Alzheimer's Disease Risk Index (ANU-ADRI) [19] and the more recent Assessment for Cognitive Health and Dementia Risk Reduction (CogDrisk) tool [9], the Brief Dementia Screening Indicator (BDSI) [20], the Study on Aging, Cognition and Dementia (AgeCoDe) prediction score [21], and the Dementia Risk Score (DRS) [22]. These tools measure the common key risk factors identified in reviews [5,7] and WHO recommendations [8], such as diabetes, smoking, obesity, hypertension, physical activity, and alcohol overconsumption and are summarized in Table 2. Two tools (ANU-ADRI and CogDrisk) allow for self-report ratings and can be completed online, whereas the others require clinical ratings and medical data. Only the CAIDE specifically targets midlife risk factors, whereas some other tools include midlife risk variables and assess midlife and/or late-life risk factors. Some tools measure Alzheimer's disease or any dementia, whereas others measure risk for both diseases. Risk prediction for the oldest-old (80+ years) is poor [22]. The risk screening tools also differ in the types of validation used to test the predictive accuracy of models. This includes split sample (internal) validation where a single dataset is split in two, with one part of the dataset used to develop the prediction model and the other part of the dataset used to test the predictive accuracy of the model [21]. In contrast, external validation involves a model that has been developed in one dataset and tested in a different dataset to determine the model's reproducibility and generalizability to different patients [13,23] (Table 3). Apart from CogDrisk, all of the other tools have been externally validated in independent datasets to demonstrate the predictive accuracy of models in different patients. Although these tools have been associated with accuracy for predicting dementia cases, most are long, require data from medical tests (eg, apoE ϵ4), and algorithms are not designed to be used in clinical settings to identify risk factors that can be targeted in treatment.

Future Directions in Risk Assessment

With the increased focus on dementia prevention strategies, new risk screening tools are being developed that can be used in clinical settings at a population scale to identify people at an increased risk for developing dementia so that any identified risk factors can be targeted in treatment. Although many of the current risk prediction models rely on costly medical data from genetic or brain imaging tests, there is emerging evidence that the inclusion of these variables may not substantially increase predictive accuracy [4]. For example, the CAIDE model did not show a substantial increase in predictive value when apoE ϵ4 was included in the model (area under the curve [AUC] increased from 0.78 to 0.79) [17]. Further, the impact on discriminative accuracy of modifying the calculation of a resource-intensive risk score (eg, apoE ϵ4, cerebral MRI, and carotid artery ultrasound) to incorporate less expensive measures resulted in a significantly decreased discrimination model (concordance-statistic reduced from 0.81 to 0.77), but the model was still able to categorize subjects as having low, moderate, or high risk of dementia with similar accuracy compared with the more resource-intensive score [15,16]. Therefore, there will likely be a move toward more clinically feasible and affordable risk screening methods in the future.

Finally, as interest in population-level screening for dementia risk is increasing, research is beginning to focus on the best approaches to broad implementation and how to overcome challenges to routine screening. One consideration that has largely been ignored is that, just like in genetic testing for other conditions such as Huntington's disease and breast cancer, not all individuals want to be informed of their risk of developing a future condition [24]. As such, dementia risk screening may not be acceptable to some people. Further, there is limited evidence about what is the best age to screen for risk for dementia, which risk factors are the most cost-effective targets, and how best to personalize risk screening and early intervention. Some important considerations include understanding

TABLE 2
Key Risk Screening Tools for Dementia Focusing on Lifestyle and Environmental Factors

Risk and Protective Factors	CAIDE	LIBRA	ANU-ADRI	CogDrisk	BDSI	AgeCoDe Prediction Score	DRS (Age 60–79)	DRS (Age 80–95)
Age	Y	Y (additional model)	Y (for males and females separately)	Y	Y	Y	Y	Y
Sex	Y	Y (additional model)	See age above	Y	N	N	Y	Y
Education	Y	Y (additional model)	Y	Y	Y	N	N	N
Diabetes	N	Y	Y	Y	Y	N	Y	Y
Smoking	N	Y	Y	Y		N	Y	Y
Depression/anti-depressants	N	Y	Y	Y	Y	N	Y	Y
Obesity/BMI	Y	Y	Y	Y	Y	N	Y	Y
Hypertension/systolic blood pressure	Y	Y		Y	N	N	N	Y
Social engagement	N	N	Y	Y	N	N	N	N
Hearing loss	N	N	N	N	N	N	N	N
Physical activity	Y	Y	Y	Y	N	N	N	N
Alcohol	N	Y	Y	N	N	N	Y	Y
Air pollution	N	N	N	N	N	N	N	N
Traumatic brain injury	N	N	Y	Y	N	N	N	N
Homocysteine	N	N	N	N	N	N	N	N
Antihypertensives	N	N	N	N	N	N	Y	Y
Atrial fibrillation	N	N	N	Y (for dementia, not AD)	N	N	Y	Y
Fish consumption	N	N	Y	Y	N	N	N	N
Statin use	N	N		N	N	N	N	N

(continued on next page)

TABLE 2 (continued)

	CAIDE	LIBRA	ANU-ADRI	CogDrisk	BDSI	AgeCoDe Prediction Score	DRS (Age 60–79)	DRS (Age 80–95)
Mediterranean/healthy diet	N	Y	N	N	N	N	N	N
Cognitive training/engagement	N	Y	Y	Y	N	N	N	N
Dyslipidaemia/lipid ratio/total cholesterol/hyperlipidemia	Y	Y	Y	Y	N	N	N	Y
apoE ε4	Y (additional model)	N	N	N	N	N	N	N
Coronary heart disease	N	Y	N	N	N	N	N	N
Renal dysfunction	N	Y	N	N	N	N	N	N
Pesticide exposure	N	N	Y	Y (for AD, not dementia)	N	N	N	N
Stroke and/or transient ischemic attack	N	N	N	Y	Y	N	Y	Y
Insomnia	N	N	N	Y (for dementia, not AD)	N	N	N	N
IADL	N	N	N	N	Y (needs help with money or medications)	Y	N	N
Subjective memory impairment	N	N	N	N	N	Y	N	N
Delayed verbal recall score	N	N	N	N	N	Y	N	N
Verbal fluency	N	N	N	N	N	Y	N	N
MMSE	N	N	N	N	N	Y	N	N
Aspirin	N	N	N	N	N	N	Y	Y
Social (neighborhood) deprivation	N	N	N	N	N	N	Y	N
Calendar year	N	N	N	N	N	N	N	Y
Anxiety/anxiolytics	N	N	N	N	N	N	Y	Y

Other nonsteroidal anti-inflammatory drugs	N	N	N	N	N	N	N	Y
Age group								
Midlife	Y	Y	Y	Y	N	N	N	N
Late-life	N	Y	Y	Y	Y	Y	Y	Y
Outcome								
AD	N	N	Y	Y	N	Y	N	N
Dementia	Y	Y	Y	Y	Y	N	Y	Y
Data requirements								
Clinicians/medical records	Y	Y	N	N	Y	Y	Y	Y
Genetic or brain imaging	Y (additional model)	N	N	N	N	N	N	N
Self-report	N	N	Y	Y	N	N	N	N
Target settings (eg., online, primary care)								
Clinicians/primary care	Y	Y	N	Y	Y	Y	Y	Y
Online/General public	N	N	Y	Y	N	N	N	N

Note. Tools include Cardiovascular Risk Factors, Aging, and Dementia (CAIDE) [17], Lifestyle for Brain Health (LIBRA) [18], Australian National University's Alzheimer's Disease Risk Index (ANU-ADRI) [19], the Assessment for Cognitive Health and Dementia Risk Reduction (CogDrisk) tool [9], the Brief Dementia Screening Indicator (BDSI) [20], the Study on Aging, Cognition and Dementia (AgeCoDe) prediction score [21], and the Dementia Risk Score (DRS) [22].

Abbreviations: AD, Alzheimer's disease; BMI, body mass index; IADL, Instrumental Activities of Daily Living [54]; MMSE, mini mental state examination [55]; N, no; Y, yes.

TABLE 3
Validation of the Predictive Accuracy of Key Risk Screening Tools for Dementia Focusing on Lifestyle and Environmental Factors

Tool	Types of Validation (Internal Split Sample and/or External)
CAIDE	External validation in Kaiser Permanente sample (c-statistic = 0.75 compared with original CAIDE c-statistic of 0.78) [23]. External validation on the Rush Memory and Aging Project, the Kungsholmen Project, and Cardiovascular Health Cognition Study. Excluding cholesterol and BMI (midlife risks) and testing on older adult samples, CAIDE ranged from c-statistics of 0.55–0.58 for AD, and from 0.55 to 0.60 for dementia [13]. Externally validated in older adults (≥65 y) in the 10/66 study including low- and middle-income countries (China, Cuba, the Dominican Republic, Mexico, Peru, Puerto Rico, and Venezuela). C-statistics 0.52–0.63 across countries [56]. External validation in ≥55-year-olds in the Rotterdam Study. C-statistic = 0.55 [57].
LIBRA	External validation in the DESCRIPA study. Risk for dementia increased with higher LIBRA scores in midlife (55–69 y): low dementia risk = reference HR, intermediate risk HR = 1.56, and high risk HR = 1.92. Risk for dementia increased with higher LIBRA scores in late life (70–79 y): low dementia risk = reference HR, intermediate risk HR = 1.25, and high risk HR = 1.38. Risk for dementia did not significantly increase with higher LIBRA scores in the oldest-old (80–97 y) [58]. Validated in Maastricht Aging Study participants (50–81 y) [59]. A one-point increase in LIBRA score related to 19% higher risk for dementia.
ANU-ADRI	External validation on the Rush Memory and Aging Project, the Kungsholmen Project, and Cardiovascular Health Cognition Study [13]. C-statistics of 0.64–0.74 for AD and from 0.65 to 0.73 for dementia. Validated an adapted Portuguese version of this instrument [60]. Participants were assessed by general practitioners and dementia specialists, demonstrating test-retest reliability in two settings (primary and secondary care). Externally validated in older adults (≥65 y) in the 10/66 study including low- and middle-income countries (China, Cuba, the Dominican Republic, Mexico, Peru, Puerto Rico, and Venezuela). C-statistics 0.66–0.78 across countries [56]. External validation in ≥55-year-olds in the Rotterdam Study. C-statistic = 0.75 [57].
CogDrisk	Validation of the CogDrisk on five external cohort studies across different populations is currently being conducted [9].
BDSI	Developed and validated using Cardiovascular Health Study (CHS), the Framingham Heart Study (FHS), the Health and Retirement Study (HRS), and the Sacramento Area Latino Study on Aging (SALSA). C-statistics: CHS, 0.68; FHS, 0.77; HRS, 0.76; SALSA, 0.78 [20]. Externally validated in older adults (≥65 y) in the 10/66 study including low- and middle-income countries (China, Cuba, the Dominican Republic, Mexico, Peru, Puerto Rico, and Venezuela). C-statistics 0.62–0.78 across countries [56]. External validation in ≥55-year-olds in the Rotterdam Study. C-statistic = 0.78 [57].
AgeCoDe prediction score	Internally validated on remaining half of GP clinic sample (AUC = 0.79) [21]. Externally validated in older adults (≥65 y) in the 10/66 study including low- and middle-income countries (China, Cuba, the Dominican Republic, Mexico, Peru, Puerto Rico, and Venezuela). C-statistics 0.57–0.74 across countries [56].
DRS	Validated on a separate GP clinic sample. Discrimination and calibration of the risk algorithm were good for the 60–79 y model: D-statistic 2.03, C-index 0.84, and calibration slope 0.98 [22]. Validated discrimination and calibration were poor for the 80–95 y model [22]. External validation in ≥55-year-olds in the Rotterdam Study. C-statistic = 0.81 [57].

Note. Tools include Cardiovascular Risk Factors, Aging, and Dementia (CAIDE) [17], Lifestyle for Brain Health (LIBRA) [18], Australian National University's Alzheimer's Disease Risk Index (ANU-ADRI) [19], the Assessment for Cognitive Health and Dementia Risk Reduction (CogDrisk) tool [9], the Brief Dementia Screening Indicator (BDSI) [20], the Study on Aging, Cognition and Dementia (AgeCoDe) prediction score [21], and the Dementia Risk Score (DRS) [22].
Abbreviations: AD, Alzheimer's disease; AUC, area under the curve; BMI, body mass index; GP, general practitioner; HR, hazard ratio.

the factors that might increase or decrease an individual's motivation to engage in risk screening and early intervention approaches. Research in preventative health has already identified that the presence of depression [25] and social isolation [26] is associated with reduced preventative health service use in older adults, and these are likely to also be relevant to risk screening and intervention for dementia. Further, given the challenges of sustained behavior change, an understanding of behavior change principles and motivational interviewing is important strategies likely to enhance effectiveness and uptake of screening and intervention approaches. These are the key areas in which psychiatry and psychology can play an important role.

CLINICAL INTERVENTIONS
Clinical Trials
A number of large clinical trials have now been conducted evaluating the efficacy multidomain lifestyle interventions for reducing dementia risk. The key trials are presented in Table 4. These trials have varied in the approaches to risk reduction used (eg, nutritional, medication, educational, behavioral), the inclusion criteria of participants (eg, age, at-risk vs universal intervention, presence of particular risk factors), and the outcomes measured over time (eg, changes in cognition, change in the presence of risk factors). The findings from these trials have been mixed; however, the most promising effects have come from the Finnish Geriatric Intervention Study to Prevent Cognitive Impairment and Disability (FINGER) [27]. This study found that a 2-year multidomain intervention could improve or maintain cognitive functioning in older adults aged 60 to 77 years with heightened risk for dementia as well as improve secondary outcomes (ie, BMI, dietary habits, and physical activity). Further, cardiovascular benefits were maintained at a 7-year follow-up [28]. Given these promising results, the Worldwide FINGERS trials are currently underway bringing together research teams from over 40 countries to share knowledge, harmonize data, and plan joint initiatives for the prevention of dementia (https://wwfingers.com/). Two other large clinical trials of multidomain interventions were not associated with favorable effects. The Prevention of Dementia by Intensive Vascular care (PreDIVA) [29] trial found that in an unselected population of older people aged 70 to 78 years, a nurse-led multidomain intervention did not result in a statistically significant reduced incidence of all-cause dementia over a 6-year period. The Multidomain Alzheimer Preventive Trial (MAPT) [30] found a

multidomain intervention, and polyunsaturated fatty acids had no significant effects on cognitive decline in older adults aged 70 years and older over a 3-year period [30]. Although MAPT used participants who reported a spontaneous memory complaint to their physician, limitations in one instrumental activity of daily living, or slow gait speed, these inclusion criteria do not capture many of the risk factors for dementia reported in reviews (as listed in Table 1) or measured by risk screening tools for dementia (as listed in Table 2). Of note, exploratory subgroup analyses of MAPT and PreDIVA also suggested cognitive benefits in subpopulations of participants with increased risk of dementia, such that it seems that the strongest effects for risk reduction might come from targeting older individuals who already show an increased risk for dementia. In a smaller trial, the Body Brain Life study that targeted at-risk adults in midlife using a personalized Web-based multidomain dementia risk reduction program was also found to be associated with reduced dementia risk and offers a promising Web-based delivery option [31].

Current Challenges for Clinical Interventions to Reduce Risk for Dementia
Despite the promising findings that risk reduction for dementia can be achieved through multidomain lifestyle interventions, there are few models of care available that adapt these interventions into routine care. Many of the multidomain trials require intensive commitments by patients, are very costly to deliver, and only target a subset of at-risk individuals who meet particular risk profiles. The most promising avenue for interventions delivered in routine care comes from a recent trial of the Body Brain Life program in General Practice (BBL-GP) [32]. In this study, dementia risk was reduced in patients aged 18 years and above in general practice who presented with body mass index ≥25 or a chronic health condition who completed the 12-week Body Brain Life Web-based personalized program coupled with face-to-face sessions with allied health practitioners targeting diet and physical activity. Given that much of the intervention content is provided online, this program provides a feasible pathway for dementia risk reduction to be delivered in primary care settings. However, this program currently only targets some of the known risk factors for dementia and requires allied health support. As such, it is not clear how programs such as this could be sustained in clinical settings to ensure affordable access, and more implementation research is needed.

When considering the feasibility and acceptability of adapting clinical interventions for dementia risk reduction into clinical care at scale, it is important to

TABLE 4
Multimodal Interventions for Dementia Risk Reduction Focusing on Lifestyle Factors

Study Name (and Locations)	Study Design Including Sample Characteristics	Key Inclusion and Exclusion Criteria	Intervention	Key Outcome Measurement and Statistical Significance
PreDIVA (Netherlands)	Open-label, pragmatic, multisite, cluster-randomized controlled trial involving 3526 community-dwelling individuals aged 70–78 y, recruited through general practices. Baseline and 2, 4, and 6-y follow-up measurements.	Inclusion: population-based approach inviting all community-dwelling people aged 70–78 y. Exclusion: dementia and other disorders likely to hinder successful long-term follow-up (eg, terminal illness and alcoholism).	Six-year nurse-led, multidomain cardiovascular intervention (smoking, diet, physical activity, weight, and blood pressure monitored, and individually tailored lifestyle advice supported by motivational interviews) (N = 63 practices, 1890 patients) or control (usual care) (N = 53 practices, 1636 patients).	Primary outcomes were cumulative incidence of dementia and disability score (ALDS) at 6 y of follow-up. The main secondary outcomes were incident cardiovascular disease and mortality. There were no statistically significant differences between groups on all outcomes.
FINGER (Finland)	Double-blind RCT involving 1260 individuals aged 60–77 y from the general population, recruited from previous national surveys. Baseline, 12-mo (midway) and 24-mo (trial completion) measurements. In addition, 7-y follow up.	Inclusion: CAIDE Dementia Risk Score of at least 6 points and cognition at mean level or slightly lower than expected for age. Exclusion: previously diagnosed or suspected dementia including MMSE < 20 points; disorders affecting safe engagement in the intervention (for example, malignant disease, symptomatic cardiovascular disease), severe loss of vision, hearing, or communicative ability disorders.	Two-year multidomain intervention (diet, exercise, cognitive training, vascular risk monitoring) (N = 631), or a control group (general health advice) (N = 629).	The primary outcome was change in cognition, measured through a comprehensive Neuropsychological Test Battery (NTB) Z score. Between-group difference in the change of NTB total score per year was significantly higher in the intervention vs control group, reflecting better cognitive outcomes. There were also significant intervention effects on secondary outcomes (BMI, dietary habits, and physical activity).

Study	Design	Inclusion/Exclusion	Intervention	Outcome
				7-y follow-up: the incidence of cerebrovascular events was lower in the intervention than the control group (combined stroke/transient ischemic attack [TIA], coronary events, total cardiovascular disease [CVD] events). Among those with history of CVD, the incidence of both total CVD events and stroke/TIA was lower in the intervention than the control group [28].
MAPT (France, Monaco)	Multicentre, randomized, placebo-controlled superiority trial with four parallel groups involving 1680 community-dwelling participants aged ≥70 y. Baseline and 6, 12, 24, and 36-mo assessment.	Inclusion: either relayed a spontaneous memory complaint to their physician, limitations in one instrumental activity of daily living, or slow gait speed. Exclusion: dementia, MMSE < 24, dependence in at least one activity of daily living, life-threatening diseases, severe vision disorders.	(1) Three-year multidomain intervention (physical activity, cognitive training, and nutritional advice) plus omega 3 polyunsaturated fatty acid supplementation (N = 417). (2) Multidomain intervention plus placebo (N = 420). (3) Omega 3 polyunsaturated fatty acid supplementation alone (N = 423). (4) Placebo alone (N = 420).	The primary outcome was change from baseline to 36 mo on a composite Z score combining four cognitive tests. The multidomain intervention and/or polyunsaturated fatty acids had no statistically significant effects on cognitive decline over 3 y.
HATICE (Netherlands, Finland, France)	Prospective, open-label, randomly assigned, blinded endpoint clinical trial among 2724 community-dwelling people age ≥65 y. Baseline, 12-mo and 18-mo measurements.	Inclusion: two or more cardiovascular risk factors (eg, hypertension, dyslipidaemia), or a history of cardiovascular disease (eg, stroke, transient ischemic attack) or diabetes, or both. Exclusion: dementia, computer illiteracy, and any condition expected to hinder successful 18-mo follow-up (eg, chronic alcohol abuse).	Remote coach-supported (motivational interviewing and lifestyle behavior advice) interactive Internet platform for self-management of cardiovascular risk factors (N = 1389) or a noninteractive (static) control platform with basic health information (N = 1335)	Primary outcome was the difference from baseline to 18 mo on a standardized composite score (Z score) of systolic blood pressure, low-density lipoprotein cholesterol, and BMI. The cardiovascular risk composite outcome improved in the intervention group compared with the control group at 18 mo.

(continued on next page)

TABLE 4
(continued)

Study Name (and Locations)	Study Design Including Sample Characteristics	Key Inclusion and Exclusion Criteria	Intervention	Key Outcome Measurement and Statistical Significance
BBL (Australia)	RCT involving 176 community-dwelling adults aged 50–60 y. Baseline, 12-wk and 26-wk assessment.	Inclusion: >2 risk factors (eg, BMI ≥ 25, hypertension), and <2 protective factors for Alzheimer's disease (eg, physical activity) assessed via brief screening instrument. Exclusion: global cognitive impairment, no computer at home, insufficient English fluency. History of neurologic or psychiatric conditions (eg, recent stroke, epilepsy, schizophrenia), uncorrected substantial hearing/vision loss, severe physical disability), other significant health problems (eg, treatment of cancer).	(1) Web-based personalized multidomain dementia risk reduction intervention (BBL) (N = 58). (2) BBL plus face-to-face with a clinical psychologist (BBL + FF, N = 58). (3) Active control involving weekly emails containing links to dementia prevention health-related websites and online content (N = 60).	Primary outcome: ANU-ADRI score was significantly lower for the BBL group than the control group at 26 wk. BBL and BBL + FF groups had improvement in ANU-ADRI scores at 12 and 26 wk compared with baseline due to an increase in protective factors.

Abbreviations: ALDS, Academic Medical Center Linear Disability Score; ANU-ADRI, Australian National University's Alzheimer's Disease Risk Index [19,61]; BBL, Body Brain Life; BMI, body mass index [31]; CAIDE, cardiovascular risk factors aging, and dementia [17]; FINGER, Finnish Geriatric Intervention Study to Prevent Cognitive Impairment and Disability [27]; HATICE, Healthy Ageing Through Internet Counselling in the Elderly [53]; MAPT, Multidomain Alzheimer Preventive Trial [30]; MMSE, mini mental state examination [55]; PreDIVA, Prevention of Dementia by Intensive Vascular care trial [29]; RCT, randomized controlled trial.

understand the barriers and facilitators to such translation. A recent UK-based literature review of midlife risk factors for dementia reported barriers and facilitators to "primary prevention," defined as "activities or measures pursued before any symptoms of dementia are manifest and, in principle, before even the asymptomatic stage" [33] (p4). The authors reported three types of barriers to primary prevention of dementia: system or organizational, clinician-related, and patient-oriented issues (Table 5). Facilitators to accessing clinical interventions for dementia prevention included time (manageable workload tools), good access to services, resources and information, system integration and management,

raising public awareness, and reducing stigma and improving patient motivation. Methods to overcome barriers and build on facilitators are needed to enable broad uptake of dementia prevention strategies.

ADVANCES IN THE FIELD
Applications for Psychiatry and Psychology for Dementia Risk Reduction

There are some clear applications for practitioners in psychiatry and psychology in treating risk factors for dementia. These include psychometric methods to improve the measurement of personalized risk profiles, developing appropriate strategies for informing individuals about their risk profiles and motivating them to engage in behavior change to reduce their risks and treating psychosocial risk factors such as depression and social isolation that may reduce engagement with health screening and early intervention strategies.

There is significant evidence that pharmacologic and psychological interventions are effective for the treatment of a range of risk factors associated with dementia including depression [34,35], with strong evidence for effectiveness of cognitive behavioral therapy and problem-solving therapy [35]. Cognitive behavioral therapy has also been shown to be effective for treating social isolation [36]. Interventions to target social isolation and depression are particularly important, not just because these are independent risk factors for the development of dementia, but also because these factors have been associated with reduced engagement and uptake of preventative health interventions in general [25,26] and so may need to be addressed early in treatment. Further, psychological therapies such as cognitive behavioral therapy, mindfulness-based interventions, and motivational interviewing are also effective for the treatment of alcohol and other substance abuse disorders [37–39], smoking cessation [40,41], and weight loss interventions (including increasing physical activity and healthy diet interventions) [42] and weight loss for type 2 diabetes management [43]. Thus, there is a large role for psychiatry and psychology to play in reducing risk factors for dementia.

Behavior change

One of the challenges to reduce the risk of dementia is being able to develop and implement interventions that enable people to modify their health behaviors and lifestyle habits over the long term. This requires an understanding of the underpinning structural and psychological determinants of behaviors that relate specifically

TABLE 5 Barriers to Primary Prevention of Dementia	
Type of Barrier	**Issues Identified**
System or Organizational	• Poor system integration • Lack of management and staff support • Practice information systems not geared to support assessment and management of lifestyle-related habits • Limited availability of referral services • Poor feedback from agencies
Clinician-related	• Time • Financing • Limited access to services • Lack of resources • Stigma associated with dementia could deter interest in dementia prevention
Patient-oriented	• Low patient motivation • Health conditions influencing the priority patients place on changing behavior • Lack of time • Financial costs • Entrenched attitudes and behaviors • Restrictions in the physical environment • Low socioeconomic status • Lack of knowledge • Impact of culture on knowledge/awareness

From Karagiannidou MW, Raphael & Knapp, Martin. Primary prevention of dementia: barriers and facilitators. In: Personal Social Services Research Unit LSoEaPS, ed. London, UK: Public Health England 2017. Contains public sector information licensed under the Open Government Licence v3.0.

to modifiable risk factors for dementia [44,45]. Several popular behavior change theories and models are relevant for understanding how to reduce dementia risk, namely the COM-B model/behavior change wheel [46], the health beliefs model [47] and revised health belief model [48], and the transtheoretical model of change [49,50].

Michie and colleagues [46] proposed the COM-B model in their Behavior Change Wheel framework which is a "behavior system" involving three essential conditions for engaging in a particular behavior (B). These conditions include being physically and psychologically capable (C), having the social and physical opportunity (O) to do the behavior, and motivation (M) to do the behavior more than competing behaviors. Thus, the COM-B model informs the key determinants of behavior change from the perspective of the individual delivering or receiving an intervention and is relevant for understanding how to engage individuals in behavior change required to reduce risk for dementia through lifestyle changes. In a recent study, the revised health belief model [48] was used as a conceptual model to develop a measurement of motivation for behavioral and lifestyle change for dementia risk reduction for middle-aged and older Australians [51]. In this study, the authors reported that the prevention of dementia is likely to require modification of several health behaviors at once and therefore it is important to establish individual motivations for addressing each individual risk as well as their knowledge of their risk [51]. The transtheoretical model of change [49,50] proposes a conceptual framework for understanding incremental behavioral change. Five stages of change include precontemplation (not considering change), contemplation (actively ambivalent about change), preparation (plan and commit to change), action (taking necessary steps to achieve change), and maintenance (working to maintain and sustain long-term change) [49,50]. Therefore, given the complexity of behavior change required by individuals to reduce their risk for dementia, a clear understanding of the foundations needed for behavior change outlined by these models is needed. In particular, a clear understanding of the role of motivation in initiating and maintaining behavior change is needed as well as knowledge of techniques and strategies to increase motivation for behavior change.

The role of motivational interviewing

Motivational interviewing is a therapeutic strategy that emphasizes a collaborative partnership between the patient and the practitioner in which patient autonomy is respected and the patient's intrinsic motivations for change are activated by the practitioner [52]. The basic skills of motivational interviewing include asking open-ended questions and responding with reflective listening to confirm understanding of what a patient means to say, making affirmations (eg, patient's strengths and efforts to change), and using periodic summarizing to link together material and reinforce what has been discussed [52]. The spirit of motivational interviewing is collaboration rather than confrontation, evocation of intrinsic motivation rather than telling patients what to do, and patient autonomy rather than practitioner authority. These techniques enhance motivation by facilitating patients to examine their own situations (precontemplation), resolve ambivalence (contemplation), develop a workable change plan and identify barriers and supports to this plan (preparation), increase self-efficacy, and reinforce accomplishments (action and maintenance) [52]. Motivational interviewing was used in the PreDIVA [29] and HATICE [53] trials to increase patient motivation to engage in behavior change needed to reduce risk for dementia. Routine clinical care that seeks to use the principles of behavior change models in regard to dementia risk screening and early intervention is likely to increase patient engagement and outcomes.

DISCUSSION

As the world's population is aging, more older adults will be at risk for developing dementia in the near future. Although the current treatments for dementia are not available, reducing the risk of developing dementia through modifying lifestyle factors has the potential to have large impacts on the prevalence of dementia. A number of large systematic reviews have now identified a range of lifestyle risk factors, and although there are some differences in the risk factors reported in each of these reviews, there is consensus on the following factors: diabetes, smoking, midlife obesity, hypertension, physical activity, and alcohol overconsumption. There is evidence from a number of clinical trials that have found that multidomain interventions that target a combination of these factors in at-risk individuals mid- to late-life resulted in reduced cognitive decline over the long term. These trials hold great promise for our ability to reduce the risk for developing dementia and as such reduce the number of people who develop dementia.

Despite the promising findings, there are significant challenges with translating these findings into routine clinical practice to achieve cost-effective and efficient dementia prevention at scale. Methods and processes to efficiently capture people's risk profiles are being developed, but changes are needed to ensure such measurement can be adapted into routine clinical practice in a way that is cost-effective, feasible, and acceptable to patients and clinicians. Importantly, more work is needed to develop approaches to risk screening that are personalized, reduce stigma, and increase patient motivation to reduce personal risk. Finally, models of translating multidomain lifestyle interventions into routine care are needed. In doing so, models need to be underpinned by principles of behavior change in order for patients to be successfully engaged with making the required lifestyle changes and sustaining them for the long term. There is a large role for psychiatry and psychology to play in all aspects of this clinical translation. In particular, these disciplines have unique skills in informing strategies to screen for psychosocial risk factors (such as depression and social isolation), informing individuals of personalized risk profiles and necessary behavior change needed to reduce risk in ways that increases motivation and engagement with lifestyle changes.

SUMMARY

There is a current international focus to reduce the risk for developing dementia by targeting modifiable lifestyle and environmental risk factors. To implement this approach at a population level, new approaches are needed to improve the feasibility, acceptability, and effectiveness of methods to screen for risk factors, inform individuals of their personalized risk, motivate patients to engage in required lifestyle changes, and maintain those changes to reduce their risk for their lifetime. Drawing on psychological principles and models of behavior change, psychiatrists and psychologists can increase the likely success of this grand challenge.

CLINICS CARE POINTS

- Psychiatry and psychology can play a large role in identifying and treating many risk factors for dementia including social isolation, depression, alcohol overconsumption, smoking cessation, and weight loss.
- Depression and social isolation may hinder uptake of preventive health strategies and need to be addressed as part of risk reduction programs.
- Pharmacologic and psychological interventions have been shown to be effective in treating a wide range of health conditions, including many conditions associated with increased risk for dementia.

- Adherence to behavior change principles and use of motivational interviewing may increase the uptake and effectiveness of risk reduction interventions.

ACKNOWLEDGEMENT

This research is supported by a Medical Research Future Fund Investigator Grant APP1197846 awarded to Viviana Wuthrich.

DISCLOSURE

The authors have nothing to disclose.

REFERENCES

[1] Dementia. World health organisation website. https://www.who.int/news-room/fact-sheets/detail/dementia Published 2022. Updated 20 September 2022. Accessed November, 2022.

[2] Hugo J, Ganguli M. Dementia and cognitive impairment: Epidemiology, diagnosis, and treatment. Clin Geriatr Med 2014;30(3):421–42.

[3] Victor CR, Rippon I, Nelis SM, et al. Prevalence and determinants of loneliness in people living with dementia: Findings from the IDEAL programme. Int J Geriatr Psychiatry 2020;35(8):851–8.

[4] Tang EY, Harrison SL, Errington L, et al. Current Developments in Dementia Risk Prediction Modelling: An Updated Systematic Review. PLoS One 2015;10(9):e0136181.

[5] Livingston G, Huntley J, Sommerlad A, et al. Dementia prevention, intervention, and care: 2020 report of the Lancet Commission. Lancet 2020;396(10248):413–46.

[6] Livingston G, Sommerlad A, Orgeta V, et al. Dementia prevention, intervention, and care. Lancet 2017; 390(10113):2673–734.

[7] Anstey KJ, Ee N, Eramudugolla R, et al. A systematic review of meta-analyses that evaluate risk factors for dementia to evaluate the quantity, quality, and global representativeness of evidence. J Alzheimers Dis 2019; 70(s1):S165–86.

[8] Risk reduction of cognitive decline and dementia: WHO guidelines geneva. World Health Organization; 2019. https://www.who.int/publications/i/item/9789241550543.

[9] Anstey KJ, Kootar S, Huque MH, et al. Development of the CogDrisk tool to assess risk factors for dementia. Alzheimers Dement (Amst) 2022;14(1):e12336.

[10] Peters R, Booth A, Rockwood K, et al. Combining modifiable risk factors and risk of dementia: a systematic review and meta-analysis. BMJ Open 2019;9(1):e022846.

[11] Kivipelto M, Rovio S, Ngandu T, et al. Apolipoprotein E epsilon4 magnifies lifestyle risks for dementia: a population-based study. J Cell Mol Med 2008;12(6b): 2762–71.

[12] Lourida I, Hannon E, Littlejohns TJ, et al. Association of lifestyle and genetic risk with incidence of dementia. JAMA 2019;322(5):430–7.

[13] Anstey KJ, Cherbuin N, Herath PM, et al. A self-report risk index to predict occurrence of dementia in three independent cohorts of older adults: the ANU-ADRI. PLoS One 2014;9(1):e86141.

[14] Stephan BCM, Kurth T, Matthews FE, et al. Dementia risk prediction in the population: are screening models accurate? Nat Rev Neurol 2010;6(6):318–26.

[15] Barnes DE, Covinsky KE, Whitmer RA, et al. Predicting risk of dementia in older adults: The late-life dementia risk index. Neurology 2009;73(3):173–9.

[16] Barnes DE, Covinsky KE, Whitmer RA, et al. Commentary on "Developing a national strategy to prevent dementia: Leon Thal Symposium 2009." Dementia risk indices: A framework for identifying individuals with a high dementia risk. Alzheimer's Dementia 2010;6(2):138–41.

[17] Kivipelto M, Ngandu T, Laatikainen T, et al. Risk score for the prediction of dementia risk in 20 years among middle aged people: a longitudinal, population-based study. Lancet Neurol 2006;5(9):735–41.

[18] Deckers K, van Boxtel MP, Schiepers OJ, et al. Target risk factors for dementia prevention: a systematic review and Delphi consensus study on the evidence from observational studies. Int J Geriatr Psychiatry 2015;30(3):234–46.

[19] Anstey KJ, Cherbuin N, Herath PM. Development of a new method for assessing global risk of Alzheimer's disease for use in population health approaches to prevention. Prev Sci 2013;14(4):411–21.

[20] Barnes DE, Beiser AS, Lee A, et al. Development and validation of a brief dementia screening indicator for primary care. Alzheimer's Dementia 2014;10(6):656–65.e1.

[21] Jessen F, Wiese B, Bickel H, et al. Prediction of dementia in primary care patients. PLoS One 2011;6(2):e16852.

[22] Walters K, Hardoon S, Petersen I, et al. Predicting dementia risk in primary care: development and validation of the Dementia Risk Score using routinely collected data. BMC Med 2016/01/21 2016;14(1):6.

[23] Exalto LG, Quesenberry CP, Barnes D, et al. Midlife risk score for the prediction of dementia four decades later. Alzheimer's Dementia 2014;10(5):562–70.

[24] Sherman KA, Miller SM, Shaw L-K, et al. Psychosocial approaches to participation in BRCA1/2 genetic risk assessment among African American women: a systematic review. J Community Genet 2014;5(2):89–98.

[25] Thorpe JM, Thorpe CT, Kennelty KA, et al. Depressive symptoms and reduced preventive care use in older adults: the mediating role of perceived access. Med Care 2012;50(4):302–10.

[26] Stafford M, von Wagner C, Perman S, et al. Social connectedness and engagement in preventive health services: an analysis of data from a prospective cohort study. Lancet Public Health 2018;3(9):e438–46.

[27] Ngandu T, Lehtisalo J, Solomon A, et al. A 2 year multidomain intervention of diet, exercise, cognitive training, and vascular risk monitoring versus control to prevent cognitive decline in at-risk elderly people (FINGER): a randomised controlled trial. Lancet 2015;385(9984):2255–63.

[28] Lehtisalo J, Rusanen M, Solomon A, et al. Effect of a multi-domain lifestyle intervention on cardiovascular risk in older people: the FINGER trial. Eur Heart J 2022;43(21):2054–61.

[29] Moll van Charante EP, Richard E, Eurelings LS, et al. Effectiveness of a 6-year multidomain vascular care intervention to prevent dementia (preDIVA): a cluster-randomised controlled trial. Lancet 2016;388(10046):797–805.

[30] Andrieu S, Guyonnet S, Coley N, et al. Effect of long-term omega 3 polyunsaturated fatty acid supplementation with or without multidomain intervention on cognitive function in elderly adults with memory complaints (MAPT): a randomised, placebo-controlled trial. Lancet Neurol 2017;16(5):377–89.

[31] Anstey KJ, Bahar-Fuchs A, Herath P, et al. Body brain life: A randomized controlled trial of an online dementia risk reduction intervention in middle-aged adults at risk of Alzheimer's disease. Alzheimer's Dementia: Translational Research & Clinical Interventions 2015;1(1):72–80.

[32] Anstey KJ, Cherbuin N, Kim S, et al. An Internet-Based Intervention Augmented With a Diet and Physical Activity Consultation to Decrease the Risk of Dementia in At-Risk Adults in a Primary Care Setting: Pragmatic Randomized Controlled Trial. J Med Internet Res 2020;22(9):e19431.

[33] Karagiannidou MW, Raphael, Knapp Martin. Primary prevention of dementia: barriers and facilitators. In: Personal social services research unit LSoEaPS. London, UK: Public Health England; 2017.

[34] Wuthrich VM, Meuldijk D, Jagiello T, et al. Efficacy and effectiveness of psychological interventions on co-occurring mood and anxiety disorders in older adults: A systematic review and meta-analysis. Int J Geriatr Psychiatry 2021;36(6):858–72.

[35] Cuijpers P, Karyotaki E, Pot AM, et al. Managing depression in older age: psychological interventions. Maturitas 2014;79(2):160–9.

[36] Zagic D, Wuthrich VM, Rapee RM, et al. Interventions to improve social connections: a systematic review and meta-analysis. Soc Psychiatr Psychiatr Epidemiol 2022;57(5):885–906.

[37] Magill M, Ray LA. Cognitive-behavioral treatment with adult alcohol and illicit drug users: a meta-analysis of randomized controlled trials. J Stud Alcohol Drugs 2009;70(4):516–27.

[38] Hettema J, Steele J, Miller WR. Motivational Interviewing. Annu Rev Clin Psychol 2004;1(1):91–111.

[39] Schonfeld L, Dupree LW, Dickson-Euhrmann E, et al. Cognitive-behavioral treatment of older veterans with

substance abuse problems. J Geriatr Psychiatry Neurol 2000;13(3):124–9.

[40] Vinci C. Cognitive behavioral and mindfulness-based interventions for smoking cessation: a review of the recent literature. Curr Oncol Rep 2020;22(6):58.

[41] de Souza IC, de Barros VV, Gomide HP, et al. Mindfulness-based interventions for the treatment of smoking: a systematic literature review. J Altern Complement Med 2015;21(3):129–40.

[42] Roche AI, Kroska EB, Denburg NL. Acceptance- and mindfulness-based interventions for health behavior change: Systematic reviews and meta-analyses. Journal of Contextual Behavioral Science 2019;13:74–93.

[43] West DS, DiLillo V, Bursac Z, et al. Motivational interviewing improves weight loss in women with type 2 diabetes. Diabetes Care 2007;30(5):1081–7.

[44] Painter JE, Borba CP, Hynes M, et al. The use of theory in health behavior research from 2000 to 2005: a systematic review. Ann Behav Med 2008;35(3):358–62.

[45] Michie S, Johnston M, Francis J, et al. From theory to intervention: Mapping theoretically derived behavioural determinants to behaviour change techniques. Appl Psychol Int Rev 2008;57:660–80.

[46] Michie S, van Stralen MM, West R. The behaviour change wheel: A new method for characterising and designing behaviour change interventions. Implement Sci 2011; 6(1):42.

[47] Hochbaum G, Rosenstock I, Kegels S. Health belief model. U.S. Public Health Service; 1952.

[48] Janz NK, Champion VL, Strecher VJ. The health belief model. In: Glanz K, Rimer B, Lewis F, editors. Health behavior and health education: theory, research, and practice. Jossey-Bass; 2002. p. 31–44.

[49] Prochaska JO, DiClemente CC, Norcross JC. In search of how people change. Applications to addictive behaviors. Am Psychol 1992;47(9):1102–14.

[50] Prochaska JO, Velicer WF. The transtheoretical model of health behavior change. Am J Health Promot 1997; 12(1):38–48.

[51] Kim S, Sargent-Cox K, Cherbuin N, et al. Development of the Motivation to Change Lifestyle and Health Behaviours for Dementia Risk Reduction Scale. Dement Geriatr Cogn Dis Extra 2014;4(2):172–83.

[52] Miller WR, Rollnick S. Motivational interviewing: preparing people for change. 2nd edition. The Guilford Press; 2002.

[53] Richard E, Moll van Charante EP, Hoevenaar-Blom MP, et al. Healthy ageing through internet counselling in the elderly (HATICE): a multinational, randomised controlled trial. Lancet Digit Health 2019;1(8):e424–34.

[54] Lawton MP, Brody EM. Assessment of older people: self-maintaining and instrumental activities of daily living. Gerontologist Autumn 1969;9(3):179–86.

[55] Folstein MF, Folstein SE, McHugh PR. Mini-mental state". A practical method for grading the cognitive state of patients for the clinician. J Psychiatr Res 1975;12(3): 189–98.

[56] Stephan BCM, Pakpahan E, Siervo M, et al. Prediction of dementia risk in low-income and middle-income countries (the 10/66 Study): an independent external validation of existing models. Lancet Glob Health 2020;8(4): e524–35.

[57] Licher S, Yilmaz P, Leening MJG, et al. External validation of four dementia prediction models for use in the general community-dwelling population: a comparative analysis from the Rotterdam Study. Eur J Epidemiol 2018;33(7):645–55.

[58] Vos SJB, van Boxtel MPJ, Schiepers OJG, et al. Modifiable risk factors for prevention of dementia in midlife, late life and the oldest-old: Validation of the LIBRA index. J Alzheimers Dis 2017;58(2):537–47.

[59] Schiepers OJG, Köhler S, Deckers K, et al. Lifestyle for Brain Health (LIBRA): a new model for dementia prevention. Int J Geriatr Psychiatry 2018;33(1):167–75.

[60] Borges MK, Jacinto AF, Citero VA. Validity and reliability of the Brazilian Portuguese version of the Australian National University - Alzheimer's Disease Risk Index (ANU-ADRI). Dement Neuropsychol 2018;12(3):235–43.

[61] Holman R, Lindeboom R, Vermeulen M, et al. The AMC Linear Disability Score project in a population requiring residential care: psychometric properties. Health Qual Life Outcome 2004;2(1):42.

Advances in Psychiatry and Behavioral Health 3 (2023) 177–186

ADVANCES IN PSYCHIATRY AND BEHAVIORAL HEALTH

Recent Trends and Developments in Suicide Prevention for Older Adults

Gayathiri Pathmanathan, MBBS[a], Anne Wand, PhD[b,c], Brian Draper, MD[d,*]

[a]Concord Centre for Mental Health, 1 Hospital Road, Concord West, New South Wales 2139, Australia; [b]Faculty of Medicine and Health, University of Sydney; [c]Faculty of Medicine and Health, UNSW Sydney & Concord Centre for Mental Health, c/o Jara Unit, Older Peoples Mental Health, Concord Hospital, Hospital Road, Concord, New South Wales 2139, Australia; [d]Faculty of Medicine and Health, UNSW Sydney & Eastern Suburbs Older Persons' Mental Health Service, Randwick, New South Wales, Australia

---

KEYWORDS

- Suicide prevention • Old age • Interventions • Ageism

KEY POINTS

- Suicide rates peak in late life yet few suicide prevention interventions have been adequately evaluated and found effective.
- Training of clinicians and gatekeepers, brief psychotherapies for at-risk older people, and aftercare for those who have self-harmed have best evidence of effect.
- Strategies to improve social connectedness have shown benefits on measures of social function and depression with limited evidence on improving suicide outcomes.
- Multi-layered multicomponent suicide prevention strategies that combine linked interventions may be the most effective approach.
- Strategies addressing ageism, coping mechanisms for men as they age, the impact of declining physical health on well-being, and the stresses upon caregivers are required.

INTRODUCTION

Suicide in older people remains a major clinical and socio-economic concern across the globe, the highest rates being among those aged 70 and older [1], particularly in men who have the highest age-specific rates of death by suicide in almost all countries [2]. There is a strong association between self-harm and suicide in older adults in that they share common risk factors, greater intent to die, and the use of higher-lethality means of suicide [3]. As a consequence, older adults frequently die on a first suicide attempt [3].

A range of important predictors and risk factors for suicide in old age have been identified, including suboptimally-treated physical or psychiatric illnesses, cognitive impairment, functional decline and disability, social isolation, and the downstream effects of ageism [1,2,4]. Although these factors may guide approaches to intervention, the extent to which they have been implemented and evaluated in terms of effectiveness for suicide prevention is less clear.

The purpose of this two-part review is to critically evaluate emerging trends and developments in suicide prevention in old age. The first part will describe the interventions and strategies that have been empirically evaluated in older adults. The second part will summarize future directions for suicide prevention research with older people.

---

*Corresponding author. Eastern Suburbs Mental Health Service, Prince of Wales Hospital, Barker Street, Randwick, NSW 2031, Australia. E-mail address: B.draper@unsw.edu.au

https://doi.org/10.1016/j.ypsc.2023.03.018
2667-3827/23/ © 2023 Elsevier Inc. All rights reserved.

Interventions Which Have Been Evaluated
Education and training

Health professionals and members of the public alike have potential roles in suicide prevention in older people [1]. Even for those routinely working with older adults, knowledge gaps exist [5]. Community members who engage with older adults, such as service providers, family, religious and community groups, may also be in a position to recognize at-risk older people and refer them to professional services. Although gatekeeper training may improve knowledge, attitudes, and skills, the referral patterns and long-term effects are unknown [6].

A few studies have examined the effect of clinician training in suicide prevention for older adults. A randomized controlled trial in primary care revealed that older patients under the care of general practitioners who were provided education about screening, diagnosing, and managing depression and self-harm in older people combined with case note audit, showed a modest improvement in depressive symptoms and self-harming behaviors at 24 months [7]. Another Australian study provided an education session for hospital- and community-based clinicians from various disciplines about self-harm in older adults [5]. Pre-post testing revealed a significant improvement in knowledge and confidence in managing suicide risk in older adults. However, outcomes for older adult patients of those clinicians were not reported.

The provision of a dedicated online adaptive learning tool for crisis supporters on late-life self-harm resulted in significant improvement in knowledge following completion of the intervention [8]. However, effects on outcomes for older callers in crisis were unknown. Although most studies of gatekeeper training of nursing home staff have been of low quality and lack outcomes related to suicidal behavior [9], one quasi-experimental study employed a multifaceted gatekeeper educational intervention for staff and found that facilities with staff training were significantly more likely to implement at least one aftercare measure (eg, means restriction, protocols for managing suicidal residents) and adopted more aftercare measures than untrained facilities [10]. Trained facilities were more likely to have protocols for managing suicidal residents and aftercare.

There is still no research focusing specifically on education and training of the general community, police, pharmacists, and paramedics about late-life suicide prevention. Limitations of existing studies of training include lack of demonstrated sustained effects, changes in clinical practice, or improved outcomes for at-risk older adults.

Psychotherapies

Psychosocial interventions are gaining increasing traction as evidence-based, clinically efficacious strategies in the multimodal prevention of suicide among older depressed adults, particularly as there is little evidence that antidepressants are effective in preventing suicidal behavior [11]. Multiple qualitative studies have illuminated common psychological themes and cognitions that drive suicidal and self-harming behaviors in older adults and which might be a focus of therapy (Box 1) [12–14].

Three modalities of psychotherapy have evidence of effectiveness on suicidal ideation in older people (Box 2). Cognitive Behavior Therapy (CBT) is effective in reducing suicidal behavior, though few studies have focused on older adults. There is randomized controlled trial (RCT) evidence that brief CBT reduces depression, anxiety, and suicidal ideation in older patients with chronic medical illness in primary care and suicidal ideation in veterans compared with enhanced usual care over a 12-month period [15,16].

Interpersonal therapy (IPT) has been proposed for older people with depression and suicidal ideation, due to its versatility in helping the person negotiate life transitions and losses, challenge pessimistic cognitions and assuage isolation. IPT proved beneficial in decreasing depressive symptoms, and contemplations of death or suicide, while simultaneously boosting psychological well-being in a cohort of older adults identified as at-risk for suicide [17].

BOX 1
Themes Underpinning Suicidal Ideation/ Behaviors in Older Adults

Functional disability
Family conflict/rejection
Fear of burdening family/carers
Feelings of hopelessness and helplessness
Increasingly poor physical health
Loss of purpose
Loss of identity/personhood
Rejection by health care professionals
Social isolation/loneliness
Sub-optimally controlled pain
Weariness of living

BOX 2

Psychotherapies Potentially Suitable for
Reducing Suicidal Behavior in Older Adults

Psychotherapies shown to reduce suicidal ideation and
   depressive symptoms
   CBT
   Interpersonal therapy (IPT)
   PST
Other psychotherapies effective in treating late-life
   depression
   Problem adaptation therapy (PATH)
   Social Engage Psychotherapy
   Behavioral Activation

Problem-Solving Therapy (PST), a derivative of CBT, focusing on guided identification assessment, and resolution of problems, was conceived as a specialized form of psychotherapy to accommodate the cognitive limitations of some older adults. A 12-week RCT found that PST was superior to supportive therapy in reducing suicidal ideation in older people with features of depression and executive dysfunction. The effect persisted at 36 weeks [18].

Thus CBT, IPT, and PST are promising interventions for suicide prevention in old age given their demonstrated efficacy in ameliorating depression and suicidal ideation. Yet they require replication and investigation of longer-term outcomes beyond suicidal ideation. Psychotherapies are seldom incorporated into collaborative care models and are therefore often inaccessible to aged populations despite patients' preferences and growing acceptance [19,20]. Limited physical and logistical accessibility to psychotherapies continues to pose barriers, although there is emerging evidence that internet- and telephone-facilitated approaches are acceptable and effective in older people [21,22].

Aftercare

Aftercare refers to coordinated follow-up and management after self-harm [23]. It is especially pertinent for suicide prevention in older adults given the close relationship between self-harm and subsequent suicide in older people [3]. Assertive aftercare for older adults who have self-harmed represents an important avenue for tertiary suicide prevention.

There has been limited evaluation of the effectiveness of aftercare interventions specifically for older people with most studies describing the processes of care including referral pathways, engagement strategies, suicide screening tools, and safety planning rather than evaluating care outcomes [24]. The Elderly Suicide Prevention Programme (ESPP) in Hong Kong was an exception. The two-tiered program included outpatient assertive specialist psychogeriatric follow-up, intensive care management, treatment of depression, regular multidisciplinary meetings, psychoeducation to older adults, and gatekeeper training. The 2-year suicide and suicide attempt outcomes were compared with the pre-intervention observational phase of the study and found that the ESPP was associated with a reduced rate of suicide but not the rate of repeat suicide attempts. Although promising, there are methodological limitations and replication is required [25].

Qualitative studies with older people with lived experience of self-harm, their caregivers and clinicians and crisis counselors [13,14,26,27], have outlined important themes which may guide optimal engagement (Box 3). Although these insights are important, they are yet to be operationalized into aftercare interventions and tested.

A few studies have evaluated screening tools for older adults following self-harm but the value of such types of risk assessment is questionable given low sensitivity, low positive predictive values, and the lack of evidence that identification of risk category reduces repeat self-harm or suicide [28,29]. Instead, an empathic person-centered clinical assessment of needs is recommended [30]. This approach, while not directly tested in older adults, accords with qualitative studies of self-harm in older people which suggest the benefits of exploring and addressing modifiable individual reasons for self-harm [26], within their psychosocial context of strengths, supports, and coping styles [28]. One

BOX 3

Themes to Guide Optimal Engagement of Older
People in Aftercare

Good communication between service providers, older
   adults, and their families
Validation of the experience and contributing reasons for
   self-harm in the older person to avoid feelings of
   rejection
Provision of practical support
Means restriction
Clinician training to improve understanding of older adult
   needs and the effects of ageism
Clinician recognition of the impact of decisions such as
   involuntary psychiatric admission or placement in long-
   term residential care

suggested method, based on an evidence-derived framework for safety planning to manage suicide risk using the '5' 'Ds' (depression, disability, disease, disconnectedness, and deadly means) in older people, although promising, has not been empirically tested [31].

Social connectedness

Social isolation, loneliness, and disconnectedness are insidious and under-appreciated risk factors for late-life suicidal behavior, particularly for older people without families, the homebound, and those living in residential care [2,4,32]. Lack of emotional social support from family and friends, as opposed to practical support, was a feature of late-life suicides in comparison with sudden death controls [33].

Research on interventions in this area has had mixed results, lacks replication, or has not focused on suicide outcomes. A much-cited study from over two decades ago demonstrated that twice-weekly contacts from a telephone support service in combination with a 24-hour emergency hotline were associated with lower suicide rates in older women over 10 years but has not been replicated [34]. Interventions that focus on improving social connection in old age lack suicide-related outcomes but deserve further attention (Box 4). In a systematic review of interventions against social isolation in older adults, various types of group interventions such as psychosocial groups, social activation, and groups that provided social support were found to reduce loneliness with long-term benefits. Other interventions that involved volunteering, befriending, health promotion, or were person-centered had limited research with little evidence of long-term benefits [35]. A pilot RCT of Social Engage psychotherapy (S-ENG) did not improve primary outcomes related to social disconnection, but was effective in secondary outcomes of alleviating depressive symptoms and improving socio-emotional quality of life [36].

A systematic review and meta-analysis found physical activity interventions improved social functioning in older adults, but did not improve loneliness, social support, or social networks [37]. An RCT that examined the impact of a specially designed computer system for older adults, the Personal Reminder Information and Social Management system, on improving social support demonstrated improvements on loneliness and social support at 6 months that were not maintained at 12 months [38].

Coping with the impacts of physical illness

There has been little empirical research targeting physical health in suicide prevention. Physical illnesses, especially if inadequately treated, are associated with late-life suicide through issues such as psychosocial disadvantage, functional disability, poor quality of life, chronic pain, premature aging, and psychiatric comorbidity. A systematic review identified that suicide risk appeared greatest among older people experiencing chronic medical problems with attendant complications of pain, disability, and sensory impairment (Table 1) [39].

Several psychotherapies have been trialed that focus on coping with aspects of physical illnesses. As noted earlier, CBT was found to be effective in reducing suicidal ideation in older people with chronic medical illnesses [16]. Problem Adaptation Therapy (PATH), which borrows some strategies from PST, has been piloted for the management of depressive symptoms and negative emotions in older people with chronic pain in primary care [40]. For individuals residing in nursing homes with more severe physical disorders and suicidal ideation, resilience training based on the 'I have, I am, I can' strategy is an intervention requiring

---

BOX 4
Social Connection Intervention Targets Requiring Evaluation with Suicide Outcomes

Improving social support, particularly emotional support,

Reducing loneliness

Increasing social connection

Improving psychosocial quality of life

Facilitating contact with family, friends, neighbors

Assisting older people to use technological solutions through telephone and Internet

---

TABLE 1
Physical Illnesses and Features Associated with Suicidal Behavior in Older Adults

Physical Illnesses Associated with Suicidal Behavior in Older Adults	Features of Physical Illness Associated with Suicidal Behavior in Older Adults
Genitourinary disorders	Functional disability
Neoplastic disease	Increasing dependence on others
Neurological disorders (eg, stroke, epilepsy)	Pain
Respiratory disorders	Personality traits (eg, lack of adaptability)
Rheumatological conditions	Poor quality of life
	Psychiatric comorbidity
	Sensory impairment

further research. An 8-week course involving 34 nursing home residents with suicidal ideation resulted in significantly lower rates of suicidal ideation and depressive symptoms at 1-month follow-up compared with 34 wait-list controls [41].

Although these approaches show promise, they require adequately powered RCTs with medium- to long-term suicide-related outcomes.

ISSUES REQUIRING EMPIRICAL EVIDENCE RELATED TO SUICIDE PREVENTION INTERVENTIONS

Universal and selective interventions in primary care settings that research protective factors such as the impact of general health promotion to optimize well-being and independent functioning for older adults with physical illness on suicide outcomes are required [42]. The extent to which depression could potentially be prevented by addressing known health and psychosocial risk factors has been calculated using a risk matrix [43]. Geriatricians have an important role in promoting high-quality geriatric care and implementing programs that improve physical and mental health [19]. A good example is resistance training, which improves depressive symptoms, physical functioning, pain, and muscle strength in older people, although suicide outcomes have not been measured [44].

Dementia, cognitive impairment, and suicidal behavior

Historically, dementia had not been regarded as a risk factor for suicide, but this was largely based on observations of people with moderate to severe dementia where cognitive impairment could be protective against suicide as an individual loses cognitive competence to carry out an intentional act of self-harm [45]. Over the last 15 years, worldwide campaigns supported by international and national organizations that have encouraged early dementia diagnosis have focused attention on early dementia [46]. There is now consistent evidence of an increased risk of suicide for up to a year after dementia diagnosis, but particularly in the first 3 months and in those with early dementia [47,48]. The risk is increased in those diagnosed at a younger age, with the greatest risk under the age of 70, and in those with psychiatric comorbidity (Box 5) [48–50].

These findings extend to other suicidal behaviors. Hospitalization rates for intentional self-harm in people aged 60 years and over with dementia were found to be double those without dementia, and associated with psychiatric comorbidity and worse outcomes [51]. Some evidence suggests that suicidal behavior

---

> **BOX 5**
> **Risk Factors for Suicide in Dementia**
>
> Replicated Risk Factors
>   Within 12 months of dementia diagnosis
>   Early dementia
>   Younger age of onset
>   Psychiatric comorbidity
>
> Other Possible Risk Factors
>   Chronic pain
>   Substance use
>   Rural residence
>   Frontotemporal dementia

---

might be more common in people with frontotemporal dementia but this requires replication as most studies to date have not examined this issue or have had inconsistent findings [52].

Strategies to prevent suicide in people with dementia have yet to be adequately tested but there is agreement that diagnostic disclosure should be handled sensitively (including the right to not know), post-diagnostic support provided routinely, and adequate treatment of psychiatric comorbidity should be the basis of interventions, particularly in those diagnosed at a younger age or pre-symptomatically with biomarkers (Box 6) [48,49,53].

Key components of post-diagnostic support for people with dementia and their support person or carer have been identified and include the timely identification and management of needs, understanding and managing dementia, a focus on psychological and emotional well-being, practical support as required,

---

> **BOX 6**
> **Suggested Strategies to Prevent Suicide in People with Cognitive Disorders**
>
> Support and monitoring of people with mild cognitive impairment
>
> Careful diagnostic disclosure of dementia
>
> Post-diagnostic support of person with dementia and carer focusing on needs, managing dementia, and psychological and emotional well-being
>
> Effective treatment of depression in dementia and cognitive impairment
>
> Integrated approaches to care
>
> Personalized assessment and management of needs

and integrated care [54]. A small quasi-experimental study of a 5-week twice-weekly suicide prevention program for people with early dementia at daycare centers in Korea incorporating a mix of the key components identified as important for post-diagnostic dementia support demonstrated improvements in measures of health status, depression, social support, and suicidal ideation from pre-to post-treatment [55]. Some specific issues that might need to be addressed in such programs are listed in Box 7.

For those with depression-complicating dementia, PATH offers a treatment modality in a context in which antidepressant medication has limited effectiveness. The therapeutic focus is on optimizing emotional regulation while simultaneously incorporating environmental factors and the involvement of carers in people with dementia. An RCT comparing 12-week PATH with supportive therapy in 74 older adults with major depression, cognitive impairment, and disability to the level of moderate dementia found that PATH had a significantly greater reduction of depression and disability as well as higher depression remission rates [56]. Although no data were provided about the effects on suicidal ideation or behaviors, PATH is a promising intervention that requires replication with measures of suicidal behavior.

Wherever possible, the involvement of the carer or supporter in these interventions is important. Carers and supporters of people with dementia have high rates of psychological distress and suicidal ideation [57]; thus the interventions should have a dual focus.

Ageism

Ageism encapsulates prejudice, discrimination, and devaluation of people of older age. Ageist attitudes toward older adults are long-standing and remain deeply

---

entrenched throughout the world and can be internalized in older people resulting in a negative view of life, which in turn may set off a cascade effect in poorer cognition and functioning, in addition to deteriorating physical and psychological health [2]. Ageism has been linked with human rights violations that together may create or exacerbate psychosocial factors which underpin suicidal behavior in older people [58]. Importantly, people with ageist attitudes are more likely to accept an older person's suicide and are more permissive in their attitudes when suicide is presented in positive terms of not prolonging life [59]. Western European societies that have more favorable attitudes toward older people and labor market inclusion of older people have lower suicide rates in older people than Eastern European societies [60]. The experience of age discrimination is associated with higher rates of suicidal ideation and suicide attempts [61,62].

Ageist stereotypes pervade health care systems. Older people face significant difficulties in terms of accessing high-quality medical and psychiatric care, especially in regional and remote regions [2,19]. Ageist views include depression and contemplations of death as normal phenomena within the spectrum of aging and have even been espoused by physicians. Such attitudes result in the under-treatment of depression and other treatable conditions in late life. Some clinicians believe that suicidal desire in an older person without a psychiatric disorder is both rational, defined as a well-thought-out decision to die by an individual who is mentally competent, and acceptable [63]. This acceptance may in itself be ageist as it implicitly endorses a view that losses associated with aging result in a 'life not worth living' as well as curtailing more detailed exploration of the issues behind the wish to die which could potentially be addressed [64,65]. With voluntary euthanasia and physician-assisted suicide being legalized in increasing numbers of jurisdictions worldwide for those who are deemed rational, fears have been expressed about an ageist approach to their application that may facilitate gerontocide [66].

Strategies that combat ageism with evidence of an impact on suicidal behavior are lacking but universal suicide prevention interventions to address ageism should be a component of multi-level strategies (Box 8).

Interventions targeting men

Despite older men having the highest suicide rates in most countries and most suicide prevention interventions being ineffective in older men [67], there has been a paucity of work focusing on male-specific interventions. Men may have difficulty assessing and

---

> **BOX 7**
> **Issues to Address in Post-Diagnostic Support of People with Cognitive Disorders**
>
> Uncertainty of whether or not a diagnosis of mild cognitive impairment will progress to dementia
>
> Anticipation of cognitive and functional decline
>
> Loss of employment
>
> Loss of driving license
>
> Loss of autonomy and dependency on others
>
> Disempowerment
>
> Loneliness and depression
>
> Perceptions of being a burden on family, friends, and the broader community

---

BOX 8
Strategies to Combat Ageism

- Develop a United Nations convention on the rights of older persons
- Adequate inclusion of older people in national suicide prevention plans
- Remove age discrimination practices in the workforce to facilitate employment of older people
- Remove age barriers to the receipt and funding of health care and social welfare
- Ensure new digital and telecommunications platforms are user-friendly for older people before being used in the mainstream
- Public and health care education about ageism

---

recognizing their emotions, and minimize or conceal suicidal ideation and plans due to stigma and feelings of shame [68]. A qualitative study involving men aged 80 years and over exploring their attitudes toward dying and suicide, found that masculine norms influenced how they coped with aging and their journey toward death, with some men regarding suicide as a rational alternative to dependence in their final years [69].

Future suicide prevention research in older people needs to include interventions that might specifically improve outcomes in men (Box 9).

Caregivers

The families, friends, and informal caregivers of older adults at risk of suicide are highly relevant in suicide prevention. They may have important information

---

BOX 9
Potential Suicide Prevention Interventions for Older Men

Interventions focusing on helping men cope with the effects of aging in the context of masculine norms, dying, and dependency

Interventions that focus on the reduction of stigma around mental health and suicidal behavior

Assertive follow-up after self-harm and other mental health crises

Interventions that address loneliness and social isolation from a male gender perspective

Firearm safety measures particularly in rural areas and in depressed men

Interventions that address anger and impulsivity

---

regarding biopsychosocial stressors and suicide risk in older adults, however, they may not recognize the significance of this information or share it with health care professionals [70]. This lack of communication represents a missed opportunity to intervene to prevent suicide in older adults. There are no dedicated interventions which test the effectiveness of formalizing this approach to seeking collateral information and sharing management of at-risk older people with their caregivers. However, the need to involve caregivers in aftercare of suicidal older adults has been identified [71].

Interpersonal difficulties and complex emotional responses of caregivers to the older person's self-harm such as anger, depression, exhaustion, and guilt, may contribute to ongoing risk of repeated suicidal behaviors [71]. Further, family caregivers of older adults with dementia may themselves be at risk of suicide, which may relate to dementia severity, care burden, and suboptimal coping strategies to respond to the needs of the person with dementia [72]. Although interventions have been suggested to target caregiver distress and burden as part of the routine response to self-harm in an older person, we are unaware of any empirical evaluation of such caregiver "first aid" or of family therapy in this context. Similarly, there are no dedicated interventions to reduce the risk of suicide in caregivers of older adults with dementia, but monitoring for depression, suicidal ideation, and employment support for caregivers (to balance work and care roles) have been suggested [72].

DISCUSSION

Given the complex array of factors contributing to suicidal behavior, no single intervention is likely to be adequate alone. Multi-layered suicide prevention strategies involve the combination of interventions in at least two of the three layers of public health interventions—universal (entire population), selective (high risk populations), and indicated (symptomatic individuals). A review of nine multi-layered multifaceted suicide prevention programs that were mostly undertaken in rural areas of Japan noted the importance of building formal and informal linkages between the layers, particularly between selective and indicated interventions, while universal approaches could more widely disseminate benefits from these interventions [73]. Evidence of reduced incidence of suicide was more frequently observed in women, speculated to be due to women being more likely to accept services than men. The authors suggest that more systematic methods may be needed for indicated mental health interventions for older men and that programs needed to address suicidal impulsivity

[73]. The extent to which multi-layered suicide prevention strategies are effective within urban settings has yet to be established, though there is some evidence that the effectiveness of government-led national suicide prevention plans in 21 organization for economic cooperation and development (OECD) countries was more pronounced in older people and in youth [74].

There are potentially many avenues to prevent suicide in older people, but most remain inadequately evaluated. The voices of older people who have lived experience of suicidal behavior might assist in the development of new interventions along with primary and secondary protective factors [27]. Many interventions addressing various risk factors for late-life suicide have been investigated but few have included suicide-related long-term outcomes. To advance the field, it is essential that investigators add such secondary outcomes to their protocols to maximize the array of trial data available and go beyond short-term proxy measures. Otherwise suicide prevention strategies in late life will likely remain inadequately evaluated.

CLINICS CARE POINTS

- Suicide prevention training relevant to older people should be mandatory for clinical staff involved in the care of older people
- Older people who have expressed suicidal ideation or have self-harmed require assertive follow-up and aftercare
- At-risk older people with anxiety and depression may benefit from a range of psychological therapies
- Lonely isolated older people may benefit from social support interventions
- Post-diagnostic psychological support after dementia diagnosis should be standard practice
- Physically ill older people with declining self-care, depressed mood, and/or pain require effective management of mood and pain

DISCLOSURE

The authors have nothing to disclose.

REFERENCES

[1] de Mendonça Lima CA, De Leo D, Ivbijaro G, et al. Suicide prevention in older adults. Asia Pac Psychiatry 2021; 13(3):e12473.

[2] De Leo D. Late-life suicide in an aging world. Nature Aging 2022;2:7–12.

[3] Troya MI, Babatunde O, Polidano K, et al. Self-harm in older adults: systematic review. Br J Psychiatry 2019; 214(4):186–200.

[4] Holm AL, Salemonsen E, Severinsson E. Suicide prevention strategies for older persons—An integrative review of empirical and theoretical papers. Nursing Open 2021;8(5):2175–93.

[5] Wand APF, Draper B, Brodaty H, et al. Evaluation of an educational intervention for clinicians on self-harm in older adults. Arch Suicide Res 2021;25(1):156–76.

[6] Isaac M, Elias B, Katz LY, et al. Gatekeeper training as a preventative intervention for suicide: a systematic review. Can J Psychiatry 2009;54(4):260–8.

[7] Almeida OP, Pirkis J, Kerse N, et al. A randomized trial to reduce the prevalence of depression and self-harm behavior in older primary care patients. Ann Fam Med 2012;10(4):347–56.

[8] Wand APF, Jessop T, Peisah C. Educating crisis supporters about self-harm and suicide in older adults. Am J Geriatr Psychiatry 2022;30(11):1212–20.

[9] Chauliac N, Leaune E, Gardette V, et al. Suicide prevention interventions for older people in nursing homes and long-term care facilities: a systematic review. J Geriatr Psychiatry Neurol 2020;33(6):307–15.

[10] Chauliac N, Brochard N, Payet C, et al. How does gatekeeper training improve suicide prevention for elderly people in nursing homes? A controlled study in 24 centres. Eur Psychiatry 2016;37:56–62.

[11] Laflamme L, Vaez M, Lundin K, et al. Prevention of suicidal behavior in older people: a systematic review of reviews. PLoS One 2022;17(1):e0262889.

[12] van Wijngaarden E, Leget C, Goossensen A. Experiences and motivations underlying wishes to die in older people who are tired of living: a research area in its infancy. Omega 2014;69(2):191–216.

[13] Wand APF, Peisah C, Draper B, et al. Why do the very old self-harm? A qualitative study. Am J Geriatr Psychiatry 2018;26(8):862–71.

[14] Wand APF, Peisah C, Draper B, et al. Understanding self-harm in older people: a systematic review of qualitative studies. Aging Ment Health 2018;22(3):289–98.

[15] Cully JA, Stanley MA, Petersen NJ, et al. Delivery of brief cognitive behavior therapy for medically ill patients in primary care: a pragmatic randomized clinical trial. J Gen Intern Med 2017;32(9):1014–24.

[16] Ecker AH, Johnson AL, Sansgiry S, et al. Brief cognitive behavioral therapy reduces suicidal ideation in veterans with chronic illnesses. Gen Hosp Psychiatry 2019;58:27–32.

[17] Heisel MJ, Talbot NL, King DA, et al. Adapting interpersonal psychotherapy for older adults at risk for suicide. Am J Geriatr Psychiatry 2015;23(1):87–98.

[18] Gustavson KA, Alexopoulos GS, Niu GC, et al. Problem-solving therapy reduces suicidal ideation in depressed older adults with executive dysfunction. Am J Geriatr Psychiatry 2016;24(1):11–7.

[19] Van Orden K. Late-life suicide prevention strategies: current status and future directions. Curr Opin Psychol 2018;22:79–83.

[20] Luck-Sikorski C, Stein J, Heilmann K, et al. Treatment preferences for depression in the elderly. Int Psychogeriatr 2017;29(3):389–98.

[21] Spek V, Nyklíček I, Smits N, et al. Internet-based cognitive behavioural therapy for subthreshold depression in people over 50 years old: a randomized controlled clinical trial. Psychol Med 2007;37(12):1797–806.

[22] Brenes GA, Miller ME, Williamson JD, et al. A randomized controlled trial of telephone-delivered cognitive-behavioral therapy for late-life anxiety disorders. Am J Geriatr Psychiatry 2012;20(8):707–16.

[23] Shand F, Vogl L, Robinson J. Improving patient care after a suicide attempt. Australas Psychiatry 2018;26(2):145–8.

[24] Wand AP, Browne R, Jessop T, et al. A systematic review of evidence-based aftercare for older adults following self-harm. Aust N Z J Psychiatry 2022;56(11):1398–420.

[25] Chan SS, Leung VP, Tsoh J, et al. Outcomes of a two-tiered multifaceted elderly suicide prevention program in a Hong Kong Chinese community. Am J Geriatr Psychiatry 2011;19(2):185–96.

[26] Wand APF, Draper B, Brodaty H, et al. Self-harm in the very old one year later: has anything changed? Int Psychogeriatr 2019;31(11):1559–68.

[27] Deuter K, Procter N, Rogers J. The emergency telephone conversation in the context of the older person in suicidal crisis. Crisis 2013;34(4):262–72.

[28] Carter G, Spittal MJ. Suicide risk assessment. Crisis 2018;39(4):229–34.

[29] Large MM, Ryan CJ, Carter G, et al. Can we usefully stratify patients according to suicide risk? BMJ 2017;359:j4627.

[30] Carter G, Page A, Large M, et al. Royal Australian and New Zealand College of Psychiatrists clinical practice guideline for the management of deliberate self-harm. Aust N Z J Psychiatry 2016;50(10):939–1000.

[31] Conti EC, Jahn DR, Simons KV, et al. Safety planning to manage suicide risk with older adults: case examples and recommendations. Clin Gerontol 2020;43(1):104–9.

[32] Fässberg MM, van Orden KA, Duberstein P, et al. A systematic review of social factors and suicidal behavior in older adulthood. Int J Environ Res Public Health 2012;9(3):722–45.

[33] De Leo D, Draper BM, Snowdon J, et al. Suicides in older adults: a case-control psychological autopsy study in Australia. J Psychiatr Res 2013;47(7):980–8.

[34] De Leo D, Dello Buono M, Dwyer J. Suicide among the elderly: the long-term impact of a telephone support and assessment intervention in northern Italy. Br J Psychiatry 2002;181:226–9.

[35] Manjunath J, Manoj N, Alchalabi T. Interventions against social isolation of older adults: a systematic review of existing literature and interventions. Geriatrics 2021;6:82.

[36] Van Orden KA, Areán PA, Conwell Y. A pilot randomized trial of engage psychotherapy to increase social connection and reduce suicide risk in later life. Am J Geriatr Psychiatry 2021;29(8):789–800.

[37] Shvedko A, Whittaker AC, Thompson JL. Physical activity interventions for treatment of social isolation, loneliness, or low social support in older adults: A systematic review and meta-analysis of randomized controlled trials. Psychol Sport Exerc 2018;34:128–37.

[38] Czaja SJ, Boot WR, Charness N, et al. Improving social support for older adults through technology: findings from the PRISM randomized controlled trial. Gerontol 2018;58(3):467–77.

[39] Fässberg MM, Cheung G, Canetto SS, et al. A systematic review of physical illness, functional disability, and suicidal behaviour among older adults. Aging Ment Health 2016;20(2):166–94.

[40] Kiosses DN, Ravdin LD, Stern A, et al. Problem adaptation therapy for pain (PATH-Pain): a psychosocial intervention for older adults with chronic pain and negative emotions in primary care. Geriatrics 2017;2(1):5.

[41] Zhang D, Tian Y, Wang R, et al. Effectiveness of a resilience-targeted intervention based on "I have, I am, I can" strategy on nursing home older adults' suicidal ideation: a randomized controlled trial. J Affect Disord 2022;308:172–80.

[42] Conwell Y. Suicide later in life: challenges and priorities for prevention. Am J Prev Med 2014;47(3 Suppl 2):S244–50.

[43] Almeida OP, Alfonso H, Pirkis J, et al. A practical approach to assess depression risk and to guide risk reduction strategies in later life. Int Psychogeriatr 2011;23(2):280–91.

[44] Khodadad Kashi S, Mirzazadeh ZS, Saatchian V. A systematic review and meta-analysis of resistance training on quality of life, depression, muscle strength, and functional exercise capacity in older adults aged 60 years or more. Biol Res Nurs 2022. https://doi.org/10.1177/10998004221120945 10998004221120945.

[45] Haw C, Harwood D, Hawton K. Dementia and suicidal behavior: a review of the literature. Int Psychogeriatr 2009;21(3):440–53.

[46] Prince M, Bryce R, Ferri C. World Alzheimer Report 2011. The benefits of early diagnosis and intervention. London: Alzheimer's Disease International; 2011.

[47] Choi JW, Lee KS, Han E. Suicide risk within 1 year of dementia diagnosis in older adults: a nationwide retrospective cohort study. J Psychiatry Neurosci 2021;46(1):E119-e27.

[48] Alothman D, Card T, Lewis S, et al. Risk of suicide after dementia diagnosis. JAMA Neurol 2022;79(11):1148–54.

[49] Schmutte T, Olfson M, Maust DT, et al. Suicide risk in first year after dementia diagnosis in older adults. Alzheimers Dement. 2022;18(2):262–71.

[50] Erlangsen A, Zarit SH, Conwell Y. Hospital-diagnosed dementia and suicide: a longitudinal study using prospective, nationwide register data. Am J Geriatr Psychiatry 2008;16(3):220–8.

[51] Mitchell R, Draper B, Harvey L, et al. The survival and characteristics of older people with and without dementia who are hospitalised following intentional self-harm. Int J Geriatr Psychiatry 2017;32(8):892–900.

[52] Lai AX, Kaup AR, Yaffe K, et al. High occurrence of psychiatric disorders and suicidal behavior across dementia subtypes. Am J Geriatr Psychiatry 2018;26(12):1191–201.

[53] Draper B, Peisah C, Snowdon J, et al. Early dementia diagnosis and the risk of suicide and euthanasia. Alzheimers. Dement. 2010;6(1):75–82.

[54] Bamford C, Wheatley A, Brunskill G, et al. Key components of post-diagnostic support for people with dementia and their carers: a qualitative study. PLoS One 2021; 16(12):e0260506.

[55] Kim JP, Yang J. Effectiveness of a community-based program for suicide prevention among elders with early-stage dementia: a controlled observational study. Geriatr Nurs 2017;38(2):97–105.

[56] Kiosses DN, Ravdin LD, Gross JJ, et al. Problem adaptation therapy for older adults with major depression and cognitive impairment: a randomized clinical trial. JAMA Psychiatr 2015;72(1):22–30.

[57] O'Dwyer ST, Moyle W, Zimmer-Gembeck M, et al. Suicidal ideation in family carers of people with dementia. Aging Ment Health 2016;20(2):222–30.

[58] Wand A, Verbeek H, Hanon C, et al. Is suicide the end point of ageism and human rights violations? Am J Geriatr Psychiatry 2021;29(10):1047–52.

[59] Gamliel E, Levi-Belz Y. To end life or to save life: ageism moderates the effect of message framing on attitudes towards older adults' suicide. Int Psychogeriatr 2016;28(8): 1383–90.

[60] Yur'yev A, Leppik L, Tooding LM, et al. Social inclusion affects elderly suicide mortality. Int Psychogeriatr 2010; 22(8):1337–43.

[61] Kim G, Lee MA. Age discrimination and suicidal ideation among korean older adults. Am J Geriatr Psychiatry 2020;28(7):748–54.

[62] Ko Y, Han SY, Jang HY. Factors influencing suicidal ideation and attempts among older korean adults: focusing on age discrimination and neglect. Int J Environ Res Public Health 2021;18(4). https://doi.org/10.3390/ijerph18 041852.

[63] Gramaglia C, Calati R, Zeppegno P. Rational suicide in late life: a systematic review of the literature. Medicina (Kaunas) 2019;55(10). https://doi.org/10.3390/medicina55100656.

[64] Dzeng E, Pantilat SZ. Social causes of rational suicide in older adults. J Am Geriatr Soc 2018;66(5):853–5.

[65] Balasubramaniam M. Rational suicide in elderly adults: a clinician's perspective. J Am Geriatr Soc 2018;66(5): 998–1001.

[66] Pope AA. Psychological history of ageism and its implications for elder Suicide. In: McCue RE, Balasubramaniam M, editors. Rational suicide in the elderly: clinical, ethical, and sociocultural aspects. Cham: Springer International Publishing; 2017. p. 63–74.

[67] Lapierre S, Erlangsen A, Waern M, et al. A systematic review of elderly suicide prevention programs. Crisis 2011; 32(2):88–98.

[68] Hinton L, Zweifach M, Oishi S, et al. Gender disparities in the treatment of late-life depression: qualitative and quantitative findings from the IMPACT trial. Am J Geriatr Psychiatry 2006;14(10):884–92.

[69] King K, Dow B, Keogh L, et al. 'Is life worth living?' The role of masculinity in the way men aged over 80 talk about living, dying and suicide. Am J Men's Health 2020;14(5):1557988320966540.

[70] Draper B, Krysinska K, Snowdon J, et al. Awareness of suicide risk and communication between health care professionals and next-of-kin of suicides in the month before suicide. Suicide Life Threat Behav 2018;48(4): 449–58.

[71] Wand APF, Peisah C, Draper B, et al. Carer insights into self-harm in the very old: a qualitative study. Int J Geriatr Psychiatry 2019;34(4):594–600.

[72] Kong JW, Park JY. Understanding suicide risk in people with dementia and family caregivers in South Korea: a systematic review. Behav Sci 2022;12(4). https://doi.org/10.3390/bs12040097.

[73] Sakashita T, Oyama H. Suicide prevention interventions and their linkages in multilayered approaches for older adults: a review and comparison. Front Public Health 2022;10:842193.

[74] Matsubayashi T, Ueda M. The effect of national suicide prevention programs on suicide rates in 21 OECD nations. Soc Sci Med 2011;73(9):1395–400.

Advances in Psychiatry and Behavioral Health 3 (2023) 187–195

ADVANCES IN PSYCHIATRY AND BEHAVIORAL HEALTH

Future Directions in Addressing Loneliness Among Older Adults

Tegan Cruwys, PhD/MClinPsy, PhB (Sci)(Hons), MAPS FCCLP

School of Medicine and Psychology, The Australian National University, 39 Science Road, ANU ACT 2601, Australia

KEYWORDS

- Loneliness • Social isolation • Social exclusion • Social identity • Geriatric • Mental health

KEY POINTS

- Older adults are at highest risk of loneliness if they are financially disadvantaged, have reduced mobility, chronic health conditions, or are among the oldest old.
- Loneliness precedes and predicts decline in mental, physical, and cognitive health—making it a prime target for public health intervention.
- Intervention might occur at the level of individual, group, or whole of community, but what effective interventions tend to have in common is that they provide a subjective sense of belonging to groups (social identification).
- Emerging topics for future study are life transitions, how to provide opportunities for meaningful contribution, and intersectional research that acknowledges the multiplicative impact of having multiple marginalized identities.

INTRODUCTION

Loneliness has long been a scourge experienced by too many people. However, perhaps because the burden of loneliness has always been borne disproportionally by those on the margins of mainstream society, it is only in the last decade that loneliness has entered public consciousness as cause for concern. Loneliness is defined as the difference between one's actual level of social connectedness and one's desired social connectedness. Of note, this differs from social isolation, which refers to an objective lack of contact with others. Although older people can experience both of these (and isolation is a risk factor for loneliness), it is loneliness that is the more distressing and distinctly linked to a swathe of negative outcomes [1].

Bob Putnam famously summarized the importance of social connection for health in his influential book *Bowling Alone* as follows: "if you smoke and belong to no groups, it's a toss-up statistically whether you should stop smoking or start joining." (p. 331) [2]. Although this statement seemed provocative at the time of publication in 2000, it has largely been confirmed by subsequent research. There are strong links between loneliness (or proxy disconnection measures, such as a lack of social integration) and health. Particularly influential was a meta-analytic review [3], which pooled studies looking at diverse risk factors for premature mortality. Across almost 150 studies and over 300,000 participants, these researchers found that being socially disconnected was the *strongest* predictor of premature death. Indeed, the odds ratios for social disconnection were comparable to smoking and larger than for obesity or alcohol. Along with all-cause mortality, loneliness has also been causally linked to specific pathologies, including heart disease, depression, and dementia [4–6]. This has led researchers to call for loneliness to be the focus of research and intervention not only to ameliorate suffering directly related to

E-mail address: tegan.cruwys@anu.edu.au

https://doi.org/10.1016/j.ypsc.2023.03.008
2667-3827/23/ © 2023 Elsevier Inc. All rights reserved.

loneliness, but as a modifiable primary risk factor for poor health [7,8].

This review has three goals. First, it starts by debunking several persistent myths about loneliness in older people. These myths have the potential to lead the field astray, in terms of both our understanding of the problem and efforts to improve it. Second, it reviews loneliness interventions for older people, with a focus on emerging evidence and new theory-driven directions. Third and finally, it identifies three topics that warrant further attention as a call to action for future research.

MYTHS ABOUT LONELINESS IN OLDER PEOPLE

The first misconception is that loneliness is an inevitable, or even common, feature of aging. In fact, many people remain (or even become) very well socially connected into their older age. Population prevalence studies across several countries have found evidence that loneliness is actually most common in young adults, with older people, on average, being relatively protected [9,10]. Nevertheless, there are several factors that can place older people at risk. Socioeconomic disadvantage can act as a barrier to forming and maintaining social connections in older age. One recent study found that one of the main reasons why financial security is important for health following retirement is because it enables people to remain socially connected over time [11]. Another risk factor for loneliness among older people is when they become *physically* isolated, either due to bereavement or because of health and capacity challenges [12]. Reduced mobility, especially driving cessation, can precipitate loneliness as a person finds it increasingly difficult to engage with their valued networks and communities [13]. For these reasons, it is not surprising that meta-analytic evidence suggests that the risk of loneliness increases in oldest age (80+), and that interindividual differences become more pronounced in this age cohort [14].

A second common myth is that technology is a *panacea* that can cure loneliness among older people if only they were trained to make use of it. Curiously, this myth is almost the mirror image of how technology is often described in the context of young people: as a *plague* which separates, rather than connects [15]. In fact, previous research has shown mixed effects of enabling older people to have greater access to and skills in using social media. Although some studies have found that increased social media use can reduce

loneliness and benefit well-being [16], others have found no effects or even negative outcomes [17–19]. Two considerations can help us to interpret these mixed results. First, social media technologies are not uniform, and nor are the ways in which we engage with them. For instance, passive consumption of social media and engaging in social comparison have shown more consistent negative effects, whereas actively sharing content seems to be more beneficial, especially when the intended audience is a valued group [20]. Second, researchers should be cautious not to uncritically accept age-related stereotypes, such as that older people are technologically illiterate. This stereotype is only becoming more inaccurate as this cohort are increasingly composed of baby boomers, who were the first generation for whom information technology was a major industry [21].

A third and final myth about loneliness in older people is that it is merely an outcome of increasing infirmity, or an inevitable later life condition. Although declining health certainly *can* precipitate loneliness, this relationship is strongly bidirectional. In fact, population studies have found that the effect of loneliness on subsequent health decline is approximately three times stronger than the effect of health decline on subsequent loneliness [22]. Another study, involving 3413 people aged 50+, found that social group connections became increasingly important as a protective factor for cognitive health as people aged [23]. This was such that being one standard deviation below the mean in social group connections at age 50 years predicted a cognitive age of 54 years (ie, 4 years older than one's chronological age). However, by the age of 80 years, this gap had widened such that lonelier participants were functioning cognitively more like 90-year-olds. These effects were replicated in a subsample of participants with above average cognitive health at baseline, suggesting that reverse causality is unlikely to account for the effects.

Therefore, loneliness represents a "canary in the coalmine" for health; an early warning sign that a person is at risk of imminent decline but that it is not too late to intervene. Even a short period of relative isolation and resulting loneliness may thus be a significant risk factor for health into the future. Unfortunately, lockdown restrictions and shielding related to the COVID-19 pandemic created the opportunity to test this hypothesis. Emerging research confirms that older people were particularly likely to experience severe loneliness during the pandemic [24], and that this, at times, could precipitate a rapid deterioration in health (including first-onset psychosis) [25].

THERAPEUTIC OPTIONS
Setbacks and Breakthroughs

In 2011, a meta-analysis of extant loneliness interventions [26] identified only 20 experimental studies, the majority of which focused on older people. The most common content of these interventions was either social skills training or "befriending," where a younger person is encouraged to form a bond with an older person, often in the context of residential care. The mean effect size was only $d = -.20$, a finding that the authors summarized as follows: "the most we can say is that these interventions achieve, at best, only modest improvement but not recovery. Thus, there is a need for improvements in interventions to reduce loneliness if clinically significant improvements are to be achieved." An updated review in 2018 [27] including only older people similarly described the evidence as weak and called for a stronger theoretical foundation in future research.

In the intervening years, rapid developments have occurred that respond to this call. Two specific developments warrant particular attention here: (1) growing evidence for the essential role of a *group environment* for intervention and (2) more sophisticated theorizing about the psychological processes underpinning loneliness. Speaking to the first of these, one characteristic of the interventions that featured prominently in the 2011 meta-analysis [26] is that they were intrapersonal or interpersonal in nature. That is, they focused either on addressing potential deficits within the individual (eg, a lack of social skills) or on forming a bond between two individuals. What was missing from these approaches is attention to the role of *social group processes* in loneliness. In the intervening decade, a growing number of interventions have used a group-based format. Indeed, despite these interventions having great diversity in their content and underlying theorizing, a group-based format is associated with greater effect sizes than interventions delivered one-on-one or in a self-help format [28,29].

A theoretical framework that can help us understand why a group format might prove particularly beneficial is the social identity approach, a framework which has had increasing influence in conceptualizing loneliness [30]. Encompassing both social identity and self-categorization theories [31,32], a central tenet of this framework is that our self-concept is composed not only of our individual qualities (the things that make us different from others), but also by the social groups of which we are a part (the things we have in common with fellow group members). A social identity is the subjective internalization of a group membership; the degree to which a group is represented psychologically and informs a person's self-definition. Although many theoretical frameworks are relevant to loneliness, the social identity approach, with its specific focus on subjective connection to social groups (rather than other kinds of social relationship), is consistent with the extant evidence that group-based interventions seem to be most effective. Furthermore, a social identity approach brings to our attention that the importance of subjective, meaningful engagement with such groups—just "showing up" is not enough to reap the benefits. Empirical evidence has borne this out, with social identification being uniquely associated with positive outcomes in diverse contexts (over and above social contact or interpersonal friendships) [33,34]. The social identity approach has also informed many of the recent developments in loneliness interventions, as described below.

Loneliness Interventions: Recent Advances

This section provides a brief overview of three kinds of interventions (at the level of the individual, group, and community) that build on these developments and may have particular promise for addressing loneliness in older adults. The first, social prescribing, has gained traction around the world but particularly in the United Kingdom, where the National Health Service has recently announced major investment in trials of social prescribing for vulnerable people [35]. Social prescribing involves people who are lonely or at risk of loneliness being referred to a dedicated *link worker*, whose role is to provide a tailored assessment of an individual's social needs, and support them to become involved in community, recreational and volunteer activities that are likely to meet those needs [36]. Also called community referral, social prescribing is typically initiated by a primary care physician. Primary care can be a good point of referral because lonely people are often frequent attenders [37].

Although social prescribing is a promising new frontier for tackling loneliness in older people, several barriers remain. The first is that high-quality evaluation trials have been few in number and thus the quality of the evidence supporting this approach lags behind its implementation in many areas [38,39]. This is particularly true for older adults [40]. In fact, one recent systematic review of social prescribing for frail older adults found *zero* eligible studies [41]. In addition, studies have found evidence that link workers experience inconsistent funding and limited professional development and peer support [42,43], which threaten their commitment to the profession and thus the viability of social prescribing as a widespread model of care. Although the simplicity of social prescribing is perhaps one of its more appealing features, it has also been criticized for lacking a sound theoretical rationale [36,44] and for struggling to adequately engage people who are in greatest need [45].

Moving to group-level interventions, the model with the strongest evidence is *Groups 4 Health* (G4H), which is suitable for implementation in clinical practice. Unlike social prescribing, the development of G4H was strongly guided by a theoretical framework: the social identity approach to health. G4H is a five-module psychotherapeutic group program that seeks to build group-based belonging by not only teaching *skills* to create social connections but also providing *opportunities* to do so in the form of the therapy group itself, which acts as a scaffold for enduring social connections after the active phase of the program is completed.

Three controlled trials of G4H have been published, all with people experiencing loneliness and accompanying psychological distress. In the phase I/pilot trial, G4H reduced loneliness ($d = -.86$), depression, and anxiety relative to a matched control group at 6 month follow-up [46]. In the phase II randomized-controlled trial (RCT), G4H reduced loneliness ($d = -1.04$), social anxiety, and health-service use relative to a treatment-as-usual control [47]. In the phase III definitive non-inferiority RCT, G4H was compared with a dose-controlled group cognitive behavior therapy (CBT) program for depression [48]. Improvements in depression were comparable across both groups, whereas improvements in loneliness ($d = -1.07$) were greater in G4H than CBT at 12-month follow-up. Speaking to the role of COVID-19 in exacerbating the risk of loneliness, a subsequent analysis of these data found that the benefits of G4H, compared with CBT, were more pronounced among those participants who completed their follow-ups during COVID-19 lockdown [49]. Although these data provide strong support for G4H, importantly, these evaluations were in younger populations, with only one of these trials having a mean age greater than 30 years. Although this somewhat tempers the case for G4H as an intervention for older people experiencing loneliness, several smaller-scale trials do provide insights into its suitability in this context.

The first of these was a small trial for G4H in a rehabilitation hospital among 21 people preparing to return to the community after a long period of hospitalization. The average age of participants in this trial was 75 years [50], and participants experienced large and significant improvements in group-based belonging and

depression. Another smaller trial, run embedded in usual care of a community organization, included older people at risk of elder abuse and their carers, who qualitatively reported social benefits [50]. Finally, experimental evidence found that an adaptation of G4H specifically designed to support people in the transition to retirement led to better adjustment and well-being than a financial planning control condition [51]. Earlier research also suggested that less structured social group interventions in residential care homes (eg, reminiscence groups, gentlemen's clubs) were effective to the degree that they led to a meaningful increase in social identification with fellow residents [52–55]. Together, this evidence suggests promise for the utility of G4H—and other group-based interventions that increase social identity—for tackling loneliness among older people, particularly those experiencing complex social or health issues.

Finally, one approach to loneliness interventions that should not be overlooked is universal ones that seek to improve social participation and inclusion at the whole-of-community level. These address a key limitation of extant social identity interventions; they have tended to be small group and resource-intensive, which limits their utility in addressing the high levels of loneliness across the population. Approaches that address these limitations need to be embedded in the community, accessible, and affordable. One model in Australia that meets these requirements is the *Neighbors Every Day* campaign: a grass-roots initiative that is organized by and for members of the general public to connect in neighborhoods. Organized around an annual day of action, Neighbors Every Day events are all distinct and tailored by the hosts to the needs of their community. Most common are activities such as community barbeques, informal yard sales, or organizing a social media page for one's street. Evidence suggests that involvement in Neighbors Every Day leads to increased social identification with one's neighborhood, which in turn supports greater social cohesion, reduced loneliness, and improved well-being up to 6 months later [56]. There was no evidence that the benefits of Neighbors Every Day were moderated by socioeconomic disadvantage, indicating that this universal approach shows benefit across the spectrum of need in the community. A separate evaluation conducted during the pandemic found that participants in Neighbors Every Day were protected against a decline in mental health across a period of extended COVID lockdowns [57]. This benefit was fully mediated via social identification, providing further evidence that this is the key ingredient that loneliness interventions should target to be most effective.

FUTURE DIRECTIONS

Need to Create Meaningful Opportunities for Older People to Contribute

Compared with the rest of the population, older people are particularly concerned with *generativity* [58], that is, with having opportunities to meaningfully contribute to society and to have these contributions respected and valued. Aligning with this is evidence from another tradition, which has suggested that conceptualizations of social support place too much emphasis on *receipt* of support from others [59]. Instead, it seems that *providing* social support is more reliably and robustly linked to positive outcomes, including reduced loneliness [60]. This has also been found in the context of older adults, where providing support to others predicted well-being but receiving it oneself did not [61].

Responding to this evidence requires that we move the dial from a focus on the lonely older person, to a focus on their social context and how it can support their meaningful inclusion. One means to doing this is by developing community and social services that facilitate people to "age in place." Community groups and not-for-profit organizations are often undervalued, seen as recreational activities and optional "extras" rather than part of the preventative public health system. This runs contrary to the evidence that such groups can deliver great personal and public health benefit, especially by offering inclusive spaces that affirm a person's value. For example, a qualitative study with members of a Bridge Club [62] found that such activities fill an essential niche for older people, providing opportunities to remain connected and to meaningfully contribute by supporting fellow members.

Need for an Increased Emphasis on Life Transitions

Another domain that warrants further consideration in interventions research is the role of life transitions. This can include both largely positive transitions that are planned and voluntary (such as retirement) and those that are more straightforwardly negative (such as a chronic illness diagnosis). All kinds of life transitions can be stressful, compromise well-being, and often precipitate loneliness [63]. However, what has often been left implicit is that the reason such transitions are experienced as stressful is often precisely *because* they fundamentally alter the nature of our social relationships and the nature of our social identities specifically [64]. Because of this, people will be relatively protected in the context of a life transition if they are able to maintain their social identities or develop new social

identities [65]. This has been verified in the context of several life transitions that are particularly relevant to older people, such as experiencing a health threat (eg, stroke or other acquired brain injury [66,67]). The domain with the most supportive evidence for this idea is retirement, where maintaining social identities and developing new ones is not only crucial to well-being, but predicts a sizable proportion of the variance in the risk of premature death [68–70]. This research speaks to the need for researchers more generally to be aware of the importance of life transitions as high-risk periods for the onset of loneliness and ideal opportunities for intervention.

Need for an Intersectional Focus

Being a member of a marginalized group, and especially multiple marginalized groups, greatly increased a person's risk of loneliness. For example, older people who are diverse in their sexuality or gender (LGBTQIA+) are more likely to experience loneliness [71,72] and are more likely to find a transition to residential care disruptive and alienating [73]. This is not only due to direct discrimination but also due to a greater likelihood of being childless and of having fractured relationships with their birth family [74]. Research in this context has found that opportunities for connection with the LGBTQIA+ community are particularly valued among older people at risk of loneliness [75].

Similarly, older people who are part of a cultural minority in their country of aging typically experience more loneliness [76]. Language proficiency can be a substantive barrier to forming new connections in this population [77] and should be taken into consideration when designing interventions for this group. Similar to the findings for other marginalized groups, research has found that opportunities to engage with groups oriented around one's heritage culture reduces loneliness and are welcomed by older people [78]. Indeed, across the board, researchers have found a need among marginalized groups for opportunities to connect with in-group members [79,80]. This also speaks to the importance of codesign as a principle for advancing our understanding of loneliness and its solutions, as a way of combating one-size-fits-all approaches that do not meet the needs of service users [81].

SUMMARY

Bringing these points together, there is a need to reorient our science and practice to include not only the lonely older person but also the context in which they are situated. When such contexts involve rapid change, do not offer opportunities for meaningful contribution or inclusion, or actively discriminate, it is perhaps no wonder that they create toxic conditions that foment loneliness and health decline. Increasingly though, there is an emerging picture of what can be done to tackle this problem, including interventions such as social prescribing, therapeutic social identity interventions, or whole-of-community social cohesion initiatives. What such approaches have in common is that they respect the agency and capacity of older people and support them to connect with groups in ways that meet their needs and provide a sense of subjective belonging. Moving forward, research on loneliness should take care to avoid myths such as overemphasizing the potential benefits or harms of technology or stereotypes about the commonality or inevitability of loneliness in older people. To the extent that we can advance our understanding and translation of evidence-based interventions, reducing the prevalence of loneliness is more within our grasp than ever.

CLINICS CARE POINTS

- Loneliness represents a "canary in the coalmine" for health. Practitioners who assess and intervene to address loneliness are thus likely to protect against health decline.
- Social exclusion, discrimination, and disadvantage are key contributors to loneliness. Effective intervention must thus go beyond the lonely individual to consider the context in which they are embedded.
- The last decade has seen progress in loneliness interventions of multiple forms: individual, group, and whole of community. Different levels of intervention will be suitable for different populations, contexts, and practitioners.

DISCLOSURES

The authors have nothing to disclose.

FUNDING

The author is supported by a National Health and Medical Research Council Fellowship (#1173270), and has received funding from Relationships Australia, the Australian Research Council, and Australian Rotary Health. The funders had no role in data analysis, manuscript preparation, or the decision to publish.

REFERENCES

[1] Perissinotto CM, Stijacic Cenzer I, Covinsky KE. Loneliness in older persons: A predictor of functional decline and death. Arch Intern Med 2012;172(14):1078–83.

[2] Putnam RD. Bowling Alone. New York: Simon & Schuster; 2000.

[3] Holt-Lunstad J, Smith TB, Layton JB. Social Relationships and Mortality Risk: A Meta-analytic Review. PLoS Med 2010;7(7):e1000316.

[4] Valtorta NK, Kanaan M, Gilbody S, et al. Loneliness and social isolation as risk factors for coronary heart disease and stroke: Systematic review and meta-analysis of longitudinal observational studies. Heart 2016;102(13):1009–16.

[5] Erzen E, Çikrikci Ö. The effect of loneliness on depression : A meta-analysis. Int J Soc Psychiatry 2018;64(5): 427–35.

[6] Akhter-Khan SC, Tao Q, Ang TFA, et al. Associations of loneliness with risk of Alzheimer's disease dementia in the Framingham Heart Study. Alzheimer's Dement 2021;17(10):1619–27.

[7] Lim MH, Eres R, Vasan S. Understanding loneliness in the twenty-first century: an update on correlates, risk factors, and potential solutions. Soc Psychiatry Psychiatr Epidemiol 2020;55(7):793–810.

[8] Cacioppo S, Grippo AJ, London S, et al. Loneliness: Clinical Import and Interventions. Perspect Psychol Sci 2015;10(2):238–49. Available at: http://pps.sagepub.com/content/10/2/238.abstract.

[9] Dykstra PA. Older adult loneliness: Myths and realities. Eur J Ageing 2009;6(2):91–100.

[10] Barreto M, Victor C, Hammond C, et al. Loneliness around the world: Age, gender, and cultural differences in loneliness. Pers Individ Dif 2021;169(January 2020): 110066.

[11] Cruwys T, Haslam C, Steffens NK, et al. Friendships that money can buy : financial security protects health in retirement by enabling social connectedness. BMC Geriatr 2019;19(319):1–9.

[12] Luhmann M, Hawkley LC. Age Differences in Loneliness From Late Adolescence to Oldest Old Age. Dev Psychol 2016;52(6):943–59.

[13] Jetten J, Pachana N. Not wanting to grow old: A Social Identity Model of Identity Change (SIMIC) analysis of driving cessation among older adults. In: Jetten J, Haslam C, Haslam SA, editors. The social cure: identity, health and well-being. New York, NY, USA: Psychology Press; 2012.

[14] Mund M, Freuding MM, Möbius K, et al. The stability and change of loneliness across the life span: A meta-analysis of longitudinal studies. Personal Soc Psychol Rev 2020;24(1):24–52.

[15] Appel M, Marker C, Gnambs T. Are social media ruining our lives? A review of meta-analytic evidence. Rev Gen Psychol 2020;24(1):60–74.

[16] Tsai HH, Tsai YF. Changes in depressive symptoms, social support, and loneliness over 1 year after a minimum

3-month videoconference program for older nursing home residents. J Med Internet Res 2011;13(4):1–12.

[17] Shah SGS, Nogueras D, van Woerden HC, et al. Evaluation of the effectiveness of digital technology interventions to reduce loneliness in older adults: Systematic review and meta-analysis. J Med Internet Res 2021; 23(6). https://doi.org/10.2196/24712.

[18] Morton TA, Wilson N, Haslam C, et al. Activating and Guiding the Engagement of Seniors With Online Social Networking: Experimental Findings From the AGES 2.0 Project. J Aging Health 2018;30(1):27–51.

[19] Aarts S, Peek STM, Wouters EJM. The relation between social network site usage and loneliness and mental health in community-dwelling older adults. Int J Geriatr Psychiatry 2015;30(9):942–9.

[20] Yang S, Huang L, Zhang Y, et al. Unraveling the links between active and passive social media usage and seniors' loneliness: a field study in aging care communities. Internet Res 2021;31(6):2167–89.

[21] LeRouge C, Van Slyke C, Seale D, et al. Baby Boomers' adoption of consumer health technologies: Survey on readiness and barriers. J Med Internet Res 2014;16(9). https://doi.org/10.2196/jmir.3049.

[22] Saeri AK, Cruwys T, Barlow FK, et al. Social connectedness improves public mental health : Investigating bidirectional relationships in the New Zealand attitudes and values survey. Aust N Z J Psychiatry 2018;52(4): 365–74.

[23] Haslam C, Cruwys T, Haslam SA. The we's have it": Evidence for the distinctive benefits of group engagement in enhancing cognitive health in aging. Soc Sci Med 2014; 120:57–66.

[24] Müller F, Röhr S, Reininghaus U, et al. Social isolation and loneliness during covid-19 lockdown: Associations with depressive symptoms in the German old-age population. Int J Environ Res Public Health 2021;18(7). https://doi.org/10.3390/ijerph18073615.

[25] Deshpande S, Livingstone A. First-onset psychosis in older adults: social isolation influence during COVID pandemic – a UK case series. Prog Neurol Psychiatry 2021;25(1):14–8.

[26] Masi CM, Chen HY, Hawkley LC, et al. A meta-analysis of interventions to reduce loneliness. Personal Soc Psychol Rev 2011;15(3):219–66.

[27] Gardiner C, Geldenhuys G, Gott M. Interventions to reduce social isolation and loneliness among older people: an integrative review. Heal Soc Care Community 2018;26(2):147–57.

[28] Cattan M, White M, Bond J, et al. Preventing social isolation and loneliness among older people: a systematic review of health promotion interventions. Ageing Soc 2005;25(1):41–67.

[29] Dickens A, Richards S, Greaves CJ, et al. Interventions targeting social isolation in older people: a systematic review. BMC Publ Health 2011;11:647.

[30] Haslam SA, Haslam C, Cruwys T, et al. Social identity makes group-based social connection possible: Implications for loneliness and mental health. Curr Opin Psychol 2022; 43(c):161–5.

[31] Tajfel H, Turner JC. An integrative theory of intergroup conflict. In: Austin WG, Worchel S, editors. The social psychology of intergroup relations. Monterey: Brooks/Cole.; 1979. p. 33–47.

[32] Turner JC, Hogg MA, Oakes PJ, et al. Rediscovering the social group: a self-categorization theory. Oxford: Blackwell; 1987.

[33] Jetten J, Branscombe NR, Haslam SA, et al. Having a lot of a good thing: Multiple important group memberships as a source of self-esteem. PLoS One 2015;10(5): e0124609.

[34] Cruwys T, Haslam SA, Dingle GA, et al. Feeling connected again: Interventions that increase social identification reduce depression symptoms in community and clinical settings. J Affect Disord 2014;159: 139–46.

[35] UK Gov. Press release: Walking, wheeling and cycling to be offered on prescription in nationwide trial. Available at: https://www.gov.uk/government/news/walking-wheeling-and-cycling-to-be-offered-on-prescription-in-nationwide-trial. Accessed August 22, 2022.

[36] Calderón-Larrañaga S, Greenhalgh T, Finer S, et al. What does the literature mean by social prescribing? A critical review using discourse analysis. Sociol Heal Illn 2022; 44(4–5):848–68.

[37] Cruwys T, Wakefield JRHH, Sani F, et al. Social isolation predicts frequent attendance in primary care. Ann Behav Med 2018;52(10):817–29.

[38] Elston J, Gradinger F, Asthana S, et al. Does a social prescribing "holistic" link-worker for older people with complex, multimorbidity improve well-being and frailty and reduce health and social care use and costs? A 12-month before-and-after evaluation. Prim Health Care Res Dev 2019;20:e135.

[39] Bickerdike L, Booth A, Wilson PM, et al. Social prescribing: Less rhetoric and more reality. A systematic review of the evidence. BMJ Open 2017;7(4). https://doi.org/10.1136/bmjopen-2016-013384.

[40] Percival A, Newton C, Mulligan K, et al. Systematic review of social prescribing and older adults: where to from here? Fam Med community Heal 2022;10:1–13.

[41] Smith TO, Jimoh OF, Cross J, et al. Social prescribing programmes to prevent or delay frailty in community-dwelling older adults. Geriatr Times 2019;4(4):4–8. https://doi.org/10.3390/geriatrics4040065.

[42] Sharman LS, McNamara N, Hayes S, et al. Social prescribing link workers—A qualitative Australian perspective. Heal Soc Care Community 2022;1–10. https://doi.org/10.1111/hsc.14079.

[43] Hamilton-West K, Milne A, Hotham S. New horizons in supporting older people's health and wellbeing: Is social prescribing a way forward? Age Ageing 2020;49(3): 319–26.

[44] Wakefield JRH, Kellezi B, Stevenson C, et al. Social Prescribing as 'Social Cure': A longitudinal study of the

health benefits of social connectedness within a Social Prescribing pathway. J Health Psychol 2020. https://doi.org/10.1177/1359105320944991.

[45] Stuart A, Stevenson C, Koschate M, et al. 'Oh no, not a group!' The factors that lonely or isolated people report as barriers to joining groups for health and well-being. Br J Health Psychol 2022;27(1):179–93.

[46] Haslam C, Cruwys T, Haslam SA, et al. Groups 4 Health: Evidence that a social-identity intervention that builds and strengthens social group membership improves mental health. J Affect Disord 2016;194:188–95.

[47] Haslam C, Cruwys T, Chang MXL, et al. GROUPS 4 HEALTH reduces loneliness and social anxiety in adults with psychological distress: Findings from a randomized controlled trial. J Consult Clin Psychol 2019;87(9):787–801.

[48] Cruwys T, Haslam C, Rathbone JA, et al. Groups 4 Health versus cognitive-behavioural therapy for depression and loneliness in young people: Randomised phase 3 non-inferiority trial with 12-month follow-up. Br J Psychiatry 2022;220:140–7.

[49] Cruwys T, Haslam C, Rathbone JA, et al. Groups 4 Health protects against unanticipated threats to mental health: Evaluating two interventions during COVID-19 lockdown among young people with a history of depression and loneliness. J Affect Disord 2021;295:316–22.

[50] Bentley S, Haslam C, Cruwys T, et al. In: Asmundson GJ, editor. Comprehensive Clinical Psychology, 2. Elsevier; 2022. p. 402–14. https://www.sciencedirect.com/referencework/9780128222324/comprehensive-clinical-psychology.

[51] LaRue CJ, Haslam C, Bentley SV, et al. GROUPS 4 HEALTH Retirement: A New Intervention that Supports Well-being in the Lead-up to Retirement by Targeting Social Identity Management. J Occup Organ Psychol 2023.

[52] Gleibs IH, Haslam C, Jones JM, et al. No country for old men? The role of a "Gentlemen's Club" in promoting social engagement and psychological well-being in residential care. Aging Ment Health 2011;15(4):456–66.

[53] Gleibs IH, Haslam C, Haslam SA, et al. Water clubs in residential care: is it the water or the club that enhances health and well-being? Psychol Health 2011;26(10):1361–77.

[54] Haslam C, Haslam SA, Ysseldyk R, et al. Social identification moderates cognitive health and well-being following story- and song-based reminiscence. Aging Ment Health 2013;1–10. https://doi.org/10.1080/13607863.2013.845871.

[55] Knight C, Haslam SA, Haslam C. In home or at home? How collective decision making in a new care facility enhances social interaction and wellbeing amongst older adults. Ageing Soc 2010;30(08):1393–418.

[56] Fong P, Cruwys T, Robinson SL, et al. Evidence that loneliness can be reduced by a whole-of-community intervention to increase neighbourhood identification. Soc Sci Med 2021;277:113909. https://doi.org/10.1016/j.socscimed.2021.113909.

[57] Cruwys T, Fong P, Evans O, et al. A community-led intervention to build neighbourhood identification predicts better wellbeing following prolonged COVID-19 lockdowns. Front Psychol 2022;1–12. https://doi.org/10.3389/fpsyg.2022.1030637.

[58] Akhter-khan SC, Prina M, Wong GH, et al. Understanding and Addressing Older Adults' Loneliness : The Social Relationship Expectations Framework. Perspect Psychol Sci 2022. https://doi.org/10.1177/17456916221127218 17456916221127218.

[59] Nurullah AS. Received and Provided Social Support: A Review of Current Evidence and Future Directions. Am J Health Stud 2012;27(3):173–88.

[60] Lanser I, et al, Lanser I, Eisenberger NI. Prosocial Behavior Reliably Reduces Loneliness : An Investigation Across Two Studies. Emotion 2022.

[61] Steffens NK, Jetten J, Haslam C, et al. Multiple social identities enhance health post-retirement because they are a basis for giving social support. Front Psychol 2016;7:15191.

[62] Fong P, Haslam C, Cruwys T, et al. There's a Bit of a Ripple-effect": A Social Identity Perspective on the Role of Third-Places and Aging in Place. Environ Behav 2020. https://doi.org/10.1177/0013916520947109.

[63] Evans O, Cruwys T, Cárdenas D, et al. Social identities mediate the relationship between isolation, life transitions, and loneliness. Behav Chang 2022;39:191–204.

[64] Praharso NF, Tear MJ, Cruwys T. Stressful life transitions and wellbeing: A comparison of the stress buffering hypothesis and the social identity model of identity change. Psychiatry Res 2017;247:265–75.

[65] Haslam C, Haslam SA, Jetten J, et al. Life Change, Social Identity, and Health. Annu Rev Psychol 2021;72:635–61.

[66] Haslam C, Holme A, Haslam SA, et al. Maintaining group memberships: social identity continuity predicts well-being after stroke. Neuropsychol Rehabil 2008;18(5–6):671–91.

[67] Jones JM, Haslam SA, Jetten J, et al. That which doesn't kill us can make us stronger (and more satisfied with life): the contribution of personal and social changes to well-being after acquired brain injury. Psychol Health 2011;26(3):353–69.

[68] Haslam C, Lam BCP, Branscombe NR, et al. Adjusting to life in retirement: The protective role of new group memberships and identification as a retiree. Eur J Work Organ Psychol 2018;27(6):822–39.

[69] Lam BCP, Haslam C, Steffens NK, et al. Longitudinal evidence for the effects of social group engagement on the cognitive and mental health of chinese retirees. Journals Gerontol - Ser B Psychol Sci Soc Sci 2020;75(10):2142–51.

[70] Steffens NK, Cruwys T, Haslam C, et al. Social group memberships in retirement are associated with reduced risk of premature death: Evidence from a longitudinal cohort study. BMJ Open 2016;6:e010164.

[71] Fish J, Weis C. All the lonely people, where do they all belong? An interpretive synthesis of loneliness and social

support in older lesbian, gay and bisexual communities. Qual Ageing Older Adults 2019;20(3):130–42.

[72] Kneale D. Connected communities? LGB older people and their risk of exclusion from decent housing and neighbourhoods. Qual Ageing Older Adults 2016; 17(2):107–18.

[73] Kneale D, Henley J, Thomas J, et al. Inequalities in older lgbt peoples health and care needs in the united kingdom: A systematic scoping review. Ageing Soc 2021;41(3):493–515.

[74] Wilkens J. Loneliness and Belongingness in Older Lesbians: The Role of Social Groups as "Community. J Lesbian Stud 2015;19(1):90–101.

[75] Perone AK, Ingersoll-Dayton B, Watkins-Dukhie K. Social Isolation Loneliness Among LGBT Older Adults: Lessons Learned from a Pilot Friendly Caller Program. Clin Soc Work J 2020;48(1):126–39.

[76] Morgan T, Wiles J, Moeke-Maxwell T, et al. 'People haven't got that close connection': meanings of loneliness and social isolation to culturally diverse older people. Aging Ment Heal 2020;24(10):1627–35.

[77] Tran TLN, Liu S, Gallois C, et al. The diversity of social connectedness experiences among older migrants in Australia. Int J Intercult Relations 2022;89:208–22.

[78] Dane S, Haslam C, Jetten J, et al. The benefits of ethnic activity group participation on older immigrant well-being and host country adjustment. Int J Intercult Relations 2020;77:119–24.

[79] Cameron JE, Voth J, Jaglal SB, et al. "In this together": Social identification predicts health outcomes (via self-efficacy) in a chronic disease self-management program. Soc Sci Med 2018;208:172–9.

[80] Walsh RS, Muldoon OT, Gallagher S, et al. Affiliative and "self-as-doer" identities: Relationships between social identity, social support, and emotional status amongst survivors of acquired brain injury (ABI). Neuropsychol Rehabil 2015;25(4):555–73.

[81] Ogrin R, Cyarto EV, Harrington KD, et al. Loneliness in older age: What is it, why is it happening and what should we do about it in Australia? Australas J Ageing 2021;40(2):202–7.

Education and Clinical Practice

Advances in Psychiatry and Behavioral Health 3 (2023) 197–208

Advances in Child Psychiatry Education and Training

Afifa Adiba, MD[a,b,c,*], Shawn Singh Sidhu, MD, DFAPA, DFAACAP[d], Deepika Shaligram, MD[e], Manal Khan, MD[f,1], Zheala Qayyum, MD, MMSc[g]

[a]Sheppard Pratt Health System, Towson, MD, USA; [b]University of Maryland, 6501 North Charles Street, Baltimore, MD 21204, USA; [c]Yale School of Medicine, New Haven, CT, USA; [d]Division of Child and Adolescent Psychiatry, Department of Psychiatry, University of California San Diego Medical Center, UCSD Medical Center, Rady Children's Hospital of San Diego, 2125 Citracado Parkwy, Escondido, CA 92029, USA; [e]Boston Children's Hospital, Harvard Medical School, 9 Hope Avenue, Waltham, MA 02453, USA; [f]University of California, 300 Medical Plaza Driveway, Los Angeles, CL 90095, USA; [g]Harvard Medical School, Yale School of Medicine, 300 Longwood Avenue, Boston, MA 02115, USA

KEYWORDS

• Child psychiatry • Training and education • Advance in child psychiatry

KEY POINTS

• The article focuses on advancing child psychiatry and child psychiatry training to prepare future child psychiatrists for the challenges of the field.

• Incorporating a holistic approach to evaluating child psychiatry fellows by emphasizing the importance of maintaining humanity in medicine and assessing competencies beyond clinical skills.

• Providing comprehensive training for child psychiatry fellows in evidence-based treatments for trauma, exposure to maternal/parental mental health and early childhood intervention clinics, cultural humility, gender-affirming interventions, and trauma-informed care principles to prepare them for the evolving field of child psychiatry.

INTRODUCTION: CHILD AND ADOLESCENT PSYCHIATRY—A FIELD OF HOPE

The field of child and adolescent psychiatry (CAP) can be summarized in a singular, powerful, and all-encompassing word: "hope." "Hope" that children and families who have been suffering emotionally for generations will finally begin to heal. "Hope" that the shackles and bondages of trauma can be released, so that people can live freely and fully. "Hope" that we can partner with communities to prevent at-risk youth from developing chronic, lifelong conditions that significantly alter the trajectory of their lives. "Hope" that we can remove barriers such as systemic racism and discrimination, such that children and their families can thrive regardless of their gender, race, ethnicity, religion, sexual preference, citizenship status, or other identifying characteristics.

If child and adolescent psychiatrists ultimately specialize in "hope," then our metaphorical stethoscope must be core values of love, emotional intelligence, empathy, compassion, equity, patience, inclusion, openness, passion, and justice. Without fully embodying these values, neither will we be able to access the inner world of a child and their family nor will we have the determination to confront recalcitrant systems or the courage to advocate for innovations that affect countless lives. We

---

[1] Present address: 300 Medical Plaza Driveway, Los Angeles, CA 90095, USA.

*Corresponding author. 6501 North Charles Street, Baltimore, MD 21204. *E-mail addresses:* afifa.adiba@sheppardpratt.org; afifa.adiba@yale.edu

also cannot do this alone. Our ability to act as change agents in our communities largely depends on our ability to build bridges and alliances with a broad range of partners, all the while challenging ourselves to improve access to care and reach children and families where they are.

The following article first summarizes the national state of affairs in CAP, before introducing advancements in theoretical frameworks, concrete recommendations for training, and future directions. It is our "hope" that this article might inspire our colleagues to push the boundaries of education and training for a better today and brighter tomorrow; meanwhile, honoring and doing justice to the youth and families whom we serve.

PRESENT STATE OF AFFAIRS

In this section, we will provide a brief historical background of CAP training in the United States, followed by an up to the minute discussion of current trends.

Brief Historical Background

The field of CAP is a relatively new medical specialty that originated in Europe and the United States during the late 1800s and early 1900s [1]. In Germany, physicians gained training in child psychiatry through schools founded by Johannes Trüper, Theodor Ziehen, and Wilhelm Strohmayer [2]. Hermann Emminghaus published the first German overview of emotional problems in children, "Mental Disorders of Childhood," in 1887, while Moritz Tramer defined CAP in terms of diagnosis, treatment, and prognosis in 1933 [3].

In the United States, Leo Kanner founded the first academic child psychiatry department in 1930 at the Johns Hopkins Hospital, where he established the first formal elective course in child psychiatry in 1936. The Institute for Juvenile Research, founded by Jane Addams and her colleagues in Chicago in 1909, became the world's first child guidance clinic [1]. In February 1923, The Maudsley, a psychiatric hospital in London dedicated to postgraduate teaching and research, established a modest psychiatry department to cater specifically to children. Similarly, the early development of child psychiatry training took place in numerous countries in between 1920 and 1930 [4].

The development and training in the subspecialty of CAP in Europe hails from diverse historical traditions, including the neuropsychiatric, remedial clinical, psychoanalytic, and empirical, epidemiologic, and statistical traditions, depending on specific countries [5]. Efforts to unify clinical practice and training across Europe date back to the first symposium of the European Child and Adolescent Psychiatrists in Switzerland

in 1954 and continue with the current European Society for Child and Adolescent Psychiatry. National organizations representing CAP are present in more than 90% of European countries, with more than half having CAP training organizations as part of general psychiatric organizations but there are still some European countries without formal CAP training programs [6].

CAP was recognized as a medical specialty in the United States in 1953 with the founding of the American Academy of Child Psychiatry and established as a board-certified medical specialty by the American Board of Psychiatry and Neurology (ABPN) in 1959. The founding of the Accreditation Council for Graduate Medical Education (ACGME) in 1981 then provided standardization of training guidelines and expectations within CAP. Although the early years of CAP were imperative and formative, they also included controversies such as prolonged institutionalization, lobotomization, paternalism without patient autonomy, overmedication within the foster care system, pathologizing of sexual and gender minorities, racism, sexism, discrimination, and overdiagnosis of bipolar disorder in child and adolescent populations.

Modern Trends Following the Turn of the Century: Media Use, COVID-19, and the National State of Emergency in Child Mental Health

The turn of the century saw the increasing utilization of broadband Internet technology [7] followed by the release of the first-generation iPhone in 2007 [8,9]. Although these 2 inventions fundamentally changed the daily lives of children and adolescents, they also shaped the trajectory of the human experience indefinitely.

Concurrently, since the turn of the century, rates of child and adolescent depression, anxiety, autism, and suicide have increased. Yet, at the same time, rates of substance use, automobile accidents, and teen pregnancy have declined. Although the causes of these trends are likely multifactorial, some have posited that the sizable presence of screen time in the lives of teens has displaced both healthy and unhealthy activities. The displacement of face-to-face contact with others and resultant social isolation and withdrawal may have contributed to increases in depression, anxiety, and suicide; meanwhile, the displacement of high-risk behaviors has resulted in a decline in substance use, automobile accidents, and teen pregnancy [10]. Although some studies have linked increased media use to social comparison and depression in teens, other data suggest that media use with real-world relationships is promoting health, and minority teens also report a sense of community online that they never had before [11]. Rates of depression, anxiety, and autism also may be increasing due to greater awareness, early identification, and decreased stigma associated with these conditions.

In 2020, the world saw its first pandemic in a century, and the COVID-19 infected almost a billion individuals globally, while claiming the lives of nearly 7 million people around the world by February of 2023 [12]. The pandemic, and associated quarantines and social isolation, only furthered the increase of depression, anxiety, school difficulties, and social difficulties in youth [13–15].

Meanwhile, there continues to be a shortage of child and adolescent psychiatrists nationally. As of 2022, there were approximately 8300 child and adolescent psychiatrists in the country, when it is estimated that 35,000 are required to meet the needs of the youth and families whom we serve (AACAP, 2022). Given the increases in rates of child and adolescent depression, anxiety, and suicide, and given the relative paucity of emergency department and inpatient CAP beds across the country, the American Academy of Child and Adolescent Psychiatry, American Academy of Pediatrics, and Children's Hospital Association declared a National State of Emergency in Child and Adolescent Mental Health in October of 2021 [16]. This prompted President Joe Biden's White House to announce a strategy to address the national mental health crisis, including an increase in mental health funding [17].

ADVANCES IN THEORETICAL FRAMEWORKS

The past 20 years have also seen a number of movements that have profoundly affected societal thought on critical social topics. Awareness of increasing rates of physician suicide in both trainees and attendings has furthered the discussion on the crisis of physician burnout. The murder of George Floyd spurred the *#BlackLivesMatter* movement, which swept the nation and the entire world, from individual households to the largest corporations. The *#MeToo* movement and advocates such as Malala Yousafzai shed light on sexual assault and human rights violations against women of all races, ages, and statuses, whereas the physician-led *#ThisIsOurLane* movement raised awareness about the physical and emotional damage caused by firearm violence. In 2018, then 15-year-old Greta Thunberg captured the world's attention when delivering a speech to the United Nations on climate change. All of these movements have been so powerful that their so-called trickle-down effect has affected all spaces, including training and education in CAP.

In this section, we will examine advances in theoretical constructs regarding CAP training, including physician burnout; prevention and access to care; diversity, equity, and inclusion (DEI); and trauma-informed care.

Physician Burnout

Unfortunately, physician levels of burnout remain high, and some reports suggest they have only increased with the COVID-19 pandemic [18].The causes of physician burnout seem multifactorial and include expectations for round-the-clock coverage, burdensome documentation, countless mandates and regulations, isolation in practice, separation from loved ones, difficulty in attaining work–life balance, moral injury, recalcitrant and bureaucratic health systems, dogmatic billing and coding practices, delayed gratification, financial debt, and a loss of meaning in medicine. As a result, rates of physician suicide far exceed those of the general population, and are especially high for female physicians who suffer from dual role stressors and decreased compensation compared with men [19,20]. Psychiatrists in particular report higher rates of substance use disorders and divorce than other specialties in medicine.

The ACGME has implemented a series of sequential changes aimed at reducing physician burnout, including both a reduction in duty hours and a mandate that all programs include wellness programming and education on topics such as burnout and sleep deprivation. However, despite these efforts, rates of burnout remain high in medical trainees.

Prevention, Early Identification, and Access to Care

Although the first few decades of CAP focused more on describing clusters of clinical symptoms and the study of evidence-based psychotherapies and pharmacology, the importance of prevention, early identification, and access to care has been an increasing presence and focus of the field in recent years. Even mainstream politicians, such as Elizabeth Warren, have begun emphasizing the importance of early childhood experiences and their downstream effects. New health systems have emerged, such as federally qualified health centers and capitated health systems (Kaiser Permanente), which not only prioritize but also reimburse physicians based on their ability to keep patients healthy and out of higher levels of care; however, the vast majority of health systems continue to operate under a fee-for-service model, which incentivizes larger payments for higher levels of care and procedures.

Diversity, Equity, and Inclusion

DEI efforts have become a clarion call in CAP training, due in part to the resounding voices of the #BlackLives-Matter and #MeToo movements. As new research aims to ensure that a diverse patient population is being reached, the ACGME is mandating that all programs provide training in health disparities. However, the lack of diversity in CAP remains a concern, with medical schools and residency programs searching for ways to attract and retain underrepresented minorities and women.

The ACGME and the Liaison Committee on Medical Education are also requiring programs to provide information about their DEI policies and procedures for interviewing and ranking applicants. This is all the more important because the US population is diverse, and a lack of diversity among physicians means that many patients do not have access to care that reflects their cultural and social backgrounds. For example, only 5.0% of physicians identify as Black [21], whereas Black Americans make up 12.2% of the US population. By embracing diversity, we can foster physician–patient relationships that yield better outcomes for minority and minoritized patients and ensure that everyone has access to the care they need.

Gender-Affirming Care

In recent years, child psychiatry has undergone a remarkable transformation, embracing gender-affirming care for transgender and gender nonbinary individuals. This groundbreaking approach acknowledges the challenges faced by these communities, from discrimination to limited access to health care [22]. Yet, despite a growing body of evidence supporting the effectiveness of these interventions, the political and legislative landscape remains fraught with obstacles. Several states have proposed or enacted laws that impede access to gender-affirming care for youth, leaving child and adolescent psychiatrists to navigate a complex and often hostile legal environment while striving to provide optimal care for their patients.

Despite these challenges, medical and psychiatric organizations have been steadfast in their advocacy, promoting access to evidence-based care and standing up for the rights of transgender and gender nonbinary individuals. As we continue to learn more about the benefits of gender-affirming care, we can envision a future in which all children and adolescents, regardless of their gender identity, receive compassionate, personalized care tailored to their specific needs.

Patient Autonomy and Trauma-Informed Care

As the era of paternalism comes to a close, the field of medicine is realigning its ethical priorities toward increases in patient autonomy and education. This coincides with the acknowledgement that many of our patients, particularly in CAP, have experienced adverse childhood experiences (ACEs) and a loss of control in their lives secondary to life-altering trauma. The principles of Trauma-Informed Care seek to empower patients so that they feel in control of their health-care experience and are treated with the basic human compassion and respect that they deserve.

CONCRETE RECOMMENDATIONS FOR ADVANCES IN CHILD AND ADOLESCENT PSYCHIATRY EDUCATION AND TRAINING

In this section, we provide concrete recommendations for advances in CAP education and training based on the aforementioned state of affairs and theoretical constructs.

Core Values and Competencies

The ACGME mandates that CAP fellowship programs systematically evaluate all fellows twice yearly, using the ACGME Milestones as a guide. The Milestones have undergone several revisions, and future directions include CAP following suit with the rest of medicine in creating Entrustable Professional Activities for which fellows can be evaluated.

However, relatively less discussion has encouraged thinking more broadly about how we evaluate CAP fellows. That is, what exactly are we wanting our fellows to be able to do for their patients and their communities when they graduate, and how are we measuring that? How do we train fellows in and evaluate core values of love, emotional intelligence, empathy, compassion, equity, patience, inclusion, openness, passion, and justice? Although the ability for fellows to navigate an electronic health record is certainly a requirement in modern medicine, should that carry the same weight as humanistic factors?

To cultivate the next generation of child and adolescent psychiatrists, our recommendation is that training programs must take a holistic approach to evaluating their fellows. It is not just about clinical competence—it is about fostering an open-minded and inclusive environment. We recommend evaluating fellows on their efforts to include others in treatment decisions and consider how they see themselves as part of a broader community. It is also important to assess their ability to break down nonverbal communication, provide validation, and create a welcoming environment for a diverse range of youth and families, peers, colleagues, and staff. Ultimately, fellows should be evaluated on their ability to maintain their humanity in the practice of medicine. By broadening the scope of evaluations, we can ensure that our fellows are truly prepared to provide the best possible care to a diverse range of patients. So let us embrace a more holistic approach to training the next generation of child and adolescent psychiatrists, one that recognizes the vital importance of empathy, inclusion, and humanity in the practice of medicine. Together, we can create a future where all patients, regardless of background or identity, receive care that is both clinically competent and deeply compassionate.

Prevention, Early Identification, and Referral to Treatment (Subheading)

The aforementioned increase in awareness about prevention and early identification should shape the way we think about education and training in CAP. At a bare minimum, fellows should understand the research conveying the importance of early childhood intervention. However, ideally training would also include critical and high-quality clinical experiences in maternal/parental mental health and early childhood intervention clinics. In this way, fellows will have direct experience working with the parents of unborn children, while also helping families with children in the 0 to 5 years age range who are struggling. These clinical experiences will help to ensure that CAP fellows are trained to care for children throughout the life span, from conception to transitional age.

Fellows should also be trained not only in the use of screening questionnaires but also in the broader systemic implications of identifying at-risk youth and families early and then subsequently linking those families to services in the community. As every child is situated within the strengths and challenges of their family system, it is essential for training in CAP to encompass skills that enable working with families to facilitate primordial and primary prevention, diagnostic processes, and therapeutic interventions (including psychopharmacology).

Trauma Informed Care—Adverse Childhood Experiences, Humanism/Compassion, Mistrust of Authority Figures

A broader awareness of ACEs in the medical community and universal rejection of paternalism has resulted in the Trauma-Informed Care movement, which is a systematic approach that assumes that both patients and staff are more likely to have a history of trauma than not, and it acknowledges the role that trauma may play in their lives [23]. It also acknowledges a mistrust in the medical system and/or authority figures that may have developed during the course of generations. The guiding principles of trauma-informed care include safety, trustworthiness or transparency, choice, collaboration, and empowerment. It involves not only the direct care of patients and their families but also reception desk staff involvement, telephonic and electronic communications, forgiving clinic policies, a clinic environment that emphasizes healing and minimizes retraumatization, and a safe, clean, and soothing physical space and esthetics.

In addition to learning about the broader systemic implications of trauma-informed care, fellows must be trained in evidence-based treatments for trauma. These include but are not limited to pharmacotherapy and cognitive behavioral therapy (CBT), eye movement desensitization and reprocessing, prolonged exposure therapy, narrative exposure therapy, trauma-focused cognitive behavioral therapy (TF-CBT), dialectical behavioral therapy (DBT), somatic experiencing, attachment-based therapy, and mindfulness-based stress reduction and trauma informed family therapy. Although CBT, TF-CBT, and DBT are commonly included in fellowship curricula, having a broader range of tools can aid in creating a sense of safety, providing choice and control, and fostering empowerment and collaboration for patients. With training in trauma therapy, child psychiatry fellows can effectively incorporate trauma-informed care into their practice, resulting in better outcomes for the patients.

Gender-Affirming Care: Gender Identity, Countertransference, Introspective Approach

Gender is a multifaceted construct influenced by biology, experiences, desires, conflicts, culture, and societal norms. Gender-affirming care provides a mosaic of social, psychological, and medical interventions to support transgender and gender nonbinary individuals [24]. Research shows that social transitioning can normalize depression and alleviate anxiety symptoms for transgender children [25].

Because more young people explore their gender identity, child and adolescent psychiatrists must be attuned to their unique challenges. Training programs should provide knowledge of pubertal suppression, hormone therapy, and surgery while encouraging a multifaceted and introspective approach. To provide the best care possible, psychiatrists must examine their own biases and countertransference reactions. By embracing a nuanced and inclusive approach to gender, we can cultivate a vibrant mosaic of individuals, all celebrated for their unique identities.

Diversity, Equity, and Inclusion —COVID Worse, Burnout Worse, Trauma, Mistrust

Unfortunately, underrepresented communities continue to be disproportionately affected by health disparities, as demonstrated by increased deaths and decreased vaccination rates during the COVID-19 pandemic. Decades of institution and systemic racism have resulted in a mistrust of authority figures and the medical community for some underrepresented individuals. Gender minorities and women also continue to have disproportionately higher rates of mental health concerns. Within medicine, women and minorities are more likely to experience discrimination and burnout while being considered for higher positions far less frequently than their counterparts. Future CAP fellows need to be aware of the impact of racism and discrimination both within medicine and in terms of the impacts on our patients.

Cultural humility is a model that should be front and center in all CAP training programs. Cultural humility is a lifelong endeavor to develop intercultural communication skills, respect, and lack of superiority regarding cross-cultural differences to enhance therapeutic relationships. It complements "structural competency," which examines forces influencing health outcomes above individual interactions [26]. To promote a culturally sensitive systems-based approach, the American Academy of Child and Adolescent Psychiatry has developed a Diversity and Cultural Competency Curriculum for Child and Adolescent Psychiatry Training and a Practice Parameter on Cultural Competence in Child and Adolescent Psychiatric Practice [27,28].

The AACAP Diversity and Cultural Competency Curriculum recommends specific skills, including effectively interviewing and communicating with children and families of different cultural backgrounds, formulating diagnoses that include cultural dimensions, formulating culturally sensitive treatment plans, providing culturally specific psychotherapeutic and psychopharmacological interventions, advocating for access to mental health services for all children in need, and understanding cross-cultural dynamics [28].

Child psychiatry training should teach the skills of assessing experiences with bias and prejudice and place these, along with the presenting symptoms, in the context of developmental stages of diverse youth. Approaches that increase cultural humility, invite dialog

about experiences of discrimination, and tailor psychoeducation to explanatory models of illness can improve family engagement and treatment outcomes [29].

Training should also include strength-based approaches to working with diverse families that recognize the protective effects of bicultural or multicultural identity to promote psychological well-being [30]. Trainees need to be aware of culturally informed child-rearing practices, behavior expectations, communication patterns, and acceptable coping skills to avoid diagnostic pitfalls and foster engagement. Adjunctive training in public health analysis, advocacy skills, and collaborative approaches with individuals with lived experience, parents, and caregivers are needed to disrupt systemic/structural barriers and create patient-friendly care systems [31].

The evaluation of developmental competencies should include competencies specific to the experiences and strengths of diverse youth and families, including the impacts of individual and institutionalized racism, implicit bias and prejudice, as well as flexibility in straddling bicultural identities [32].

In addition to implementation and training in cultural humility, both trainees and practicing child and adolescent psychiatrists need to directly engage and involve underrepresented minorities in discussions regarding mental health services. This means creating collaborative relationships with local cultural grassroots and nonprofit organizations, including churches, schools, legal centers, cultural centers, job training centers, immigration centers, health-care clinics, or other entities committed to underrepresented groups. This type of collaboration elevates the voices of underrepresented minorities as true stakeholders with the ability to make decisions that affect their health care and communities.

Access to Care and Integrated Care— Including Telehealth, Integrated Care

Given the shortage of child and adolescent psychiatrists, training is the optimal place and time in professional development to engage learners in solutions to address access to care. A myriad of solutions have been proposed, and some have been studied, to provide a greater amount of support to a larger number of youth and families in need. Broadly, these solutions can be broken down into (1) providing direct services to children who have reduced access, and (2) utilizing a "multiplier effect" to extend the knowledge and expertise of child and adolescent psychiatrists to other providers.

Efforts to provide direct services to children who have reduced access include the utilization of telehealth and integrating with other child-facing systems. The COVID-19 pandemic paved the way for many health-care institutions, organizations, and private practices to modernize in telepsychiatry, and the majority of training programs now provide clinical experiences in telehealth. Similarly, in working closely with schools, juvenile justice, foster care, group homes, child protective services, and other child-facing programs, child and adolescent psychiatrists can remove barriers to treatment by visiting the children where they are.

The greatest effort to use a "multiplier effect" is through training and consulting with other health-care providers who can then go on to treat an exponentially larger sum of youth. Given the shortage of child psychiatrists, pediatric primary care providers (PPCPs) are increasingly at the forefront of managing mental health conditions [33]. Collaborative care models (CCMs) between PPCPs and child psychiatrists can provide PPCPs with the necessary support to deliver mental health services [34].

The standard framework for levels of integrated care, developed by the Substance Abuse and Mental Health Services Administration and the Health Resources and Services Administration, conceptualizes integration as a continuum ranging from separate mental health and primary care systems with minimal coordination to integrated systems, in which mental health clinicians and PPCPs function as a team in a shared practice setting. Elements used to characterize the level of integration include (1) communication (frequency and type), (2) practice location (on-site, off-site, and remote), and (3) practice change (eg, shared workflows and medical records systems) [35].

The US Surgeon General's report in 2021 recognizes the importance of CCMs and recommends the expansion of Pediatric Mental Health Care Access (PMHCA) programs, which provide PPCPs with teleconsultations, training, technical assistance, and care coordination to support the diagnosis, treatment, and referral of children with mental health and substance use needs [36]. Integrated care, especially CCMs, has been shown to improve mental health outcomes for children and adolescents when compared with standard care [37]. The most commonly reported components of effective pediatric integrated mental health care models associated with the clinical improvement of mental health symptoms are (1) population-based care, (2) measurement-based care, and (3) delivery of evidence-based mental health services [38].

Thus, in CCMs, child and adolescent psychiatrists (CAPs) are called on to build the knowledge and skills of PPCPs to manage mild-to-moderate pediatric mental health issues in primary care and conserve the scarce child psychiatry resources for patients with more complex and severe conditions. The first PMHCA program, Massachusetts Child Psychiatry Access Program, was established in 2004 and covers more than 95% of the state's youth [39,40]. It has since been replicated in 46 states across the United States and seen increased utilization during the pandemic [41].

Because CCMs differ from traditional mental health practice and require robust consultative skills that are not routinely taught in current child psychiatry training [42], it is essential to formalize a child psychiatry curriculum and establish competency requirements [43]. Approximately one-third of US child psychiatry fellows receive didactic teaching and/or clinical exposure to integrated care models. During these rotations, trainees learn to function as a consultant to multidisciplinary professionals while building their communication, consulting, and system analysis skills [44]. The triple board and postpediatric portal program trainees, due to their inherent combined pediatric/psychiatric training, are well prepared for leadership positions on integrated care teams [45]. A novel integrated behavioral health rotation for CAP fellows described by Njoroge and colleagues [46] illustrates the application of the 6 ACGME core competencies to the practice of integrated care in child psychiatry in Table 1.

Interdisciplinary training experiences are recommended for trainees in the medical and psychiatric fields to complement their competency areas. To optimize pediatric mental health care and promote collaboration between child psychiatrists and PCPs, a standardized, case-based curriculum covering important topics in the management of medical and psychiatric comorbidity was developed with the support from the American Academy of Child and Adolescent Psychiatry and the American Academy of Pediatrics (AAP). This curriculum consists of 3 case-based educational modules that were pilot-tested and evaluated as a part of the "Collaborative Essentials for Pediatric and Child and Adolescent Psychiatry residents: Working Together to Treat the Child" project [47].

One child psychiatry fellowship program based in Massachusetts mandates a 10-week integrated care rotation (half-day per week) during their first year of training. Fellows engage in-person and virtual consultations in the primary care clinic and perform electronic chart reviews to develop the skills of conducting a focused, time-limited evaluation that informs assessment, treatment plan documentation, teaching, and case review with PPCPs. The rotation emphasizes the unique skills of CAPs in integrated care models, such

TABLE 1
Application of Accreditation Council for Graduate Medical Education Core Competencies to Integrated Care in Child Psychiatry

Competency	Description
Interprofessional communication	Encouraging shared decision-making for effective team-based care
Professionalism	Establishing ethical and professional guidelines
Integrated care systems practice	Understanding primary care context and professional roles
Practice-based learning	Collaborating with other disciplines, evidence-based practice, quality improvement
Preventive screening and assessment	Identifying emerging behavioral health conditions and assessing patient outcomes
Cultural competence	Collaborating within diverse communities, understanding barriers to treatment, and the psychosocial determinants of health

as measurement-based care, short-term and goal-oriented treatment, and partnering with PPCPs, which may not be the focus of training in other settings [48].

Advocacy and Leadership

Child and adolescent psychiatrists are optimally positioned to become change agents in their communities. Although psychopharmacology and psychotherapy are certainly the mainstays of basic child psychiatry training, and while the fundamentals of assessing a broad range of patients and creating an evidence-based treatment are the building blocks of our practice, trainees should be encouraged and empowered to see themselves as capable of making transformative changes that can reach many more patients than they could ever see individually in their offices.

Child and adolescent psychiatrists are trained to understand not only children and their family units but also the myriad of systems, which are exposed to children and their families. These include but are not limited to health care, school/education, juvenile justice, foster care, child protective services, developmental disability services, immigration settings. As a result, child psychiatry input is relevant to anything and everything that involves social change in the fabric of our society.

One vehicle through which child psychiatrists can affect change is public education. CAP trainees often take their breadth and depth of knowledge for granted, and may feel "imposter syndrome" or a sense that they do not have anything to offer to the public. Yet, most children and their families have never been given this same knowledge, and many may think as if they are throwing proverbial darts in the dark. Thus, even the most basic knowledge about core topics in child psychiatry can be highly valuable to the public. This could include anything from simply explaining why it is important for parents to spend face-to-face, one-on-one time with their children in the busy digital age to a nuanced explanation of neuronal circuits.

Media collaborations can be an efficient and effective means to deliver public education. There are a multitude of media formats that remain relevant today, and thus child psychiatrists can tailor their messaging to forms of the media that enhance their strengths. Those who are strong writers can write for their local institution's blog or newsletter, the local newspaper, or even national outlets. Those who are strong speakers can contact their local news channels and pitch poignant and compelling news stories. Those who are connected in social media can begin spreading awareness and collectively reach broader audiences. Ultimately, most patients do not read scientific journals independently but they do universally consume media. Thus, if we are to reach the greatest number of families who need our help, the media has to be a part of the solution.

Another means to delivering public education is through advocacy efforts. As with the media, many trainees may think that they do not have enough knowledge or experience to inform elected officials about policies that influence children and families. However, in truth, trainees have dedicated thousands of hours of their lives to knowing and understanding the lives of their patients. Many trainees also have lived experience of family members who have suffered with their own emotional concerns or traumas. Thus, trainees are well positioned to engage in advocacy efforts, and doing so while in-training may pave the way for a lifelong career in advocacy. Local legislative conferences for regional medical organizations can be a gradual and low-pressure initiation into advocacy. Most regional medical organizations have dedicated positions and roles for trainees. National advocacy opportunities are also available in the form of visiting Washington D.C. to meet with national leaders and joining committees that write professional amicus briefs and position statements in response to current events.

If trainees question why public education and advocacy are important, in addition to helping the youth and families that we serve, it is that they are an antidote to burnout. Trainees and child psychiatrists can often feel a sense of burnout and a loss of meaning in medicine when faced with larger systems that are not trauma-informed, culturally sensitive, and patient-centered. This can feel disempowering to providers, who think that their hands are figuratively tied. Advocacy is the opportunity to change those very systems, such that they are more patient facing, and engaging in this effort can instill resilience and inspiration in trainees to combat burnout.

FUTURE DIRECTIONS
In this section, we explore some future directions in CAP training based on recent developments in the field.

Interventional Psychiatry
Interventional child psychiatry is a rapidly developing field and involves the use of various interventional procedures to treat children with psychiatric conditions when traditional treatments have been unsuccessful.

One common interventional procedure is electroconvulsive therapy, which involves the use of electrical currents to stimulate the brain and alleviate symptoms of severe depression or other mental health conditions [49]. Another procedure is transcranial magnetic stimulation (TMS), which uses magnetic fields to stimulate specific areas of the brain that are involved in mood regulation.

Other interventional procedures used in child psychiatry include deep brain stimulation, vagus nerve stimulation, and repetitive TMS. These procedures are typically reserved for severe or treatment-resistant cases of conditions such as obsessive-compulsive disorder or Tourette syndrome. Ketamine therapy is another treatment option that has shown promise in addressing treatment-resistant depression, anxiety, and other mental health conditions for children.

The field has also grown with respect to wearable devices, such as a trigeminal nerve stimulator for attention-deficit hyperactivity disorder, and multiple technologies to assist youth with autism spectrum disorder in social communication.

As the field of child psychiatry expands, it is crucial for fellows to gain knowledge of interventional child psychiatry. Therefore, it is recommended that programs incorporate this topic into their curriculum, enabling fellows to stay up-to-date on the latest research regarding the effectiveness and safety of these interventions in children and adolescents.

Application of Psychedelics and Cannabidiol Therapeutics
Although there remains little in the way of consistent evidence for use in child and adolescent populations, innovations in the use of ketamine, psilocybin, and cannabidiol (CBD) in adults with mental health concerns bear tracking for near-term implications in child and adolescent education and training.

The Role of Media in the Lives of Youth
Given the ever-expanding role of media in the lives of both youth and family units, fellows should be provided with education and training regarding the effective screening and management of media-based concerns in youth. This includes taking a comprehensive media history when evaluating child and adolescent population that addresses the amount of screen use, types of media and/or apps used, whether or not the child posts original content, and how the child uses media socially. Youth, families, and communities should also be provided with psychoeducation on the impacts of extended screen time, high-risk media behavior, and strategies that parents can use to keep their children safe. This also includes the creation of media curricula for schools.

Sex Education
The #MeToo has highlighted that among many other things, the concept of consent is at best misunderstood by much of society. Yet, teenagers do not routinely receive education on what consent means when it comes to intimacy and safe sexual practices. Child and adolescent psychiatrists should be at the forefront of leading community-based efforts to inform all children about the importance of consent, with the hope of reducing rates of sexual assault.

Maintenance of CERTIFICATION
The oral boards in CAP gave way to recertification examinations, which have now again given way to the Article-Based Continuing Certification Pathway of the

ABPN. Programs should utilize journal clubs not only to review the latest evidence-based literature but also to train fellows in how to navigate the ABPN website and take article-based quizzes to maintain board certification.

Recruitment and Retention

It is clear that addressing the workforce shortage for child and adolescent mental health will require innovative ways to target the pipeline, enhance recruitment, and retain diverse clinicians who can meet the needs of the children and families they serve.

Targeting the pipeline through mentorship programs and early exposure to CAP can generate interest in students and inspire toward a career in CAP. The influence of lengthy training of career choice for students requires creative ways to provide optimal training in CAP in a shorter period. To address workforce development, alternatives to the traditional training pathways have been proposed and being considered by professional organizations at various stages of development [50]. These pathway strategies include early commitment through the "Child Track" in the Match program, shortened training, with 3-year CAP training only or a 4-year combined general and CAP training model. Another broadening recruitment from other primary specialties (eg, 3-year postfamily medicine fellowship model). Some of these models are based on the triple board training experience, where general (18 months) and child and adolescent (18 months) psychiatry training is completed in a 3-year period [31].

Additionally, recruitment strategies require support and commitment from government and administration in the form of national strategies focusing on equitable pay, capacity building and providing stipends or loan forgiveness options to offset training expenses. An investment in the health-care force that is striving to meet the ever-increasing demands during a national crisis in children's mental health is critical.

Supporting and retaining child and adolescent psychiatrists from diverse backgrounds, trained in contemporary issues in CAP is key to meet the needs of children and their families. This requires mentorship, investment in career progression, research, scholarship, and academic enhancement opportunities.

SUMMARY

In this article, we first summarized the present state of affairs in CAP, including a brief historical background, the impact of the COVID-19 pandemic, and the proclamation of a National State of Emergency in Child and Adolescent Mental Health. We then reviewed advances in theoretical frameworks involving physician burnout, prevention, access to care, DEI, and trauma-informed care. We provided concrete recommendations for training regarding core values and competencies, prevention and early identification, DEI, trauma-informed care, advocacy, leadership, and systems of care including schools, juvenile justice, foster care, and child protective services. Finally, we shifted to future directions and anticipated upcoming changes within the field, including interventional psychiatry, psychedelics and CBD, the role of media in the lives of youth, sex education, and maintenance of certification. In closing, it is our "hope" that this article has inspired our colleagues to push the boundaries of education and training for a better today and brighter tomorrow; meanwhile, honoring and doing justice to the youth and families whom we serve.

CLINICS CARE POINTS

- CAP fellows should receive clinical experience in maternal/parental mental health and early childhood intervention clinics to care for children throughout their life span.
- Fellows should be trained to identify at-risk youth and families and link them to community services, including skills to work with families for prevention, diagnosis, and intervention.
- Incorporate training on Trauma-Informed Care principles and practices, including creating a safe and healing environment, fostering collaboration and empowerment, and addressing mistrust in medical authority figures and systems.
- Provide comprehensive training on evidence-based treatments for trauma, to equip child psychiatry fellows with a range of tools for providing effective care to patients who have experienced trauma.
- CAP fellowship programs should take a holistic approach to evaluating their fellows.
- Emphasis should be placed on maintaining humanity in the practice of medicine and Programs should go beyond just assessing clinical competence and embrace a more comprehensive approach to evaluating fellows.
- Training programs should provide education on a wide range of gender-affirming interventions, including pubertal suppression, hormone therapy, and surgery, while emphasizing the importance of a multifaceted and introspective approach to care that involves examining and addressing personal biases and countertransference reactions.

- Incorporate cultural humility training as a core component of CAP training programs, including developing intercultural communication skills and respect for cross-cultural differences to enhance therapeutic relationships.
- Empower trainees to be change agents in their communities through public education and advocacy. Provide opportunities for skill development in media collaborations and advocacy, emphasizing their importance in combating burnout and promoting impactful careers in CAP.
- Include interventional psychiatry, psychedelics, and CBD therapeutics in the curriculum of child psychiatry training programs.

DISCLOSURE

The authors have nothing to disclose.

REFERENCES

[1] Mian AI, Milavić G, Skokauskas N. Child and adolescent psychiatry training: a global perspective. Child Adolesc Psychiatr Clin 2015;24(4):699–714.

[2] Gerhard UJ, Schönberg A, Blanz B. Johannes Trüper–mediator between child and adolescent psychiatry and pedagogy. Zeitschrift Fur Kinder-Und Jugendpsychiatrie Und Psychotherapie 2008;36(1):55–63.

[3] Nissen G. Hermann Emminghaus. Founder of scientific child and adolescent psychiatry. Zeitschrift fur Kinder-und Jugendpsychiatrie 1986;14(1):81–7.

[4] Evans B, Rahman S, Jones E. Managing theunmanageable': interwar child psychiatry at the Maudsley Hospital, London. Hist Psychiatry 2008;19(4):454–75.

[5] Forman MA. Child and adolescent psychiatry in europe. In: Remschmidt H, van Engeland H, editors. Historical development, current situation, future perspectives. Berlin: Springer-Verlag; 2000 1999, pp 409. US $56.95 ISBN 3798511705. Developmental Medicine and Child Neurology, 42(7), 501–501.

[6] Simmons M, Pacherova L, Barrett E, Child, E. F. P. T., & Adolescent Psychiatry Working Group. Training in child and adolescent psychiatry (CAP) in Europe: 2010–11 survey by the European Federation of psychiatric trainees CAP working group. Eur Psychiatry 2011;26(S2):582.

[7] Broadband Technology. (n.d.). In The New Dictionary of Cultural Literacy, 3rd ed. Available at: https://www.encyclopedia.com/economics/encyclopedias-almanacs-transcripts-and-maps/broadband-technology

[8] Wingfield, N. (2007, June 27). Comcast Blocks Web Traffic, Drawing Ire. The Wall Street Journal. Available at: https://www.wsj.com/articles/SB118289311361649057/. Accessed June 27, 2007.

[9] Cloud, J. (2007, October 22). Teens in Tech: Building Gadgets, Tinkering with Software and Generally Messing Around. Time. Available at: https://content.time.com/time/specials/2007/article/0,28804,1677329_1678542,00.html. Accessed November 01, 2007.

[10] Loades ME, Chatburn E, Higson-Sweeney N, et al. Rapid systematic review: the impact of social isolation and loneliness on the mental health of children and adolescents in the context of COVID-19. J Am Acad Child Adolesc Psychiatry 2020;59(11):1218–39.e3.

[11] Kelly Y, Zilanawala A, Booker C, et al. Social media use and adolescent mental health: Findings from the UK Millennium Cohort Study. EClinicalMedicine 2018;6:59–68.

[12] World Health Organization. (2023). COVID-19 weekly epidemiological update. Available at: https://covid19.who.int/?mapFilter=deaths. Accessed April 12, 2023.

[13] Golberstein E, Wen H, Miller BF. Coronavirus disease 2019 (COVID-19) and mental health for children and adolescents. JAMA Pediatr 2021;175(9):817–8.

[14] Patrick SW, Henkhaus LE, Zickafoose JS, et al. Well-being of parents and children during the COVID-19 pandemic: a national survey. Pediatrics 2020;146(4):e2020016824.

[15] Ravens-Sieberer U, Kaman A, Erhart M, et al. Impact of the COVID-19 pandemic on quality of life and mental health in children and adolescents in Germany. Eur Child Adolesc Psychiatry 2021;30(5):27–37.

[16] American Academy of Pediatrics, American Academy of Child and Adolescent Psychiatry, Children's Hospital Association. (2022). Declaration of a national emergency in child and adolescent mental health. Available at: https://www.aap.org/en/advocacy/child-and-adolescent-healthy-mental-development/aap-aacap-cha-declaration-of-a-national-emergency-in-child-and-adolescent-mental-health/. Accessed December 22, 2022.

[17] The White House. (2022, March 1). Fact sheet: President Biden to announce strategy to address our national mental health crisis as part of unity agenda in his first State of the Union. Available at: https://www.whitehouse.gov/briefing-room/statements-releases/2022/03/01/fact-sheet-president-biden-to-announce-strategy-to-address-our-national-mental-health-crisis-as-part-of-unity-agenda-in-his-first-state-of-the-union/. Accessed March 01, 2022.

[18] Shanafelt TD, Hasan O, Dyrbye LN, et al. Intensive care unit physician burnout and clinician support during COVID-19. J Am Med Assoc 2020;324(20):2007–9.

[19] Schernhammer ES, Colditz GA. Suicide rates among physicians: a quantitative and gender assessment (meta-analysis). Am J Psychiatry 2004;161(12):2295–302.

[20] Moriates C, Dohan D, Spetz J. Women Physicians in the United States in 2020: COVID-19 Pandemic Impacts and Initial Insights. J Womens Health 2021;30(4):482–6.

[21] AAMC. (2019). Diversities in Medicine: Facts and Figures 2019. Available at: https://www.aamc.org/data-reports/workforce/interactive-data/figure-18-percentage-all-active-physicians-race/ethnicity-2018. Accessed December 22, 2022.

[22] Winter S, Diamond M, Green J, et al. Transgender people: health at the margins of society. Lancet 2016;388(10042):390–400.

[23] Feder KA, Smith C. Addressing adverse childhood experiences: implications for health care providers. J Womens Health 2018;27(10):1218–25.

[24] Poteat T, Scheim AI, Xavier J, et al. Global health burden and needs of transgender populations: A review. Lancet 2019;394(10192):412–36.

[25] De Vries AL, McGuire JK, Steensma TD, et al. Young adult psychological outcome after puberty suppression and gender reassignment. Pediatrics 2014;134(4):696–704.

[26] Metzl JM, Hansen H. Structural competency: theorizing a new medical engagement with stigma and inequality. Soc Sci Med 2014;103:126–33.

[27] Pumariega AJ, Rothe E, Mian A, et al, American Academy of Child and Adolescent Psychiatry (AACAP) Committee on Quality Issues (CQI). Practice parameter for cultural competence in child and adolescent psychiatric practice. J Am Acad Child Adolesc Psychiatry 2013;52(10):1101–15.

[28] American Academy of Child and Adolescent Psychiatry. (n.d.). Diversity and Cultural Competency Curriculum for Child and Adolescent Psychiatry Training. Available at: https://www.aacap.org/App_Themes/AACAP/Docs/resource_centers/cultural_diversity/Diversity_and_Cultural_Competency_Curriculum_for_CAP_Training.pdf. Accessed December 25, 2022.

[29] Cama SF, Sehgal P. Racial and ethnic considerations across child and adolescent development. Acad Psychiatry 2021;45(1):106–9.

[30] Tikhonov AA, Espinosa A, Huynh QL, et al. Bicultural identity harmony and American identity are associated with positive mental health in US racial and ethnic minority immigrants. Cultur Divers Ethnic Minor Psychol 2019;25(4):494–504.

[31] Shaligram D, Bernstein B, DeJong SM, et al. "Building" the 21st century child and adolescent psychiatrist. Acad Psychiatry 2022. https://doi.org/10.1007/s40596-022-01543-3.

[32] García Coll C, Lamberty G, Jenkins R, et al. An integrative model for the study of developmental competencies in minority children. Child Dev 1996;67:1891–914.

[33] Olfson M, Blanco C, Wang S, et al. National trends in the mental health care of children, adolescents, and adults by office-based physicians. JAMA Psychiatry 2014;71:81–90.

[34] American Academy of Pediatrics. Committee on Psychosocial Aspects of Child and Family Health and Task Force on Mental Health. The future of pediatrics: mental health competencies for pediatric primary care. Pediatrics 2009; 124:410–21.

[35] Heath, B, Wise Romero, P, & Reynolds, K. (2013). A review and proposed standard framework for levels of integrated healthcare. SAMHSA-HRSA Center for Integrated Health Solutions. Available at: https://www.integration.samhsa.gov/integrated-care-models/A_Review_and_Proposed_Standard_Framework_for_Levels_of_Integrated_Healthcare.pdf.

[36] Office of the Surgeon General (OSG). (2021). Protecting Youth Mental Health: The U.S. Surgeon General's Advisory. U.S. Department of Health and Human Services. Available at: https://www.hhs.gov/surgeongeneral/priorities/youth-mental-health/index.html/ Accessed 2021.

[37] Asarnow JR, Rozenman M, Wiblin J, et al. Integrated medical-behavioral care compared with usual primary care for child and adolescent behavioral health: A meta-analysis. JAMA Pediatr 2015;169(10):929–37.

[38] Yonek J, Lee CM, Harrison A, et al. Key components of effective pediatric integrated mental health care models: A systematic review. JAMA Pediatr 2020;174(5):487–98.

[39] Sarvet B, Gold J, Bostic JQ, et al. Improving access to mental health care for children: the massachusetts child psychiatry access project. Pediatrics 2010;126(6):1191–200.

[40] Straus JH, Sarvet B. Behavioral health care for children: the massachusetts child psychiatry access project. Health Aff 2014;33(12):2153–61.

[41] Dvir Y, Ryan C, Straus JH, et al. Comparison of use of the Massachusetts Child Psychiatry Access Program and patient characteristics before vs during the COVID-19 pandemic. JAMA Netw Open 2022;5(2):e2146618.

[42] Pomerantz AS, Corson JA, Detzer MJ. The challenge of integrated care for mental health: leaving the 50-minute hour and other sacred things. J Clin Psychol Med Settings 2009;16(1):40–6.

[43] American Academy of Child and Adolescent Psychiatry (AACAP) Committee on Collaborative and Integrated Care and AACAP Committee on Quality Issues. Clinical Update: collaborative mental health care for children and adolescents in pediatric primary care. J Am Acad Child Adolesc Psychiatry 2022. https://doi.org/10.1016/j.jaac.2022.06.007.

[44] Burkey MD, Kaye DL, Frosch E. Training in integrated mental health-primary care models: a national survey of child psychiatry program directors. Acad Psychiatry 2014;38(4):485–8.

[45] Gleason MM, Sexson S. Preparing trainees for integrated care: triple board and the postpediatric portal program. Child Adolesc Psychiatr Clin N Am 2017;26:689–702.

[46] Njoroge WFM, Williamson A, Mautone JA, et al. Competencies and training guidelines for behavioral health providers in pediatric primary care. Child Adolesc Psychiatr Clin N Am 2017;26:717–31.

[47] D.R. DeMaso, J.R. Knight, et al., Collaboration essentials for pediatric & child and adolescent psychiatry residents: working together to treat the child. Available at: https://www.aacap.org/App_Themes/AACAP/docs/clinical_practice_center/systems_of_care/Collaboration_Essentials_2013.pdf. Accessed December 27, 2022.

[48] Shaligram D, Skokauskas N, Aragones E, et al. Staff of the Texas Child Mental Health Care Consortium, Watkins M, Leventhal B. International perspective on integrated care models in child and adult mental health. Int Rev Psychiatry 2022;34(2):101–17.

[49] Imberti C, Hertecant J, van den Broek A, et al. Electroconvulsive therapy in children and adolescents: a systematic review of clinical and safety issues. Child Psychiatry Hum Dev 2014;45(4):1–10.

[50] Guerrero APS, Beresin EV, Balon R, et al. New concepts and new strategies for the future. Acad Psychiatry 2022; 46(1):6–10.

Advances in Psychiatry and Behavioral Health 3 (2023) 209–218

ADVANCES IN PSYCHIATRY AND BEHAVIORAL HEALTH

Clinician Well-Being: Addressing Distress and Burnout

Lisa MacLean, MD

Department of Behavioral Services, Michigan State University, Henry Ford Health, One Ford Place, 1C, Detroit, MI 48202, USA

KEYWORDS
• Burnout • Depression • Suicide • Well-being • Distress

KEY POINTS
- Self-perceived wellness is known to worsen during medical education and training.
- Mitigation strategies should have a bifocal approach addressing individual as well as system-level factors.
- Organizations can better support well-being for their workforce by having leadership structure in place to drive well-being strategy and program development.
- Wellness programs need to have a multipronged strategy and should be focused on four key areas: healthy work environments, efficient processes, healthy people, and safe teams.

CONSEQUENCES OF DISTRESS IN MEDICINE

Reflecting on medical school experiences, no doubt many recall a mixture of feelings from high stress, distress, and a sense of inadequacy to the wonder and awe of seeing your first patient and feeling like you had the capacity to use your knowledge and skills to truly impact the lives of others. Medicine attracts a robust, high-performing group of people [1]. At entry, medical students are less depressed, less burned out and have better quality of life but in 2 short years this begins to shift [2,3]. So what happens to students and what can we learn about the medical education learning trajectory and its impact on learners and our faculty (Table 1)? Why, as it was first recognized as a major health issue and despite many efforts, have we had so little success in reducing clinician burnout and distress? [4].

For most, medical school and then residency is one of the most difficult challenges a person can face. Yet, so many choose medicine as their calling due to their deep desire to truly help people [5]. For many clinicians,

the act of caring for others is truly altruistic and results in great professional and personal fulfillment [6]. Indeed, many clinicians would consider it a privilege to care for others and worthy of great personal sacrifice [7]. Unfortunately, sustained self-sacrifice may lead to burnout [8]. Indeed, nearly half of US medical students, residents, and faculty experience symptoms of burnout such as feeling emotionally exhausted, detached from patients, and apathy regarding their impact on patient care [9–12]. Burnout has been branded an epidemic, with societal, human, economic, and personal costs [13,14]. This phenomenon of burnout cannot be ignored, as it places at risk the clinician's quality of life with potential grave individual outcomes as well as long-term downstream adverse consequence for patients [15]. For the clinician suffering from burnout, recovery can seem daunting or even impossible but must not be ignored.

In addition to burnout, many studies have also found a high prevalence of psychological distress among medical students, residents, and faculty both in the United

---

E-mail address: lmaclea1@hfhs.org

https://doi.org/10.1016/j.ypsc.2023.03.005
2667-3827/23/ © 2023 Elsevier Inc. All rights reserved.

TABLE 1
Consequences of Distress in Medicine

	Consequence	Description	Study
1	Depression	Individuals report worsening depression as they go through medical education and residency training. This effect is independent of level of training.	Dyrbye et al [9] 2008 Dyrbye et al [10] 2018 Shanafelt et al [11] 2019 Rosen et al [12] 2006
2	Burnout	All clinical groups (physicians, residents, and medical students) demonstrate an increase in burnout over time.	Gengoux & Roberts [8] 2018
3	Psychological distress	Increased distress is measured using the Mayo Well-Being Index. These findings impact all learners and faculty.	Dyrbye et al [16] 2006 Shanafelt et al [17] 2012
4	Quality of life (QOL)	Using a QOL measurement tool, there is a decline in QOL after 2 y in medical students, and this persists into training.	Dyrbye 2006
5	Empathy	There is a loss of empathy and increased apathy over time. More and more clinicians report a gradual hardening as the stress of medicine increases over the learning trajectory.	Dyrbye et al [16] 2006 Shanafelt et al [17] 2012
6	Patient satisfaction	Clinician burnout can negatively impact quality of care and ultimately patient satisfaction.	Halbesleben et al [15] 2008
7	Medical errors	Both the perception of error and actual error are increased. In addition, physicians who screen positive for depression are at higher risk for medical error.	Dyrbye et al [16] 2006 Shanafelt et al [17] 2012 Pereira-Lima et al [18] 2019
8	Teamwork/Ethics	Psychological distress is linked to dysfunctional interactions between colleague's secondary ethical misconduct.	Dyrbye et al [16]2006 Shanafelt et al [17] 2012
9	Substance use	Individuals report an increase in stress resulting in substance abuse and self-medication	Dyrbye et al [16] 2006 Shanafelt et al [17] 2012
10	Physician suicide ideation/suicide	Regardless of where a physician is at in the educational trajectory, there is not only an increase in suicidal ideation, but also completed suicide.	Dyrbye et al [16] 2006 Shanafelt et al [17] 2012 Dong et al [19] 2022

States and abroad [16,17]. This distress has serious long-term negative professional consequences impacting empathy levels, patient satisfaction, medical error [18], interactions between colleagues and ethical misconduct, as well as personal consequences such as increased substance use/self-medication, depression, and even suicidal ideation and suicide [16,17,19]. Addressing these concerns is important not only for our students, residents and faculty but also for patients and society leading to better outcomes and improved patient satisfaction [20]. What can be more important for the public good than clinical providers who are engaged, effective, and fulfilled?

Individual and Organizational Factors Associated with Distress and Burnout

There are a variety of factors both within and beyond the control of medical school and hospital administrators that contribute to the distress and burnout of our students, trainees, and faculty (Table 2). Unhealthy work environments, long hours resulting in sleep deprivation, disorganized rotations and clinics, broken health care policies and processes, and poor colleague and leader support can all affect the mental health and professional development of these groups [12,21,22]. More and more organizations are recognizing that there are many outside forces that contribute

TABLE 2
Individual and Organizational Factors Associated with Distress and Burnout

	Individual Factors	Impact	Study
1	Conditioning	The clinician personality is one of self-sacrifice and perfectionism. Sustained self-sacrifice over time can link to burnout.	van Nistelrooy [7] 2014 Gengoux et al [8] 2018
2	Work–life balance	An inability to integrate work–life balance into daily life contributes to a lack of overall well-being. To rejuvenate and invest in the work, providers need time outside of medicine to invest in themselves. Clinicians must also have time to invest in personal life events.	Shanafelt et al [38] 2017
3	Values	A misalignment in the individual's personal values and that of the organization can create a disconnect and be a driver of burnout. This misalignment can also be an organizational factor contributing to distress.	Kane [23] 2021 Shanafelt et al [24] 2016; Shanafelt et al [38] 2017
	Organizational Factors	**Impact**	**Study**
1	Work environments	Working in learning environments that are not caring and supportive impacts all team members regardless of their role on the medical team. Hostile work environments are also associated with negative outcomes.	Dyrbye 2010 Rosen et al [12] 2006 Spickard et al [22] 2022 Shanafelt et al [24] 2016 Shanafelt et al [38] 2017
2	Works hours	Long hours without rest and opportunities to invest in personal self-care, such as sleep and exercise, can create increased distress.	Dyrbye 2010 Rosen et al [12] 2006 Spickard et al [22] 2022 Shanafelt et al [24] 2016 Shanafelt et al [38] 2017
3	Efficient processes	The ease of how work is conducted and whether individuals consistently work at the top of their license is directly linked with provider satisfaction.	Kane [23] 2021 Shanafelt et al [24] 2016; Shanafelt et al [38] 2017
4	Culture/policies	A culture that demonstrates that they truly care through transparent leadership messaging and policies that support well-being can improve their workforce well-being.	Dyrbye (2010) Rosen et al [12] 2006 Spickard et al [22] 2022 Shanafelt et al [38] 2017
5	EHR	With the implementation of EHR, there has been increased burnout. The EHR, though important for the delivery of quality and safe care, can take away from the provider's ability to connect at a human level with their patient.	Kane [23] 2021 Shanafelt et al [24] 2016 Alexander et al [25] 2018 Friedberg et al [26] 2014
6	Productivity expectations	A disconnect between messages from leadership that say, "we care about you," and productivity expectations can create a dilemma leaders must navigate.	Kane [23] 2021
7	Resources	Not having the resources a provider needs (like not having a medical assistant to support outpatient work) contributes to distress and burnout.	Shanafelt et al [38] 2017

Abbreviation: EHR, electronic health record.

to burnout. Indeed, the responses to the yearly Medscape survey now lists only organizational and environmental causes for burnout such as bureaucratic tasks, long work hours, electronic health records, lack of autonomy, and a focus on productivity over patient outcomes [23]. Research further supports that these identified burnout drivers do indeed contribute to higher rates of burnout [24]. The electronic health record, for example, results in less clinical time spent with the patient and more time spent interacting with a computer. This movement away from "why people went into medicine" results in a slow degradation of humanism over time, a decrease in job satisfaction, and an overall net harm to physicians [25,26]. Moreover, burnout may also be contagious and burned out clinicians may negatively impact others creating an overall negative work environment and putting the whole team at risk for becoming burned out [27]. The increasing medical regulatory and administrative demands, decreasing reimbursements and the challenge of adopting new and evolving systems only adds to the burden. Additional research by Shanafelt and colleagues also showed that the loss of one clinician or support staff can disrupt a clinical team, with changes in workflow, demand, decreased productivity and morale, until the role is replaced, and that clinician is operating at full work effort. In some cases, this can be longer than a year, resulting in lost revenue of $0.5–$2 million depending on the provider type [28]. We also know that physicians suffering from burnout are significantly more likely to leave health care [29]. Moreover, burnout will also exacerbate the challenges associated with inadequate physician supply, which is projected to get worse; by 2034, demand for all doctors will exceed supply by as many as 37,800 to 124,000—creating a growing gap between supply and demand, according to the Association of American Medical Colleges [30]. Furthermore, an estimated 400 US physician take their lives every year. This loss is profound for our physicians, their families, their patients, and society [31].

Furthermore, beyond the immediate control medical schools and hospital systems, major personal life events such as personal or family illness, having children, financial strain, and relationship issues can occur and impact a person's experience of distress and burnout [21,32]. Burnout places at risk both the clinician's personal and work life can result in significant adverse consequences for patients. Burnout has widespread consequences, including poor quality of care, increased medical errors, patient and provider dissatisfaction, and attrition from medical practice [14]. In addition to personal life events, there is also the psychological impact of working with patients especially after an unexpected adverse event [33]. Clinicians can become second victims after medical errors that result in poor patient outcomes [34]. Society sets a zero-mistake standard for physicians [33]. This standard may isolate those who make mistakes leaving them without healthy ways to cope, resulting in dysfunctional approaches to recovery [33,35]. Poor responses such as isolation, anger, sadness, substance abuse, and callousness toward patients and colleagues place the clinician at increased risk for burnout [35]. Secondarily, burnout can result in increased risk of making additional medical errors and this cycle may result in worsening symptoms causing depression or even suicide [35,36].

Historically, medicine saw burnout as a sign of personal weakness or being ill-suited to the profession [37]. However, later research by Shanafelt and Noseworthy [38] indicated that the origin of the problem is not the personal characteristics of individuals, but instead is deeply rooted to the culture of medicine and a broken care delivery system. To effectively mitigate burnout, we must acknowledge that there are numerous external forces that are real while still empowering clinicians to control what they can, their internal condition. However, clinicians must work collaboratively with leaders to confront, control, and improve external forces as much as possible.

Responding to Distress and Burnout

Despite the Liaison Committee on Medical Education (Accreditation Standard MS-26) [39], the Accreditation Committee for Graduate Medical Education (Section VI.C) [40] and the Joint Commission [41] recognizing clinician distress and burnout and mandating health and wellness programming for all learners and faculty, the high prevalence of distress and burnout has serious personal and professional ramifications. The 80-h work week requirements have not reduced distress, changes in resident lifestyle, or improved patient well-being but may have contributed to learner isolation and reduced opportunity to build community with colleagues [42]. Furthermore, clinician distress and burnout has only become more complex during the COVID-19 pandemic [43].

Initially, many well-being initiatives focused on the individual. We now know that is not the right approach. We also know that though individual characteristics contribute to burnout susceptibility, strategies such as using exercise, battle buddies, and meditation to cope have not had sustained impact on the level of burnout [14,44]. We must also address the hidden curriculum embedded in medicine. The covert messages of the curriculum often role model cynicism by faculty and other teachers and continue to convey the message that only the weak struggle or need help [45]. Concerned about confidentiality and future employment, those in distress often do not seek help [45]. Medicine needs to acknowledge that well-being goes beyond teaching people self-care skills to promote resilience. Indeed, reinforcing these skills without establishing an appropriate organization culture and policies that strive to improve the work environment will be viewed by others as setting a double standard that will only increase cynicism and contribute to anger. This creates messaging that physicians must sacrifice everything to the greater good but should not let themselves get burned out, which puts the onus on clinicians to fix the problem.

Moreover, there is increased evidence that organizational factors (see Table 2) contribute to clinician distress and burnout [38]. Understanding the burnout drivers that are causing the distress and burnout is likely to improve the work environment and support healthy self-care behaviors [38]. We must think outside the box and consider how physicians can consistently work at the top of their license. Health care needs to own the environments it creates and the mixed messages it sends. If we are to have success at mitigating burnout and reducing distress, the primary focus needs to be on the current policies, the organizational culture, and the broken processes that impact how we practice. We must work collaboratively to remove the pebbles and boulders that impact how we do the work.

There are many similarities between the US health care systems current clinician well-being journey and its quality/safety transformation. For example, well-being awareness, and the national call to action, tracks similarly beginning with the Institute of Medicine "To Err is Human" [46] and "Crossing the Quality Chasm." [47] It was then that awareness of and the scope and impact of safety lapses became apparent. In 2000, the Leapfrog Group was formed by large employers and purchasers driving a movement forward in safety and quality. Today, the public, payers, and health care workers know harm can be prevented. The reframing of safety and quality in US health care was not met with support initially, and yet, over time global changes has happened spurred by transparency, measurement, and payment. Now every US health system board measures quality and safety. To fall behind, places the organization at significant reputational and financial risk. There is alignment with the safety and quality journey with clinician well-being.

In their 2019 consensus study report on clinician burnout, the National Academy of Medicine (formerly the Institute of Medicine) stated that health care organizations should "create, implement and evaluate their own interventions using a systematic approach to reducing clinician burnout and burnout risk, and share lessons learned with other health care organizations." [48] The National Academy of Medicine understands, just as in the quality journey, the science of clinician well-being improvement is rapidly developing. So now is the time to accelerate the journey to improve clinician well-being, especially given the impact of the COVID-19 pandemic. Therefore, the National Academy of Medicine recommends that health care organizations conduct small tests of change and pilot research on organizational interventions to improve clinician well-being. Also, they should measure the impact on outcomes and clinical care and share those findings broadly so that together we can transform the health care system into one that serves those who care for others, helps them to be their best self in the workplace, and consistently delivers the highest standards of safety and quality.

So, as we strive to mitigate burnout and reduce distress, we need to approach this work accepting it for the complex problem that it is. The primary cause of burnout is systemic and organizational, and health care organizations should embrace accountability for mitigating the factors driving this epidemic [13,28]. Similar to our quality journey where central resources support local work units and are responsible for their own outcomes, so too should well-being work be developed [49]. These efforts should align with organizational priorities. An effective approach would not simply focus on interventions geared toward the individual but would include an organization multifactorial approach. One suggested that the approach includes these four prongs: healthy work environments, efficient processes, healthy people, and safe teams. Central to the framework is patient well-being. Putting this at the center supports the patient centricity of medicine and recognizes that when hospital systems are well, then patients are more likely to be well (Fig. 1).

Healthy Work Environments

The first prong focuses on the culture of medicine and promotes healthy work environments. When achieved, this healthy culture enables clinicians to be their best selves. It aligns organizational policies with the values of those who work there. In this prong, focusing on "why" we do the work can be very powerful in sustaining professionals during times of stress. A strong sense

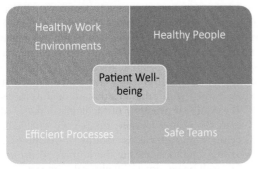

FIG. 1 Clinician well-being strategy.

of meaning and purpose that many clinicians believe about their work can be harnessed as a buffer against burnout [50]. Creating healthy work environments that foster clinician's strengths can facilitate this inherently difficult and challenging work to enable clinicians to be resilient, compassionate, and ultimately fulfill their role in society. Also striving to create work environments where clinicians are allowed to be human. This means recognizing that different people have different life stressors and working to create flexible environments that support everyone no matter where they are in life or what personal demands they have. Through creating programming that teaches about financial concerns, strives for diversity and inclusion, promotes psychological safety, and recognizes childcare challenges, we can show our clinicians that we respect and trust them. The key is developing a cultural attitude that not only supports people but cares for them as individuals.

Efficient Processes
The second prong focuses on "how" the work is done. In this prong, running listening sessions across the organization to better understand the processes of work and how easy or onerous it is to complete daily work can clarify the pebbles that get in the way of the process of work. These listening sessions, much like a focus group, allows leaders to understand the burnout drivers so that targeted interventions can be created. This work aligns nicely with quality improvement work, as new processes need to be created, tested, retested, and improved on. Organizational-level interventions need to be created to reduce overload and enhance autonomy. A sense of control and autonomy can reduce the feelings of helplessness that fuel burnout [50]. Hours worked and administrative paperwork seem greater contributors to burnout than the actual number of patients seen [51]. This suggests that targeted system-level support could

be effective without reducing capacity for care [51]. Other system-based interventions could focus on the limitations of the electronic health records, long work hours, and substantial educational debt all in a culture where we must be always perfect. Regardless of the intervention, every health system is unique in terms of the stressors clinicians face. This supports that the clinician must be involved in the design of the program to enhance their own wellness as they are the closest to understanding the specific drivers that result in distress [52].

Healthy People
The healthy people prong focuses on support for clinicians. For this prong, one must consider the development of well-being programs that focus not only on reacting to stress but also on preventing it. When considering healthy people, one must consider the physical, social, psychological, spiritual, and financial aspects of a person's life and target programming designed to lift the individual in those areas. At the core of any programming must be the philosophy that self-care is a fundamental component of professionalism. Indeed, clinicians must be aware of the stressors that impact them and intentionally create coping strategies that improve their well-being. Self-care will not happen by accident. To be healthy, people must actively create a plan to manage their nutrition, sleep patterns, and exercise [53]. Regardless of life circumstances, there is increasing evidence that well-being can be actively cultivated through intentional happiness-inducing practices [54]. This concept of intentional self-care aligns with the idea that our mental well-being is about much more than the absence of disease [55]. We need to strive to create "cultures" that explicitly values self-care as a norm.

In addition, well-being programs need to consider that life stressors happen beyond the control of an individual. Thus, in addition to prevention, one must also have robust programming that addresses the mental health care needs of this population with a core goal of improving access to treatment. We know that burned out physicians are unlikely to seek professional treatment and may attempt to deal with substance abuse, depression, and suicidal ideation alone [14]. Indeed, a 2014 survey found that nearly 40% of physicians would be reluctant to seek care for mental health due to licensure concerns [56]. Efforts need to be made to reduce stigma and encourage help-seeking behavior as a sign of strength and courage. We need to emphasize that inevitable stressful life events may not lead to impairment but could result in building resilience and fulfillment. This construct allows us to focus on programming that not only reduces burnout but creates professionals who are engaged, experience high energy, feel included and have an increased sense of personal accomplishment. Resilience programming teaching about positive psychology, gratitude, and mindfulness need to be required curriculum [50]. The core goal of this prong is to create programming such that professionals do not just survive their work lives, but flourish [57]. We need to slow down, press pause, and be present for all the moments in our lives, not just for work.

Safe Teams

The final prong is the creation of safe teams. Within this prong, a focus needs to be on how we work as teams with key priorities focused on effective communication and promoting psychological safety. There needs to be space for humanness within medicine. We are not perfect. Indeed, we are imperfect people practicing medicine in an imperfect environment. We can build cohesiveness through peer support especially after critical events but also as a matter of routine. We know that blame and isolation in the face of medical errors and poor outcomes may lead to emotional injury, which is both a contributor to and a consequence of burnout [36]. Whether people request support or not, we should create cultures in which it is expected that people need support during times of stress. These interventions should be designed to be opt out versus opt in and integrated into the daily fabric of the practice of medicine. Within medicine, we need to take steps to address stigma and provide a safe place for supportive healing conversations to happen. Underappreciation, a major contributor to burnout, can also be targeted by health care systems [58]. Creating opportunities to build social community is just one way to show appreciation. Physician affinity groups that demonstrate physicians' value and build community have shown evidence of efficacy [59]. Finally, there is a correlation between strong and effective leadership and the mitigation of burnout. Programming that targets leadership development would be helpful in providing the tools leaders need to provide support, encouragement, and role modeling [60].

Challenges

There are many challenges wellness work faces, but two main issues stand out and will continue to delay the advancement of the work if not addressed. The first is the methodological challenges as there are no standard measurements of wellness that have been developed. When we speak of physician wellness, what do we really mean? What metrics should organizations be using to measure the well-being of their workforce? Organizations need to decide what they are measuring: burnout, distress, resilience, or fulfillment and create a process to incorporate their findings into the culture of who they are. For the science of physician wellness to advance, organizations need to show that they prioritize the well-being of their workforce through annual measurement and tracking. Ideally, the metrics used should allow external benchmarking against like professionals by specialty and job type [38]. Health systems need to show through measurement that they value well-being as much as they value financial and productivity targets. Measurement also enables the organization to deploy attention, energy, and resources to the most challenged work units so that limited resources can be targeted at the people who need it the most [38].

Depending on your goals for measurement, different instruments offer diverse benefits. If the focus is on creating an opportunity for medical students, trainees, and physicians to self-assess distress, the Well-Being Index [61–63] is one tool that gives the individual immediate feedback showing them how they compare with others in their same role. The Mayo Well-Being Index is a validated 9-question self-assessment tool. It is 100% anonymous and provides an immediate feedback dashboard indicating areas of vulnerability and linking directly to local organizational and national resources. In addition, three process improvement questions are asked at the end of each assessment, allowing users to share their feedback on topics such as the drivers of stress in the workplace and additional resources desired. The collection of both qualitative and quantitative data helps systems to identify teams in high distress as well as opportunities for improvement. There are many other tools an organization could choose, understanding your purpose in measuring can allow the organization to pick the tool that best aligns with their goals.

Secondarily, measurement also provides information for targeted program development. For example, when using the Well-Being Index, the administrator of the tool can create reports that not only show the overall or program-specific distress, but also what resources participants are using and how often. In the context of rising national concern regarding physician suicide [31], our organization expanded our emotional support resources with a goal of reducing mental health stigma, encouraging help-seeking behaviors, providing support, and increasing access to care. How often participants access our embedded resources in combination with their overall distress provides information regarding the effectiveness of interventions. Specifically, we reduced stigma and encouraged help-seeking behavior by incorporating education about depression and physician suicide into our required wellness institutional curriculum. We provided support through the development of a buddy program and second victim peer support. We increased access to care by hiring a physician-designated mental health professional into our employee assistance program. Since the creation of these interventions, we have had no physicians within our health system die by suicide and we have gradually and dramatically increased our physician mental health appointments. The utilization of our suicide resources has increased. Unfortunately, the overall distress has persisted. This may, in part, be due to the impact of the COVID-19 pandemic.

In addition to measurement, health systems need to create leadership structure that supports the people within the organization that do the work. There is a good body of evidence to support a leadership structure with a Chief Wellness Officer as the right approach [64]. At minimum, there needs to be a C-suite leader who has a sense of ownership for this body of work for the organization and advocates for and advances well-being work. This person can help drive change, support initiatives, and influence the right people so that developed strategies and tactics have a higher likelihood of success. This person should be a health care professional with extensive experience providing clinical care and should report directly to senior leadership [64]. In addition to a designated wellness leader, to advance the work, there needs to be adequate and dedicated resources including people and funds. This program should not function in a silo but develop intimate collaborations with other institutional efforts and align with stakeholders across an organization [64]. Until a wellness leader is identified and supported, well-being programs will continue to struggle and not likely have the impact they seek.

SUMMARY

Just as distress and burnout in medicine are real and complex, so too are health care systems. There are multiple reasons why health care leaders need to build well-being programs. The first and most important is because it is morally and ethically right to care for those who care for others. In addition, it is expensive to organizations if even one physician leaves [28]. We also know that to ignore this crisis could lead to further crisis, such as physician suicide, and finally, because it is required by regulatory bodies. The ultimate reason is because clinician distress and burnout could harm patients [28].

To have impact and mitigate suffering, health care systems need to have an identified wellness leader and identified metrics, which are used to drive change. Organizations need to approach well-being work similarly to how quality and safety work has been navigated. Systems need to start their well-being work by asking, listening, codeveloping, implementing, measuring impact, and asking again. To have success, organizations need to have a comprehensive strategic model that includes all aspects of the work. People, processes, work environments, and team dynamics need to be part of the overall strategy. Within these areas, tactics need to be developed and customized based on the needs of the organization and the unique challenges each group faces. Organizations need to strive to minimize the stressors that cause burnout but also work to identify and bolster protective factors like creating opportunities for building community and showing appreciation.

In addition to organizational strategies where the bulk of the work should be focused, health care systems should strive to create a culture where there is infrastructure in place that helps clinicians know that their well-being is prioritized by the organization. Investing in personal strategies to improve well-being is a shared responsibility between the clinician and the organization. Programs targeted toward leader development that promotes self-awareness can help to identify areas of vulnerability and provide support and skills to leaders. Leaders, in turn, can strive to create work environments where people are heard, validated, and supported. The recognition that self-care will not happen by accident is key. Clinicians need to invest in themselves and strive to role model healthy behaviors, connectivity, and satisfying work–life integration. In addition, a culture that emphasizes meaning and purpose can help sustain clinicians during times of stress. In the end, we have a moral obligation not only to our patients but also to our colleagues, to strive to optimize each other's wellness. The same compassion we hold for our patients should extend to our colleagues and, finally, to ourselves.

CLINICS CARE POINTS

- Clinician burnout can negatively impact quality of care and patient satisfaction.
- Investing in strategies which connect clinicians with their values can help to reduce distress and burnout.
- For burnout mitigation, organizations need to work continuously on improving the efficiency and delivery of care.

DISCLOSURE

The authors have nothing to disclose.

REFERENCES

[1] Ferguson E, James D, Madeley L. Factors associated with success in medical school: systematic review of the literature. BMJ 2002;324:952–7.

[2] Dyrbye LN, Thomas MR, Huschka MM, et al. A multicenter study of burnout, depression, and quality of life in minority and nonminority US medical students. Mayo Clin Proc 2006;81:1435–42.

[3] Dyrbye LN, Harper W, Moutier C, et al. A multi-institutional study exploring the impact of positive mental health on medical students' professionalism in an era of high burnout. Acad Med 2012;87:1024–31.

[4] Battle CU. The iatrogenic disease called burnout. J Am Med Women's Assoc 1981;36:357–9.

[5] Borges NJ, Manuel RS, Duffy RD. Specialty interests and career calling to medicine among first-year medical students. Perspect Med Educ 2013;2:14–7.

[6] Feldman MD. Altruism and medical practice. J Gen Intern Med 2017;32:719–20.

[7] van Nistelrooy I. Self-sacrifice and self-affirmation within care-giving. Med Health Care Philos 2014;17:519–28.

[8] Gengoux GW, Roberts LW. Enhancing wellness and engagement among healthcare professionals. Acad Psychiatry 2018;42:1–4.

[9] Dyrbye LN, Thomas MR, Massie FS, et al. Burnout and suicidal ideation among U.S. medical students. Ann Intern Med 2008;149:334–41.

[10] Dyrbye LN, Burke SE, Hardeman RR, et al. Association of clinical specialty with symptoms of burnout and career choice regret among US resident physicians. JAMA 2018;320:1114–30.

[11] Shanafelt TD, West CP, Sinsky C, et al. Changes in burnout and satisfaction with work-life integration in physicians and the general US working population between 2011 and 2017. Mayo Clin Proc 2019;94:1681–94.

[12] Rosen IM, Gimotty PA, Shea JA, et al. Evolution of sleep quantity, sleep deprivation, mood disturbances, empathy and burnout among interns. Acad Med 2006;81:82–5.

[13] West CP, Dyrbye LM, Erwin PJ, et al. Interventions to prevent and reduce physician burnout: a systematic review and meta-analysis. Lancet 2016;388:2272–81.

[14] West CP, Dyrbye LN, Shanafelt TD. Physician burnout: contributors, consequences and solutions. J Intern Med 2018;283:516–29.

[15] Halbesleben JR, Rathert C. Linking physician burnout and patient outcomes: exploring the dyadic relationship between physicians and patients. Health Care Manage Rev 2008;331:29–39.

[16] Dyrbye LN, Thomas MR, Shanafelt TD. Systematic review of depression, anxiety and other indicators of psychological distress among U.S. and Canadian medical students. Acad Med 2006;81:354–73.

[17] Shanafelt TD, Boone S, Tan L, et al. Burnout and satisfaction with work-life balance among US physicians relative to the general US population. Arch Intern Med 2012;172:1377–85.

[18] Pereira-Lima K, Mata DA, Loureiro SR, et al. Association between physician depressive symptoms and medical errors: a systematic review and meta-analysis. JAMA Netw Open 2019;2:e1916097.

[19] Dong M, Zhou FC, Xu SW, et al. Prevalence of suicide-related behaviors among physicians: a systematic review and meta-analysis. Suicide Life Threat Behav 2020;50:1264–75.

[20] Haas JS, Cook EF, Puopolo AL, et al. Is the professional satisfaction of general internists associated with patient satisfaction? J Gen Intern Med 2000;15:122–8.

[21] Dyrbye LN, Power DV, Massie FS, et al. Factors associated with resilience and recovery from burnout: a prospective, multi-institutional study of U.S. medical students. Med Educ 2010;44:1016–26.

[22] Spickard A Jr, Gabbe SG, Christensen JF. Mid-career burnout in generalist and specialist physicians. JAMA 2022;288:1447–50.

[23] Kane L. 'Death by 1000 Cuts': Medscape National Physician Burnout & Suicide Report 2021. January 22, 2021. Available at: https://www.medscape.com/slideshow/2021-lifestyle-burnout-6013456. Accessed May 11, 2022.

[24] Shanafelt TD, Dyrbye L, Sinsky C, et al. Relationship between clerical burden and characteristics of the electronic environment with physician burnout and professional satisfaction. Mayo Clin Proc 2016;91:836–48.

[25] Alexander AG, Ballou KA. Work-life balance, burnout, and the electronic health record. Am J Med 2018;131:857–8.

[26] Friedberg MW, Chen PG, Van Busum KR, et al. Factors affecting physician professional satisfaction and their implications for patient care, health systems, and health policy. Rand Health Q 2014;3:1.

[27] Christakis NA, Fowler JH. Social contagion theory: examining dynamic social networks and human behavior. Stat Med 2013;32:556–77.

[28] Shanafelt T, Goh J, Sinsky C. The business case for investing in physician well-being. JAMA Intern Med 2017;177:1826–32.

[29] Sinsky CA, Dyrbye LM, West CP, et al. Professional satisfaction and the career plans of US physicians. Mayo Clin Proc 2017;92:1625–35.

[30] IHS Markit Ltd. The complexities of physician supply and demand: projections from 2019 to 2034. 2021. Available at: https://www.aamc.org/media/54681/download?attachment. Assessed November 19, 2022.

[31] Kishore S, Dandurand DE, Mathew A, et al. Breaking the culture of silence on physician suicide. June 3, 2016. Available at: https://nam.edu/breaking-the-culture-of-silence-on-physician-suicide/. Accessed May 10, 2022.

[32] Dyrbye LN, Thomas MR, Huntington JL, et al. Personal life events and medical student burnout: a multicenter study. Acad Med 2006;81:374–84.

[33] Wu AW. Medical error: the second victim. The doctor who makes the mistakes needs help too. BMJ 2000; 320:726–7.

[34] Lam R. Bouncing back: the struggle of second victim syndrome. Emerg Med News 2018;40:16.

[35] Tamburri LM. Creating healthy work environments for second victims of adverse events. AACN Adv Crit Care 2017;28:366–74.

[36] Shanafelt TD, Balch CM, Bechamps G, et al. Burnout and medical errors among American surgeons. Ann Surg 2010;251:995–1000.

[37] Suran BG, Sheridan EP. Management of burnout: training psychologists in professional life span perspectives. Prof Psychol Res Pr 1985;16:741–52.

[38] Shanafelt TD, Noseworthy JH. Executive leadership and physician well-being: nine organizational strategies to promote engagement and reduce burnout. Mayo Clin Proc 2017;92:129–46.

[39] Liaison Committee on Medical Education. Standards, publications, & notification forms. Available at: https://lcme.org/publications/#Standards. Accessed May 9, 2022.

[40] Accreditation Council for Graduate Medical Education. ACGME Common Program Requirements. 2022. Available at: http://www.acgme.org/What-We-Do/Accreditation/Common-Program-Requirements. Accessed November 18, 2022.

[41] The Joint Commission. Quick Safety Issue 54: Promoting psychosocial well-being of health care staff during crisis. June 3, 2020. Available at: https://www.jointcommission.org/resources/news-and-multimedia/newsletters/newsletters/quick-safety/quick-safety-issue-54/. Accessed November 18, 2022.

[42] Schenarts PJ, Anderson Schenarts KD, Rotondo MF. Myths and realities of the 80-hour work week. Curr Surg 2006;63:269–74.

[43] Dobson H, Malpas CB, Burrell AJ, et al. Burnout and psychological distress amongst Australian healthcare workers during the COVID-19 pandemic. Australas Psychiatry 2021;29:26–30.

[44] Deary IJ, Blenkin H, Agius RM, et al. Models of job-related stress and personal achievement among consultant doctors. Br J Psychol 1996;87:3–29.

[45] Schwenk TL, Davis L, Wimsatt LA. Depression, stigma, and suicidal ideation in medical students. JAMA 2010; 304:1181–90.

[46] Kohn KT, Corrigan JM, Donaldson MS, Institute of Medicine Committee on Quality of Health Care in America. To err is human: building a safer health system. Washington, DC: National Academy Press; 2000.

[47] Institute of Medicine Committee on Quality of Health Care in America. Crossing the quality chiasm: a new health system for the 21st Century. Washington, DC: National Academy Press; 2001.

[48] National Academy of Medicine Committee on System Approaches to Improve Patient Care by Supporting Clinical Well-Being. Taking action against clinician burnout: a systems approach to professional well-being. Washington, DC: National Academies Press; 2019.

[49] Salyers MP, Bonfils KA, Luther L, et al. The relationship between professional burnout and quality and safety in healthcare: a meta-analysis. J Gen Intern Med 2016;32: 475–82.

[50] MacKinnon M, Murray S. Reframing physician burnout as an organizational problem: a novel pragmatic approach to physician burnout. Acad Psychiatry 2018; 42:123–8.

[51] Moy AJ, Schwartz JM, Chen R, et al. Measurement of clinical documentation burden among physicians and nurses using electronic health records: a scoping review. J Am Med Inform Assoc 2021;28:998–1008.

[52] Nasirzadeh Y, Chertkow L, Smith S, et al. What do residents want from wellness? A needs assessment of psychiatry residents to inform a residency wellness strategy. Acad Psychiatry 2022;46:254–8.

[53] Brennan J, McGrady A. Designing and implementing a resiliency program for family medicine residents. Int J Psychiatry Med 2015;50:104–14.

[54] Lyubomirsky S, Sheldon KM, Schkate D. Pursuing happiness: the architecture of sustainable change. Rev Gen Psychol 2005;9:111–31.

[55] Dunn HL. High-level wellness for man and society. Am J Public Health Nation's Health 1959;49:786–92.

[56] Dyrbye LN, West CP, Sinsky CA, et al. Medical licensure questions and physician reluctance to see care for mental health conditions. Mayo Clin Proc 2017;92:1486–93.

[57] Wise EH, Hersh MA, Gibson CM. Ethics, self-care and well-being for psychologists: reenvisionaing the stress-distress continuum. Prof Psychol Res Pr 2012;43: 487–94.

[58] Palamara K, Sinsky C. Four key questions leaders can ask to support clinicians during the COVID-19 pandemic recovery phase. Mayo Clin Proc 2022;97:22–5.

[59] West CP, Dyrbye LN, Satele DV, et al. Colleagues meeting to promote and sustain satisfaction (COMPASS) groups for physician well-being: a randomized clinical trial. Mayo Clin Proc 2021;96:2606–14.

[60] Shanafelt TD, Gorringe G, Menaker R, et al. Impact of organizational leadership on physician burnout and satisfaction. Mayo Clin Proc 2015;90:432–40.

[61] Dyrbye LN, Satele D, Sloan J, et al. Utility of a brief screening tool to identify physicians in distress. J Gen Intern Med 2013;28:421–7.

[62] Dyrbye LN, Satele D, Sloan J, et al. Ability of the physician well-being index to identify residents in distress. J Grad Med Educ 2014;6:78–84.

[63] Dyrbye LN, Szydlo DW, Downing SM, et al. Development and preliminary psychometric properties of a well-being index for medical students. BMC Med Educ 2010;10:8.

[64] Shanafelt TD, Trockel M, Ripp J, et al. Building a program on well-being: key design considerations to meet the unique needs of each organization. Acad Med 2019;94: 156–61.

Advances in Psychiatry and Behavioral Health 3 (2023) 219–227

ADVANCES IN PSYCHIATRY AND BEHAVIORAL HEALTH

Current Landscape, Obstacles, and Opportunities in the Teaching of Psychotherapy in Psychiatric Residency

Christopher W.T. Miller, MD*, Hinda F. Dubin, MD, Mark J. Ehrenreich, MD

Department of Psychiatry, University of Maryland School of Medicine, 701 West Pratt Street, 4th Floor, Baltimore, MD 21201, USA

KEYWORDS

- Psychotherapy • Psychiatry • Residency • Education

KEY POINTS

- Providing the best possible care to patients requires training in psychotherapy with a clear understanding of the different modalities.
- A comprehensive psychotherapy curriculum encompasses didactics, clinical experiences, and supervision that are consistent with residents' evolving competencies.
- Ideally, training programs will promote a culture that highly values psychotherapy, underlining its relevance across acute care and ambulatory settings.

INTRODUCTION

Psychotherapy is a key component of psychiatric residency training. Many medical students who gravitate toward this specialty do so in the hopes of becoming adept, or at least acquiring a foundation, in the different psychotherapeutic modalities [1]. The Accreditation Council for Graduate Medical Education (ACGME) has included demonstrating competency in psychotherapy among the program requirements for psychiatric residencies.

Among the core competencies expected from trainees, the ACGME states that residents must be able to treat patients "using pharmacological regimens, including concurrent use of medications and psychotherapy" as well as use "both brief and long-term supportive, psychodynamic, and cognitive-behavioral psychotherapies" [2]. During the ambulatory year, the ACGME indicates that residents must have significant experience treating outpatients for at least 1 year, including "initial evaluation and treatment of ongoing individual psychotherapy patients, some of whom should be seen weekly" [2]. Although it is clear that psychotherapy training is an important component of residency, there is ample room for interpretation by program leadership in terms of how much exposure trainees have longitudinally to the precepts of therapy, as well as how much didactic, clinical, and supervisory experience should be incorporated beyond the "bare minimum" requirements.

In 2013, the ACGME—in collaboration with the American Board of Psychiatry and Neurology—issued the Milestones project for all accredited specialties and subspecialties in an effort to track resident progression in different domains of competency. The first use of the Milestones in psychiatry was in the 2014 to 2015 academic year, and a 2.0 version was implemented in July, 2021. The Milestones specify two sub-competencies that apply directly to the provision of psychotherapy—Patient Care 4 (PC4) and Medical Knowledge 4 (MK4) [3]. Within PC4, progressive competence is

---

*Corresponding author, *E-mail address:* chmiller@som.umaryland.edu

https://doi.org/10.1016/j.ypsc.2023.03.021
2667-3827/23/

expected in the realms of establishing a therapeutic alliance and respecting boundaries with patients, identifying core feelings within sessions, and selecting and implementing particular forms of therapy ("including supportive, psychodynamic, and cognitive-behavioral"—PC4, level 3) based on patient needs and determination of one's own skill set. PC4 outlines an increasing degree of sophistication in observing the frame and acting in/out around it as well as showing an ability to connect dynamics within sessions to deeper-seated conflicts/schemas for patients. The description of MK4 is focused primarily on understanding the technique, evidence base, and criteria for implementation of the three core individual psychotherapies (ie, the three mentioned in PC4).

Even if these guideposts for training and progression are closely observed, there is a fair amount of variability to be expected in residents' education and clinical exposure, as there are factors pertaining to the reality of different programs that may influence the training experience (Table 1). These include (1) the individual "philosophies" of residency programs, with leadership (eg, program director and director of psychotherapy education) possibly favoring one modality over another; (2)

uneven presence of faculty with content expertise, with programs often relying on voluntary faculty members with psychotherapy practices in the community to provide didactics and supervision; (3) a dearth of psychotherapy supervisors, who are typically not remunerated for their services and who may find it challenging to consistently provide one weekly hour of supervision to a trainee over the course of a year [4]; (4) divergence in the approach to presenting psychotherapy topics in didactics and seminars, with the personal orientation of educators potentially biasing the trainees to align with their own ways of practicing; and (5) uneven commitment to educating residents on the utility of psychotherapy, which may be a factor in programs emphasizing the biological/medical framework of psychiatric practice, deemphasizing the need to learn how to conduct psychotherapy, and possibly resulting in residents becoming discouraged from deepening their engagement with this form of treatment. As Clemens and Notman stated regarding department leadership attitudes toward psychotherapy, "if the leaders were overtly or subtly disparaging toward psychotherapy, they seriously undermined efforts to help the residents develop psychotherapy awareness and skills" (p. 441)

TABLE 1
Factors Limiting Psychotherapy Training

Domain	Relevant Factors
Administrative	• Inconsistent commitment to psychotherapy on the part of residency/departmental leadership • Recruitment of new faculty with psychotherapy expertise may not be a priority for the department or institution
Clinical	• Rotation structure may be geared toward gaining proficiency in acute care or psychopharmacologic management with limited time allotted for psychotherapy sessions • Limited case numbers and insufficiently diverse patient populations can restrict clinical exposure and skill acquisition • Lack of resident interest or of preceptor encouragement may skew trainee away from seeking cases or maintaining sufficient clinical contact for long-term therapeutic processes to develop
Didactic/educational	• "Philosophy" of programs can be highly variable, potentially deemphasizing need for psychotherapy teaching in didactics or seminars • Teaching through virtual platforms can pose unique challenges for psychotherapy educators • Lack of integrative approaches on different services, "cordoning off" the relevance of therapy to outpatient sessions, as opposed to emphasizing its importance and applicability across clinical settings
Supervisory	• Insufficient number of psychotherapy supervisors with content and clinical expertise • Lack of remuneration for educational services and limited availability of outpatient practitioners can limit recruitment of voluntary faculty to augment supervisor pool • Lack of standardization in supervisor approaches can lead to widely disparate resident experiences regarding the psychotherapeutic frameworks being modeled

[5]. Such positions may be rationalized as "real-world preparation" for efficiency-oriented practice settings, minimizing time spent with patients and finding ways to compress assessment, documentation, and refills into minimal timeframes. Such distancing might be part and parcel of the increasing adoption of the electronic medical record, with professionals oftentimes acknowledging they write notes *while* talking to patients. Also, tele-psychiatry has gained impressive momentum (partly due to pandemic-related pressures), but it is a modality that offers manifold distractions, as compared with in-person meetings.

The considerable emphasis in training programs on gaining proficiency in acute care settings may also skew perception of how patients are thought about and treated, focusing on immediate stabilization through psychopharmacology. This framework may have led to individual and group psychotherapy on inpatient units being deemphasized as part of the treatment approach [4]. Also, given the decreasing rates of psychiatrists who provide psychotherapy [6], trainees might be discouraged from learning about psychotherapy, as it may be posited as "a thing of the past" in light of the split-model approach to care. A trend that has been described in some programs is a *declining* interest in psychotherapy over the course of the 4 years of residency training [1], perhaps a reflection of training models that emphasize the non-psychotherapy dimensions of psychiatric practice and do not incorporate psychotherapeutic interventions as a skillset that is part of the identity of the practitioner. Indeed, post-graduate year one residents (PGY-1s) may identify more strongly as psychotherapists, as compared with senior residents [7]. This stands in contrast to the increasing interest in providing therapy by primary care providers (PCPs) [8], the presence of programs to train PCPs in psychotherapy [9], and the fact that a national sample reported that 19% of all psychotherapy visits were provided by PCPs [10].

EDUCATIONAL MODELS

Surveys gauging didactic training, supervised clinical experience, and patient volume in the three core modalities of psychotherapy within US programs showed a wide range of educational experiences [11]. As an example of this, Clemens and Notman investigated psychotherapy exposure at 11 programs in the United States. Over the 4-year span of residency, for psychodynamic therapy, the range of hours of formal education (ie, lectures, seminars, and case conferences) varied from 2 to 200; for supervision, the range was also 2 to

200; and for therapy hours with patients, 8 to 500 [5]. The investigators stated "the low-end figures are consistent with a single training program's admitted lack of intent to train residents to competence in psychodynamic therapy" (p. 439) [5]. In another survey, which investigated residents' perception of the adequacy of psychotherapy education, 14 ACGME-accredited programs were queried in New Jersey, Pennsylvania, and Delaware [12], receiving a 40.5% response rate ($n = 133$ of 328 residents). Median hours of psychodynamic and cognitive behavioral therapy (CBT) were found to be below expert recommendations. In the PGY-3, a year that often focuses on ambulatory work and the learning of psychotherapy, the range of reported hours for conducting CBT, psychodynamic therapy, and supportive therapy was from "none or less than 1 h" to "20+h" per month; a median total reported time was 15 to 21 hours. There was additional dissatisfaction with the time dedicated to interpersonal therapy, dialectical behavior therapy (DBT), and couples, family, group, and child psychotherapies—indeed, in the survey, 82.1% of PGY-4 residents reported "none or less than 1 h" per month of couples and family cases. In this same survey, median monthly hours of supervision for PGY-3s and -4s was 4 to 6 hours, which is below the ACGME requirement for at least two supervisory hours per week. Finally, only nine PGY-3 and -4 residents reported seven or more monthly hours of psychodynamic therapy didactics, whereas none reported more than 7 hours per month of supportive or CBT didactics [12]. Another survey of US programs ($n = 79$ programs responding) indicated that 15% of programs did *not require* didactics in the three core modalities as part of their curricula, and 25% of programs reported that they do not require supervised work in the three modalities [13]. Part of such variability may stem from a lack of consensus among residency leadership as to the importance of incorporating psychotherapy education in training. In an electronic survey of 15 US residency programs ($n = 249$ residents), approximately one-third indicated that key departmental leaders did not seem supportive of psychotherapy training [14].

There can be tremendous variability in how supervision is provided as well. One survey of US programs indicated that approximately 10% of supervisors use audio, video, or direct observation during sessions with trainees [15]. The accessibility of such tools has increased with the emergence of recording and transcription applications, which can create an audio and written account of the session while unencumbering the resident from having to write *at all* during a session. (Although it should be stated, checking for typos and run-on sentences is imperative afterward, lest the supervisory hour be overly consumed with attempting to decipher content.) Beyond this, however, is the immense role of subjectivity and conceptual/philosophical bias that can impact the course of therapy supervision. A psychotherapy supervisor will have preferred methods of fostering a therapeutic alliance and deepening the process in sessions [16]. Such recommendations will be conveyed to the relatively undifferentiated resident, who will likely be learning these skills for the first time, with the anxiety about "doing it right" and not prematurely having a patient quit therapy adding further pressure. This likely will inform an allegiance to and adoption of the supervisors' suggestions. Such guidance is optimally provided in an open, flexible manner, reminding the residents that they are the ones in the room with the patients, and that suggestions made are ultimately just that - suggestions. What is eventually used in the sessions needs to make sense to the trainees and be delivered in ways that are ego-syntonic and in keeping with a resident's individuality. There is, however, the risk of overly biasing the resident toward the conceptual approach of the supervisor, who may make subtle (or outright) criticisms toward other modalities of therapy. Such disparagement can broaden the gap between different modalities, a departure from teaching strategies that would seek to underline common factors and ease the "one or other" way of doing therapy, which is oftentimes more "idealistic" than the reality of what actually happens in sessions, wherein elements from different models are commonly incorporated.

Different approaches have been adopted by programs in attempts to streamline and standardize educational models, for instance by favoring psychotherapies with a more robust and clear evidence base. This may translate to an emphasis on manualized forms of treatment, given the inherency of such modalities for replicability and standardization, as well as the demonstrable effect sizes associated with manualized interventions [17]. This approach could also facilitate supervisor monitoring of trainee acquisition of skills and proficiency. However, as Crocker and Brenner stated (and in alignment with the progression through PC4), "experts and the most effective therapists use and borrow interventions from various types of therapy in a flexible manner in order to best meet the needs of each individual patient" (p. 210) [18]. The investigators go on to state that strict adherence to manualized approaches may be overly simplistic and limit adoption of a flexible, spontaneous therapeutic stance by the trainee. Attentiveness to the rapport is a critical element in optimizing psychotherapy

outcomes, given the demonstrable benefit of a working alliance in shaping successful treatment courses [19,20]. The quality of the therapy provided is also not guaranteed just because a manualized approach is being favored [17]. As Pagano and colleagues stated, "Regardless of the level of specificity of the manual, […] it is unlikely a treatment manual alone will allow a therapist to provide the treatment adequately without supervision and training" (p. 287) [17]. Indeed, the lack of supervisor expertise may limit integration of manualized psychotherapies into training curricula. Also, selective attention to the evidence base of manualized forms of therapy can bias educators away from the equally extant evidence supporting open-ended, less structured modalities. Such an approach can be fueled by the spurious argument that psychodynamic psychotherapy has less of an evidence base than manualized interventions, when indeed research has shown equally successful outcomes with psychodynamic work [21–23].

This landscape relaunches the difficult (possibly insoluble) question of how to find a balance between adherence to specific forms of treatment (which would allow for trainees to appreciate how following a disciplined technical course can lead to particular outcomes) and the necessary flexibility in sessions to tailor one's approach to the needs of individual patients. Solutions that have been suggested include finding common elements within different frameworks of psychotherapies [18], as opposed to emphasizing schisms that can seem unbridgeable over the course of training. Such an integrative approach can allow for different elements from seemingly disparate modalities to be harmonized, indeed taking some pressure off the trainee to "pick a lane" as far as pure technical allegiance is concerned. This would include underlining factors such as therapeutic alliance, the importance of empathy, and instilling positive expectations [1]. Emphasizing the overlapping elements of psychotherapeutic frameworks, drawing useful aspects from each, can reconcile approaches and make the clinical situation less restrictively organized by a particular lens. One example was emphasized by Kay and Myers: "It is often a missed opportunity that dynamically informed supportive therapy is not emphasized. It tends to provide a broad-based perspective in the treatment of more marginally functioning patients and in those with recent circumscribed trauma" (p. 567) [4].

A comprehensive psychotherapy curriculum includes an integrated model based on evidence-based treatments (with an open and ever-expansive understanding of what constitutes the evidence base). Ideally, this curriculum should present introductory level materials in the first year and gain depth over the next three. To the extent possible, clinical corollaries and broad application of psychotherapeutic precepts should be underlined in parallel to didactic experiences. Practitioners with different perspectives should model a collaborative, mutually respectful, and inquisitive approach to patient care, modeling to residents that seemingly disparate treatment frameworks can enrich one another.

BROADENING THE RELEVANCE OF PSYCHOTHERAPY

If psychotherapy is to remain a key component of residency training, its critical place in how *any* psychiatrist (and, arguably, any *provider*) thinks about and interacts with patients needs to be reinforced. Even curricula that ostensibly emphasize the neurosciences should include psychotherapy, particularly given the expansive body of research showing that therapy leads to clear biological changes [24,25]. As Morrissette and Fleisher stated, "Providing education to psychiatry residents in the early years of residency around the neurobiological underpinnings of psychotherapeutic treatment may enhance the preservation of interest in psychotherapy throughout residency training, especially for residents who intend on practicing psychiatry with a chiefly 'biological' treatment model" (p. 492) [1].

The evidence base for the effectiveness of psychotherapy is undeniable [26]. In some conditions (eg, forms of depressive disorder), combining medications *with* psychotherapy is preferable, as opposed to using either modality on its own [27,28]. There are other reports indicating psychotherapy may be *more* effective than medications in certain conditions (eg, one meta-analysis gauging treatments for post-traumatic stress disorder) [29]. There are some conditions (eg, subtypes of adjustment disorder) in which medications may not be clinically indicated, with the literature favoring psychotherapy as the *preferred* intervention [30]. Even when medications are used as the primary intervention, there is evidence that psychopharmacologic agents work *better* when there is a good therapeutic alliance with the prescriber [31,32]. In one study assessing the elements impacting antidepressant responses in patients, it was shown that the *prescribers themselves* were factors that influenced outcomes [33]. The investigators concluded, "it may be that the most effective psychiatrists augment the neurochemical effects of the drug. (…) [T]he *person* of the psychiatrist makes a difference in the response to anti-depressant medication. Therefore, the health care community would be wise to consider the psychiatrist not only as a *provider* of treatment, but also as a *means* of treatment" (p. 290, emphasis in original) [33]. It has also been noted that, as the number of psychiatrists who practice psychotherapy has decreased, the use of polypharmacy has concurrently *increased* [6,18]. This may reflect the difficulty in utilizing non-pharmacologic tools when interacting with patients, leading to an overreliance on medications to address the symptoms being presented. Just as the similarities between modalities of therapy should be better emphasized, outlining the applicability of psychotherapeutic principles to "non-psychotherapy settings" (eg, inpatient units, emergency rooms, consultation–liaison services, and outpatient medication management sessions) could reinforce the relevance of interpersonal dimensions in shaping patient outcomes (Table 2). (The reader is referred to the references listed in this table for additional background [34–41].)

It has been argued that psychotherapy education should be introduced in the first year of training [1]. Having a working understanding of how psychodynamic factors apply to clinical care beyond the outpatient psychotherapy encounter has also been underlined as an important element in residency training. This knowledge can allow providers to recognize the relevance of psychotherapeutic dimensions across clinical settings, including (but not limited to) patients' affective/emotional responses, defense mechanisms, developmental factors informing adult life, and interpersonal functioning (including transference–countertransference dynamics) [42]. As Welton and colleagues stated regarding psychodynamic factors, "A thorough understanding of these principles can benefit psychiatrists in a broad variety of treatment venues" (p. 507) [42]. As one of the present authors has suggested, "we can always *think* psychodynamically about a patient, even if we cannot always *intervene* psychodynamically" (p. 55; emphasis in original) [43].

FUTURE DIRECTIONS

There are several strategies that can address the varying levels of psychotherapy expertise in residency programs. In addition to using voluntary faculty as supervisors, residency programs can partner with one another, sharing their expertise in different forms of therapy via joint didactic classes and case conferences (which are increasingly being done in a virtual format). Programs that function in departments or medical centers that house psychology internships can procure partnership opportunities for didactic and clinical enrichment.

TABLE 2
Interpersonal Elements and Outcomes in Acute Care and Medication Management

Setting	Element/Dimension	Finding
Acute care	Therapeutic alliance	• Therapeutic alliance is associated with better inpatient experiences and improvement at discharge [34] • Positive alliance is associated with fewer rehospitalizations [35]
	Transference/countertransference	• Patients perceived as "difficult" may show less improvement on inpatient units [36] • Diagnoses in emergency settings can be quite inconsistent across providers, suggesting that clinician subjectivity may influence diagnostic assessment [39]
Medication management	Therapeutic alliance	• Alliance can improve clinical outcomes with psychopharmacological interventions [31,32] • Positive alliance improves patient attitudes toward medications, including in populations with severe and persistent mental illness [37] • Alliance is associated with greater medication adherence, including in long-term treatment courses [38,40] • Some conditions do not have a compelling evidence base for medication use, with psychotherapeutic support being the first-line treatment [30]
	Transference/countertransference	• "Attitude" of provider may differentiate outcome, at times more than the specific medication selected [33] • Personal beliefs and preferences of prescribers can be risk factors for polypharmacy [41]

Programs can encourage their trainees to enter fellowship programs that are provided by local analytic institutes, some of which are free of charge. Encouraging residents to engage in personal psychotherapy (while respecting individual choice) can underline the importance programs place on this modality in the development of a psychiatrist. Programs may engage with community providers to compile a list of therapists who might be willing to see trainees on a sliding fee basis or who partner with the residents' insurance. Interestingly, it has been shown that residents who are engaged in their own psychotherapy (as compared with those who are not) place greater value in the "experiential aspects" of psychotherapy training (eg, personal psychotherapy, supervision, hours of therapy conducted) over more instructive aspects such as didactics and readings [12].

Tiered psychotherapy pathways or tracks have also been proposed as a way of tailoring training to nurture individual interest in therapy, permitting residents to advance their experience through additional patient care and specialized didactics, beyond what is provided in the core curriculum [44]. A survey was conducted with US general psychiatry programs in 2018 (with 79

programs responding), finding that 74% of programs did not have a psychotherapy track, 22% did have one in place, and 4% were developing one [13]. Of note, of the programs that did not have a track, 81% indicated that they did not want one. Factors listed as barriers to such an endeavor included a lack of: time, specialized personnel, interest on the part of residents, and funding. (Programs with tracks in place did not feel that additional personnel or funding were necessary for implementing the track.) Given the variability of curricular offerings in non-track programs, the investigators conjectured if having a track was a proxy for the emphasis/priority that a program places (in a broader sense) on psychotherapy as part of the trainees' education [13].

Investment in educational and didactic material can also provide faculty and residents with tools to facilitate content assimilation. The use of book chapters and journal articles relating to psychotherapy can be used in different rotations, allowing for the relevance of such principles to be regularly discussed and applied to patient care in more acute and "medication-oriented" settings. This can broaden the perspective of both preceptor and resident, as these topics oftentimes benefit from discussion to better appreciate their relevance. Maintaining a discipline of engagement with psychotherapeutic literature also empowers a bidirectional education model, as residents can bring queries to preceptors and supervisors about *how* these ideas can be applied to the patients they are treating together, as opposed to wondering *if* these principles are relevant. This reinforces the utility of psychotherapy across settings. Numerous resources are widely available and can be of great use in initial and ongoing engagement with clinically relevant precepts, such as (1) the basic tenets of psychotherapy [45], (2) the psychodynamic dimensions of diagnoses frequently used in psychiatric practice [46], (3) psychotherapeutic aspects of prescribing medications [47,48], (4) psychodynamic constructs of personality disorders [49], and (5) developing a psychodynamic formulation (which can be a useful adjunct to the biopsychosocial model) [50]. Importantly, as residents can benefit from seeing experienced clinicians conduct psychotherapy (either in short snippets or full sessions), some resources include online video access to session material, for instance, select works by Gabbard and Beck [51,52]. The use of annotated bibliographies and model curricula (eg, through the American Association of Directors of Psychiatric Residency Training [AADPRT] and journals such as *Academic Psychiatry*) can provide supplementary material to be used in classrooms and clinical settings.

For those programs lacking expertise in psychodynamic therapy, the American Academy of Psychodynamic Psychiatry and Psychoanalysis and AADPRT offer an annual award (the Victor J. Teichner Award), which sponsors a three-day visit to the program by a scholar to enhance its psychotherapy program. In order to robustly and longitudinally invest in the psychotherapy resources in a residency, the department and/or training program can financially support junior faculty members to obtain additional therapy training. This could take the form of financial assistance to obtain additional education in, for instance, CBT, psychodynamic therapy, DBT, transference-focused therapy, or others of individual interest that might also serve the program's educational needs. If financial support is not an option, providing protected time to undergo additional training could also make a significant difference, particularly for faculty members with compressed clinical and administrative schedules.

SUMMARY

Given the evidence base for the effectiveness of psychotherapy, it is essential that psychiatry residency training

programs provide unequivocal support to allow for comprehensive educational models to be implemented. It is essential for psychiatrists to emerge from residency programs skilled in the full range of treatments that can be offered to patients, while keeping in mind that the interpersonal dimensions of the encounter are in themselves both diagnostic and therapeutic. Integrated curricula are those that seek to bridge psychological and biological domains, underlining common qualities as opposed to reinforcing distinctions. Such an approach will hopefully foster continued interest and proficiency in psychotherapy skills in trainees and educators.

CLINICS CARE POINTS

- Psychotherapeutic principles are relevant beyond outpatient therapy sessions, influencing clinical outcomes on inpatient units and medication management encounters.
- Maintaining ongoing educational engagement over the course of the residents' training can help illustrate the relevance of therapy in experience-near and gradual ways, helping with progressive assimilation of content.
- Integrating material from the extant psychotherapy literature in clinical rotations can encourage bidirectional learning, broadening both preceptor and trainee conceptualization of patient presentations and treatment planning.
- Educational models should seek to underline common elements between modalities of psychotherapy, as well as between pharmacologic and psychological interventions, given their synergistic potential and converging relevance in determining treatment efficacy.

DISCLOSURE

Dr Miller and Dr Ehrenreich have nothing to disclose. Dr Dubin is a principal investigator with Pharmasite Research.

REFERENCES

[1] Morrissette M, Fleisher W. Some Essential Steps for Keeping Psychotherapy at the Core of Psychiatry Training: A Response to Belcher. Acad Psychiatry 2021;45:491–3.

[2] ACGME. ACGME Program Requirements for Graduate Medical Education in Psychiatry. 2022.

[3] ACGME. Psychiatry Milestones - Second Revision. 2020.

[4] Kay J, Myers MF. Current state of psychotherapy training: preparing for the future. Psychodyn Psychiatry 2014;42: 557–73.

[5] Clemens NA, Notman MT. Psychotherapy and psychoanalysts in psychiatric residency training. J Psychiatr Pract 2012;18:438–43.

[6] Mojtabai R, Olfson M. National trends in psychotherapy by office-based psychiatrists. Arch Gen Psychiatry 2008; 65:962–70.

[7] Lanouette NM, Calabrese C, Sciolla AF, Bitner R, Mustata G, Haak J, et al. Do psychiatry residents identify as psychotherapists? A multisite survey. Ann Clin Psychiatry 2011;23:30–9.

[8] Judd F, Weissman M, Davis J, et al. Interpersonal counselling in general practice. Aust Fam Physician 2004;33: 332–7.

[9] Hegel MT, Dietrich AJ, Seville JL, et al. Training residents in problem-solving treatment of depression: a pilot feasibility and impact study. Fam Med 2004;36:204–8.

[10] Himelhoch S, Ehrenreich M. Psychotherapy by primary-care providers: results of a national sample. Psychosomatics 2007;48:325–30.

[11] Sudak DM, Goldberg DA. Trends in psychotherapy training: a national survey of psychiatry residency training. Acad Psychiatry 2012;36:369–73.

[12] Kovach JG, Dubin WR, Combs CJ. Psychotherapy Training: Residents' Perceptions and Experiences. Acad Psychiatry 2015;39:567–74.

[13] Rim JI, Cabaniss DL, Topor D. Psychotherapy Tracks in US General Psychiatry Residency Programs: A Proxy for Trends in Psychotherapy Education? Acad Psychiatry 2020;44:423–6.

[14] Calabrese C, Sciolla A, Zisook S, et al. Psychiatric residents' views of quality of psychotherapy training and psychotherapy competencies: a multisite survey. Acad Psychiatry 2010;34:13–20.

[15] Rodenhauser P. Psychiatry residency programs: trends in psychotherapy supervision. Am J Psychother 1992;46: 240–9.

[16] Miller CWT. In: Starting psychotherapy supervision, The object relations lens: a psychodynamic framework for the beginning therapist. Washington, DC: American Psychiatric Association Publishing; 2023. p. 19–31.

[17] Pagano J, Kyle BN, Johnson TL, et al. Training Psychiatry Residents in Psychotherapy: The Role of Manualized Treatments. Psychiatr Q 2017;88:285–94.

[18] Crocker EM, Brenner AM. Teaching Psychotherapy. Psychiatr Clin North Am 2021;44:207–16.

[19] Flückiger C, Del Re AC, Wampold BE, et al. The alliance in adult psychotherapy: A meta-analytic synthesis. Psychotherapy 2018;55:316–40.

[20] Horvath AO, Del Re AC, Flückiger C, et al. Alliance in individual psychotherapy. Psychotherapy 2011;48:9–16.

[21] Steinert C, Munder T, Rabung S, et al. Psychodynamic Therapy: As Efficacious as Other Empirically Supported Treatments? A Meta-Analysis Testing Equivalence of Outcomes. Am J Psychiatry 2017;174:943–53.

[22] Shedler J. The efficacy of psychodynamic psychotherapy. Am Psychol 2010;65:98–109.

[23] Leichsenring F, Leibing E. Psychodynamic psychotherapy: a systematic review of techniques, indications and empirical evidence. Psychol Psychother 2007;80:217–28.

[24] Miller CWT. Epigenetic and Neural Circuitry Landscape of Psychotherapeutic Interventions. Psychiatry J 2017; 2017:5491812.

[25] Miller CWT, Ross DA, Novick AM. Not Dead Yet!" - Confronting the Legacy of Dualism in Modern Psychiatry. Biol Psychiatry 2020;87:e15–7.

[26] Cuijpers P, Berking M, Andersson G, et al. A meta-analysis of cognitive-behavioural therapy for adult depression, alone and in comparison with other treatments. Can J Psychiatry 2013;58:376–85.

[27] Keller MB, McCullough JP, Klein DN, et al. A comparison of nefazodone, the cognitive behavioral-analysis system of psychotherapy, and their combination for the treatment of chronic depression. N Engl J Med 2000;342: 1462–70.

[28] Thase ME, Greenhouse JB, Frank E, et al. Treatment of major depression with psychotherapy or psychotherapy-pharmacotherapy combinations. Arch Gen Psychiatry 1997;54:1009–15.

[29] Lee DJ, Schnitzlein CW, Wolf JP, et al. Psychotherapy versus Pharmacotherapy for Posttraumatic Stress Disorder: Systemic Review and Meta-analyses to Determine First-line Treatments. Depress Anxiety 2016;33:792–806.

[30] O'Donnell ML, Metcalf O, Watson L, et al. A Systematic Review of Psychological and Pharmacological Treatments for Adjustment Disorder in Adults. J Trauma Stress 2018;31:321–31.

[31] Cohen JN, Drabick DAG, Blanco C, et al. Pharmacotherapy for social anxiety disorder: Interpersonal predictors of outcome and the mediating role of the working alliance. J Anxiety Disord 2017;52:79–87.

[32] Zilcha-Mano S, Roose SP, Barber JP, et al. Therapeutic alliance in antidepressant treatment: cause or effect of symptomatic levels? Psychother Psychosom 2015;84: 177–82.

[33] McKay KM, Imel ZE, Wampold BE. Psychiatrist effects in the psychopharmacological treatment of depression. J Affect Disord 2006;92:287–90.

[34] Clarkin JF, Hurt SW, Crilly JL. Therapeutic alliance and hospital treatment outcome. Hosp Community Psychiatry 1987;38:871–5.

[35] Priebe S, Gruyters T. The role of the helping alliance in psychiatric community care. A prospective study. J Nerv Ment Dis 1993;181:552–7.

[36] Colson DB, Cornsweet C, Murphy T, et al. Perceived treatment difficulty and therapeutic alliance on an adolescent psychiatric hospital unit. Am J Orthopsychiatry 1991;61:221–9.

[37] Lim M, Li Z, Xie H, et al. The Effect of Therapeutic Alliance on Attitudes Toward Psychiatric Medications in Schizophrenia. J Clin Psychopharmacol 2021;41:551–60.

[38] Frank E. Enhancing patient outcomes: treatment adherence. J Clin Psychiatry 1997;58(Suppl 1):11–4.

[39] Lieberman PB, Baker FM. The reliability of psychiatric diagnosis in the emergency room. Hosp Community Psychiatry 1985;36:291–3.

[40] Howgego IM, Yellowlees P, Owen C, et al. The therapeutic alliance: the key to effective patient outcome? A descriptive review of the evidence in community mental health case management. Aust N Z J Psychiatry 2003;37:169–83.

[41] Guillot J, Maumus-Robert S, Bezin J. Polypharmacy: A general review of definitions, descriptions and determinants. Therapie 2020;75:407–16.

[42] Welton RS, Cowan AE, Ferrari RM. You Still Do That? Training Residents to Use Psychodynamic Theory. Acad Psychiatry 2020;44:507–8.

[43] Miller CWT. Words and silence. In: The object relations lens: a psychodynamic framework for the beginning therapist. Washington, DC: American Psychiatric Association Publishing; 2023. p. 51–65.

[44] Pellegrino LD, Chang SK, Alexander C, et al. Supplementing Psychiatry Resident Training with a Tiered Psychotherapy Pathway. Acad Psychiatry 2021;45:200–2.

[45] Bender S, Messner E. Becoming a therapist: what do I say, and why?. 2nd edition. New York: The Guilford Press; 2022.

[46] Gabbard G. Psychodynamic psychiatry in clinical practice. 5th edition. Washington, DC: American Psychiatric Publishing; 2014.

[47] Mintz D. Psychodynamic psychopharmacology: caring for the treatment-resistant patient. Washington, DC: American Psychiatric Publishing; 2022.

[48] Cabaniss D. Shifting Gears: The Challenge to Teach Students to think Psychodynamically and Psychopharmacologically at the Same Time. Psychoanal Inq 1998;639–56.

[49] McWilliams N. Psychoanalytic diagnosis, second edition: understanding personality structure in the clinical process. 2nd edition. New York: The Guilford Press; 2020.

[50] Cabaniss D, Cherry S, Douglas C, et al. Psychodynamic formulation. West Sussex (UK): Wiley-Blackwell; 2013.

[51] Beck J. Cognitive behavior therapy: basics and beyond. 3rd edition. New York: The Guilford Press; 2021.

[52] Gabbard G. Long-term psychodynamic psychotherapy: a basic text. 3rd edition. Arlington (VA): American Psychiatric Publishing; 2017.

Advances in Psychiatry and Behavioral Health 3 (2023) 229–237

ADVANCES IN PSYCHIATRY AND BEHAVIORAL HEALTH

Crisis Management in Psychiatry

Overview and Training

Vedrana Hodzic, MD[a,b,c,*], **Sarah E. Johnson, MD, JD**[d]

[a]American Psychiatric Association Foundation - 800 Maine Avenue, S.outhwest, Suite 900, Washington, DC 20024, USA; [b]University of Maryland School of Medicine, Department of Psychiatry, Baltimore, MD 21201, USA; [c]Psychiatric Urgent Care – Sheppard Pratt, 6501 North, Charles Street, Towson, MD 21204, USA; [d]University of Maryland/Sheppard Pratt Psychiatry Residency Program, 701 West Pratt Street, 4th Floor, Baltimore, MD 21201, USA

KEYWORDS
- Emergency psychiatry • Crisis management • Behavioral emergency • Residency • Training

KEY POINTS

- Principles of effective psychiatric crisis management include thorough clinical assessment, judicial use of pharmacology, verbal de-escalation, prioritization of trauma-informed care, and safety and disposition planning.
- Emergency psychiatric management is a crucial competency that must be acquired during residency training, requires proficiency in a range of advanced skills, and may be learned in many settings.
- Evidence suggests that residency training in emergency psychiatry can be enhanced to better prepare future psychiatrists to manage mental health crises skillfully and safely.

INTRODUCTION

A mental health crisis is considered to be a situation where a person's behavior places them at risk of hurting themselves or others, and/or prevents them from being able to care for themselves or function in the community [1]. A significant and growing proportion of emergency department encounters constitute a behavioral emergency [2]. Psychiatrists therefore frequently confront and must adeptly manage such crises. Effective management requires a range of complex skills that should be developed and honed during residency training. This article summarizes key principles of psychiatric crisis management and current perspectives on training residents to skillfully navigate those emergencies.

PRINCIPLES OF MANAGEMENT OF PSYCHIATRIC CRISES

The main goals of evaluating and treating individuals in a mental health crisis are to make sure they are medically stable, evaluate for safety, relieve the patient's distress, and form a safe and well-communicated plan that gets the patient to the least restrictive environment [2], all as rapidly as possible in a supportive and collaborative manner with the ultimate intent of achieving stabilization and preventing a return of crisis-level symptoms [2].

The Substance Abuse and Mental Health Services Administration (SAMHSA) identified "10 essential values" to guide management of a mental health crisis [3].
- "Avoiding harm";
- "Intervening in person-centered ways";

---

*Corresponding author. 800 Maine Avenue, Southwest, Suite 900, Washington, DC 20024. *E-mail address:* vhodzic@psych.org

https://doi.org/10.1016/j.ypsc.2023.03.020
2667-3827/23/

- "Shared responsibility";
- "Addressing trauma";
- "Establishing feelings of personal safety";
- "Based on strengths";
- "The whole person";
- "The person as credible source";
- "Recovery, resilience, and natural supports"; and
- "Prevention."

SAMHSA similarly elucidated principles for honoring the essential values in the delivery of emergency mental health care [3].

Effectively managing a psychiatric emergency requires physicians to thoroughly evaluate and treat a variety of high-stakes concerns: suicidal ideation, homicidal ideation, agitation, aggression, acute psychosis, acute mania, and acute psychological trauma. Providers must simultaneously manage safety risk while the patient is in the emergency setting and assess the patient's ability to safely return to the community. The crucial efforts to ensure safety and prevent danger to self and others need to be done concurrently with the work to alleviate the patient's suffering [2]. Additionally, physicians must be familiar with the nuances of the governing laws and regulations in their state of practice, which ultimately dictate the options and standards for involuntary treatment if indicated.

Behavioral Emergencies

While seeking or receiving psychiatric emergency care, it is not uncommon for patients to display behavior that deviates from their baseline and may pose a safety concern to themselves or others [4]. Effectively managing patient agitation while maintaining safety is a critical skill required of emergency psychiatric providers.

The American Association for Emergency Psychiatry (AAEP) issued guidelines as a result of Project BETA (Best Practices in Evaluation and Treatment of Agitation), an effort undertaken in October 2010 to reconcile discrepancies in treatment approaches and ensure the service of the patient's best interests [4]. Project BETA provided general recommendations to guide the treatment of agitation [5].

- Avoiding the use of medication for restraint purposes,
- Preference for and attempting nonpharmacologic intervention before the use of medication,
- When used, medication dosing should aim to manage symptoms rather than sedate patients,
- If possible, patient involvement in medication selection should be solicited and encouraged, and

- Preference for oral over intramuscular medications.

Psychiatrists should strive to identify the cause of the agitation, promptly evaluate and treat any underlying medical causes, and tailor the choice of any medication, if indicated, accordingly [5]. Indeed, understanding the cause and mechanism of agitation facilitates the appropriate selection of medication and avoids the overuse of pharmacologic interventions that are unlikely to be optimally effective [6]. Specifically, Wilson and colleagues advise the use of the following agents if agitation cannot be adequately resolved by nonpharmacologic means [5].

- Benzodiazepines for agitation due to intoxication with a recreational drug or withdrawal from alcohol or benzodiazepines;
- Antipsychotics, and in particular haloperidol, for agitation due to intoxication with alcohol;
- Second-generation antipsychotics for agitation due to psychiatric illness with oral risperidone particularly noted for safety and efficacy and preference for intramuscular ziprasidone or olanzapine if oral medication is not feasible;
- Second-generation antipsychotics for agitation due to delirium that is not attributable to alcohol or benzodiazepine withdrawal or sleep deprivation;
- Benzodiazepines for agitation of unknown cause without psychotic features and antipsychotics for agitation of unknown cause with psychotic features.

Subsequent research suggests that psychiatry residents' practices are more aligned with Project BETA guidelines than those of attending psychiatrists or psychiatric nurses [7]. Tangu and colleagues concluded that for the management of acute agitation, compared with psychiatry residents, a significantly larger percentage of attending psychiatrists and psychiatric nurses do not perceive second generation antipsychotics to be as effective as first generation antipsychotics [7]. Notably, notwithstanding Project BETA guidelines, all 3 groups opted for intramuscular haloperidol, lorazepam, and diphenhydramine to manage severe agitation [7].

Medical Management of Psychiatric Emergencies

Patients presenting with a behavioral disturbance must be evaluated for a potential underlying medical cause, which may pose an imminent threat to life [8]. Project BETA issued guidance on the medical assessment of agitated patients [8]. Certain presentations are particularly concerning and merit emergent evaluation: loss of memory, disorientation, severe headache, extreme muscle stiffness or weakness, heat intolerance, unintentional weight loss, new onset psychosis, difficulty breathing, abnormal vital signs, frank trauma, anisocoria, slurred speech, lack of coordination, seizures, or hemiparesis [8]. Collateral informants can be invaluable in gathering a thorough history, which has been noted to have far greater utility than a physical examination for accurate medical diagnosis of patients with psychiatric presentations [8]. A targeted assessment to exclude acute medical issues should be performed for patients with a history of psychiatric illness and a consistent current presentation [8]. If the patient does not have a history of psychiatric illness, he or she requires a fulsome medical evaluation, including laboratory and imaging diagnostic tests as indicated [8]. Diagnostic testing should be targeted to the most heavily suspected causes on the differential [8]. Until otherwise excluded, a medical cause should be assumed for patients presenting with new-onset agitation, a complex medical history, or at an age that is atypical for a novel psychiatric illness [8].

Verbal De-escalation

As previously discussed, nonpharmacologic methods for agitation management are always preferred provided they can be safely undertaken. Verbal de-escalation includes "a range of nonphysical verbal and environmental interventions whose goal is redirection of the agitated patient to a calmer state of mind" [9].

With respect to agitation management, Project BETA outlined four main objectives: "(1) ensure the safety of the patient, staff, and others in the area; (2) help the patient manage his emotions and distress and maintain or regain control of his behavior; (3) avoid the use of restraint when at all possible; and (4) avoid coercive interventions that escalate agitation" [10]. Richmond and colleagues observed a relative dearth of literature detailing successful verbal de-escalation approaches [10]. Project BETA issued guidelines to guide clinicians' use of verbal de-escalation [10].

- Arranging physical space to optimize safety,
- Staff should be well suited for the complexity of agitation management,
- Staff should be appropriately trained in de-escalation,
- Employ appropriate numbers of staff,
- Use objective agitation measurement scales, and
- Clinical staff should monitor their emotions and ensure their own comfort in interacting with the patient.

Project BETA also outlined "10 domains of de-escalation" to guide clinical management of agitation [10].

- Ensure adequate personal space;
- Use nonthreatening nonverbal communication that fosters a sense of safety;
- Verbal engagement of the patient by a single staff member, who orients and reassures the patient;
- Use simple and brief communication, repeating as necessary and allowing adequate processing time;
- Solicit patient's wishes and emotions;
- Actively listen and adhere to Miller's Law[a];
- Agree wherever possible;
- Communicate expectations, including boundaries and consequences, respectfully and guide the patient on self-control;
- Present options, including for medication;
- Convey hopefulness while communicating realistic expectations;
- Debrief with the patient and staff.

Lavelle and colleagues found that successful de-escalation resulted in fewer and less aggressive events, suggesting that optimal de-escalation efforts should occur early in the sequence of behavioral emergency management [11]. In a British study, Price and colleagues described a range of intervention from support to nonphysical control to physical control and collected staff input on staff, patient, and environmental factors that led to success or failure of de-escalation efforts [12]. They noted that "more authoritative 'nonphysical control' techniques" may increase aggression and were often used due to "moral judgements regarding the function of the aggression, trial-and-error, and ingrained local customs" rather than based on an assessment of increased risk [12]. Knowing the individual patient was key to choosing an effective de-escalation method [12]. Of concern, staff identified inadequate staffing and staff anxiety were the reasons that more restrictive interventions were pursued [12]. A similar study explored patient feedback and observed that the majority of participants believed that restrictive practices rather than de-escalation techniques are used in response to escalating aggression [13]. Price and

---

[a]"To understand what another person is saying, you must assume that it is true and try to imagine what it could be true of." Richmond JS, Berlin JS, Fishkind AB, Holloman GH Jr, Zeller SL, Wilson MP, et al. Verbal de-escalation of the agitated patient: consensus statement of the American Association for Emergency Psychiatry project BETA de-escalation workgroup. West J Emerg Med 2012;13(1):17-25 (quoting Elgin SH. *Language in Emergency Medicine: A Verbal Self-Defense Handbook.* Bloomington, IN: XLibris Corporation; 1999).

colleagues concluded that to use de-escalation more effectively, it may be required to increase accountability for misuse of restrictive practices and disrespect of patients; address ward rule culture; and reduce the social distance between patients and staff [13].

Krull and colleagues found that multidisciplinary staff participating in a simulation involving verbal de-escalation and physical restraint reported significant positive change in 5 domains (knowledge, skills, ability, confidence, and preparedness to manage a violent patient) on a pretest/posttest survey [14]. Thompson and colleagues reported a significant increase in oncology nurses' confidence managing agitation 3 months after a virtual de-escalation training [15]. Story and colleagues similarly found a significant increase in medical and surgical nurses' confidence 3 months after a classroom-based workplace violence prevention training [16]. A systematic review concluded that multicomponent interventions are the most effective means to impact rates of workplace violence [17].

Commercial courses are available for purchase by health-care facilities to train their staff in de-escalation techniques [18,19]. Well-known options include the Crisis Prevention Institute's Nonviolent Crisis Intervention (NCI) program, which teaches staff de-escalation techniques and both restrictive and nonrestrictive interventions [20], and The Mandt System, which teaches evidence-based conflict resolution and de-escalation techniques to help prevent workplace violence [21]. Beaulieu and colleagues concluded that NCI training failed to reduce the use of restraints or pro re nata medication on an inpatient brain injury unit and observed that, at certain times, their use increased after training [19]. Gillam found that as more emergency department staff were NCI-trained, the monthly incidence of behavioral codes during a year-long period increased overall but significantly decreased during the prior 90 to 150 day period [18]. Those findings suggest that the benefits of NCI training may be relatively short-lived and require periodic retraining in order to maintain gains in violence prevention [18,19]. A noteworthy limitation of both the Beaulieu and Gillam studies was the lack of physician inclusion among study subjects.

Therapeutic Alliance

Patients seeking emergency psychiatric care often have histories of personal trauma [2]. Physicians should approach all patients from a trauma-informed perspective in order to avoid retraumatization [2]. The *trauma-informed* approach to emergency psychiatric care includes therapeutic alliance, avoiding coercion, and treatment in the least restrictive setting [2]. A positive

therapeutic alliance may lower the risk of patient aggression [2]. Avoiding coercion involves providing informed consent and the administration of oral medications willingly, instead of by forcible injections; utilizing verbal de-escalation techniques rather than physical restraints to bring agitated individuals to calmness; and having little or no infringement on a patient's rights [2]. Project BETA advised the use of the least restrictive seclusion or restraint when required due to dangerousness and in conjunction with ongoing verbal de-escalation and medication with a goal of ending seclusion and restraint as quickly as safely possible [22].

SAMHSA identified 4 assumptions and 6 principles governing the delivery of trauma-informed care [23]. The assumptions include the following [23]:

- "[A]ll people at all levels of the organization or system have a basic *realization* about trauma and understand how trauma can affect families, groups, organizations, and communities as well as individuals."
- "People in the organization or system are also able to *recognize* the signs of trauma."
- "The program, organization, or system *responds* by applying the principles of a trauma-informed approach to all areas of functioning."
- "A trauma-informed approach seeks to *resist retraumatization* of clients as well as staff."
  The principles emphasize [23].
- "Safety";
- "Trustworthiness and transparency";
- "Peer support";
- "Collaboration and mutuality";
- "Empowerment, voice, and choice"; and
- "Cultural, historical, and gender issues."

Kosman and Levy-Carrick observed that there is a dearth of literature for the development of a trauma curriculum for psychiatry residents [24]. They advocated multifaceted benefits of educating residents on trauma-informed care [24]:

First, residency training provides the educational venue for residents to learn this material, for residents to join trauma-informed care activities, and for senior staff to model and guide trainees on trauma-informed care principles in practice. Second, residency training comes rife with challenging cases, exposure to traumas and death, and bearing witness to emotional narratives, all in the context of residents also undergoing personal and professional life changes.

Disposition

Studies and clinical practice indicate that with prompt intervention, 60% to 80% of psychiatric emergencies can be resolved in under 24 hours and without the need for inpatient admission [25]. Providers must therefore be prepared to connect patients with crucial services before discharge from the emergency setting and should hone their familiarity with available community resources. Disposition planning includes referrals to mental health clinics and/or substance abuse treatment programs, scheduling outpatient appointments when possible, and providing instructions on what to do if crisis symptoms reoccur [2]. For many individuals, the lack of access to reliable housing is a concomitant issue affecting the patient's well-being and prognosis. Such patients may benefit from a referral to a crisis bed or residential substance abuse treatment when there is a co-occurring substance abuse disorder present. For example, at the University of Maryland Medical Center (UMMC), a Screening, Brief Intervention, and Referral to Treatment team is an invaluable collaborator in executing successful disposition plans for patients for whom substance abuse treatment is indicated and desired. Discharging from the emergency setting with an appointment scheduled may substantially reduce a patient's chance of subsequent psychiatric hospitalization [2].

TRAINING PRINCIPLES FOR PSYCHIATRIC CRISES

Guidelines for Resident Education and Training in Emergency Psychiatry

The Accreditation Council for Graduate Medical Education (ACGME) mandates that resident experience in emergency psychiatry "must be conducted in an organized, supervised psychiatric emergency service" that does not consist solely of on-call experience and does not count toward the separate requirement of 12 months of outpatient work [26]. These resident experiences must include the triage of psychiatric patients and crisis evaluation and management [26]. Interestingly, although the overwhelming majority of chief residents in US psychiatry residency programs who responded to a 2010 survey reported adequate emergency psychiatry training, 58.5% of them acknowledged a lack of awareness of ACGME requirements regarding emergency psychiatry [27]. Nearly a third (28.8%) of study participants reported receiving less than half of their emergency psychiatry training from experiences other than on-call service [27]. Direct supervision was reported to occur less frequently during on-call emergency psychiatry service [27]. Those findings call into question the degree to which all psychiatry residency programs are in full compliance with ACGME requirements for emergency psychiatry training [27].

In 2004, the AAEP issued guidelines for residency training in emergency psychiatry, acknowledging that psychiatric emergency service delivery had shifted from a triage model to a treatment model, where definitive treatment based on a reliable and specific diagnosis is initiated in the psychiatric emergency service prior to disposition being arranged [28]. The AAEP recommended a minimum of 2 months of full-time work on an emergency psychiatry rotation during the PGY-1 or PGY-2 years [28]. The preferred setting is a multidisciplinary psychiatric emergency service (PES) that is affiliated with a medical emergency department providing 24-hour service [28]. Settings such as crisis clinics, crisis residential units, mobile crisis units, and medical emergency departments, which also involve exposure to walk-in visit, brief assessments, and a high level of urgency and severity of presentation and intervention, offer alternative training sites if exposure to a PES is not feasible [28].

The AAEP outlined 10 training objectives for psychiatry residents: prioritization skills, patient assessment and management skills, crisis telephone call skills, professional communication skills, time management skills, leadership skills, medicolegal knowledge, systems knowledge, self-knowledge, and child and adolescent emergency psychiatry [28]. The AAEP also emphasized the need for direct supervision by attending psychiatrists free from the burden of cross-coverage responsibilities that would likely compete with and limit effort devoted to resident education [28]. Aspects of adequate supervision include observation by the resident of assessments by senior psychiatrists and other clinicians; the opportunity to interview patients with others; delivery of feedback to the resident on observed interviews; daily supervision; review and cosigning of the resident's documentation; and gradual assumption of responsibility [28]. The AAEP guidelines also specified a comprehensive list of curriculum topics to be covered during residency [28].

Training Settings

As previously discussed, a PES is an ideal training ground for psychiatry residents. A PES also allows for many opportunities for exposure to the medicolegal aspects of psychiatry, which include assessing consent, capacity, and navigating laws related to involuntary assessment and treatment [29]. Additionally, a PES setting also provides advanced training opportunities in emergency psychiatry through electives, chief resident positions, and fellowships [28].

Resident training on daytime shifts in PES offers multiple benefits, including more direct supervision and the opportunity for gradual assumption of increasing responsibility [29]. Successful handoff of patient care at shift change is essential to ensuring patient safety and challenges trainees to exercise and hone this professional skill [29]. Morning report offers another opportunity for teaching, although it should not significantly delay the dismissal of overnight residents or hamper the day team from efficiently proceeding with patient care [29].

A Canadian study of resident experiences in PES identified challenges such as *"hectic pace and workload,"* *clinical challenges* related to managing critically ill patients in unpredictable situations, feeling *"disrespected and misunderstood* by the ER doctors and nurses," and challenges in safety and risk associated with a 24-hour PES shift requirement [30]. Nevertheless, residents recognized the invaluable education opportunity provided by the PES [30]. Residents reported variable quality of relationships with members of the PES multidisciplinary team, which influenced their satisfaction with the PES experience [30]. McIlwrick and Lockyer proposed that those relationships could be improved through collaboration during morning rounds; multidisciplinary participation in journal clubs, staff meetings, and critical incident reviews; joint presentations of grand rounds or morbidity and mortality rounds; resident leadership in medical student education; and supervision by senior PES team members of resident-driven quality improvement projects [30].

Outside from a dedicated PES, patients experiencing a mental health crisis may be evaluated by a consulting psychiatrist in the medical emergency department or via telepsychiatry, in a mental health wing of the medical emergency department, or in a variety of psychiatric emergency facilities such as psychiatric urgent care centers, crisis stabilization units, and emergency psychiatric assessment treatment and healing (EmPath) units [2]. Psychiatric emergency facilities may be embedded in a hospital or health system or independent and, as such, the extent of their screening, diagnostic, and treatment capabilities varies with the setting and available resources [2]. All of those settings provide potentially rich training experiences in emergency psychiatry. Bennett and colleagues reported on first-year residents' positive experience in an acute care psychiatric clinic of a community mental health center [31]. Trainees particularly appreciated the opportunity for and quality of direct supervision in this setting [31].

Safety Training

Learning to manage safety risk is a crucial aspect of resident training in emergency psychiatry. Concerns about maintaining personal safety while on duty may provoke significant anxiety among clinical staff and particularly trainees—unfortunately, with good reason. Although the experience of assault against residents in all specialties is alarming, residents in psychiatry are at the highest risk [32]. In a 2012 systematic review, Kwok and colleagues reported a prevalence rate of assaults against psychiatry residents ranging from 25% to 64% compared with 38% for surgical residents, 26% for emergency medicine residents, 16% to 40% for internal medicine residents, and 5% to 9% for pediatric residents [32]. Earlier study suggested that 72% to 96% of psychiatric residents have received a verbal threat and 36% to 56% have been physically assaulted on the job [33]. Dvir and colleagues found that 1 in 4 of responding residents had been physically assaulted, and the majority had been "threatened, physically intimidated, or subjected to unwanted advances" during their training, but only 36% reported that their program provided adequate training and under half thought that the facilities they had for patient assessment were safe [34].

Identifying patients at risk for violence rapidly provides the opportunity to implement preventative measures to reduce the risk of injury and minimize escalation [35]. Physical and behavioral indicators portend agitation [35]. Unfortunately, there is no definitive instrument for violence assessment [9], yet a clinician's ability to anticipate and, where possible, defuse and prevent violence is critical to maintain the safety of both patients and staff. Kwok and colleagues found that while the percent of psychiatry residents receiving formal training on managing patient violence varied widely, only a minority believed they received adequate training [32]. Others have noted similar concern that psychiatry residents receive inadequate training on violence management [33,36].

Not surprisingly, research suggests that the ability to accurately assess violence risk depends on experience [36,37]. Wong and colleagues found significant differences in the number of risk factors about which staff psychiatrists and psychiatric residents asked during a hypothetical violence risk assessment [37]. Seniority, including among residents, directly correlated with the number of risk factors elicited on interview [37]. The Historical, Clinical and Risk Managemnt - 20 (HCR-20) is a structured tool to assess the risk of violence. A study found that the number of HCR-20 items identified by a resident was significantly related to the number of suicidal and violent patient encounters the resident had and the number of patients the resident had discharged with a duty to warn during their training, as well as ascending years of residency training [37]. There was a significant positive correlation between both informal and formal education on risk and the number of risk factors elicited on interview [37]. Teo and colleagues similarly found that the risk assessments of highly experienced attending psychiatrists had a moderate degree of predictive validity, while those of junior psychiatry residents (evaluating patients with similar characteristics) were no better than chance [36]. The authors concluded that the increased reliance on a formal instrument such as the HCR-20 might enhance the accuracy of residents' violence risk assessments [36]. Simulated patient encounters may also enhance resident training in handling behavioral emergencies [38]. A pilot study of PGY-1 and PGY-2 psychiatry residents who participated in simulations with agitated standardized patients reported increased knowledge and feelings of comfort and competence in managing agitation [38]. Most of the participants had completed an emergency psychiatry rotation and some reported continuing anxiety after the simulation [38]. This suggests that simulation can be useful for ongoing education and skill development outside of the formal training experience [38].

Nursing staff play a critical role in ensuring resident safety and teaching residents about best practices for maintaining safety. Nursing staff frequently have more consistent exposure to patient agitation in the emergency setting than resident physicians, who rotate through a variety of clinical sites and call schedules and may therefore have extended periods without clinical experiences in emergency psychiatry. As a result, nursing input on a patient's clinical status and behavior is invaluable to the treating physician and can alert the physician to potential safety issues. At UMMC, PES nurses continually monitor the patient care areas with regular rounding and continuous observation through large glass windows and with the aid of security cameras. Nurses proactively train new residents to avoid positioning themselves in the few "blind spots" in the clinical area. Shift changes for nurses and physicians are staggered to promote safety, allowing an oncoming resident to obtain feedback about a patient's behavior from a nurse who is already involved in the patient's care and may have cared for that patient over multiple days.

Security staff can also promote safety and may even play a supportive role in multidisciplinary efforts to de-escalate agitated patients. At UMMC, for example, security officers with appropriate training in mental health crises are omnipresent in the PES. Resident physicians are trained to seek accompaniment from security during all patient interactions without exception. Security staff are introduced to the patient as an integral part of the care team whose presence promotes the safety of patient and staff alike. Security staff are stationed in an area immediately outside the entrance to the locked area of the PES, ensuring that they can monitor staff entry and exit and proactively accompany clinical staff during patient interactions.

SUMMARY

Management of a psychiatric crisis is a multifaceted and demanding clinical task that requires first-rate assessment abilities, keen judgment, and interpersonal skills. Particularly in the wake of Project BETA, guidance on best practices is readily available for many aspects of crisis management. Rich, hands-on training in emergency psychiatry, however, is necessary to fully prepare residents to meet the challenge of treating acute mental health crises. Recent research highlights the potential to refine educational efforts and further hone the next generation of psychiatrists who will meet the increasing need for emergency psychiatric management. Prioritizing interprofessional collaboration in the emergency setting, violence risk assessment, and trauma-informed verbal de-escalation skills will enhance resident training and improve patient care.

CLINICS CARE POINTS

- Psychiatrists managing emergencies should familiarize themselves with Project BETA's best practice guidelines for agitation management.
- Effectively managing a psychiatric crisis involves excluding potentially serious medical causes.
- Where it can safely be undertaken, verbal de-escalation of agitation is ideal.
- Staff training may enhance verbal de-escalation efforts.
- Fostering a trauma-informed therapeutic alliance optimizes patient care.
- Effective disposition planning involves many key considerations.

DISCLOSURE

The authors have nothing to disclose.

REFERENCES

[1] NAMI. Understanding mental health crises. In: Navigating a Mental Health Crisis. 2018. Available at: https://www.nami.org/Support-Education/Publications-Reports/Guides/Navigating-a-Mental-Health-Crisis/Navigating-A-Mental-Health-Crisis?utm_source=website&utm_medium=cta&utm_campaign=crisisguide. Accessed November 28, 2022.

[2] Zeller SL, Cerny JC. Delivery models of emergency psychiatric care. In: Glick RL, Zeller SL, Berlin JS, editors. Emergency psychiatry: principles and practice. 2nd edition. Philadelphia: Wolters Kluwer; 2021. p. 3–15.

[3] U.S. Department of Health and Human Services, Substance Abuse and Mental Health Services Administration, Center for Mental Health Services. Responding to a mental health crisis. In: Practice Guidelines: Core Elements in Responding to Mental Health Crises. 2009. Available at: https://store.samhsa.gov/sites/default/files/d7/priv/sma09-4427.pdf. Accessed November 23, 2022.

[4] Holloman GH Jr, Zeller SL. Overview of project BETA: best practices in evaluation and treatment of agitation. West J Emerg Med 2012;13(1):1–2.

[5] Wilson MP, Pepper D, Currier GW, et al. The psychopharmacology of agitation: consensus statement of the american association for emergency psychiatry project Beta psychopharmacology workgroup. West J Emerg Med 2012;13(1):26–34.

[6] Miller CWT, Hodzic V, Weintraub E. Current understanding of the neurobiology of agitation. West J Emerg Med 2020;21(4):841–8.

[7] Tangu K, Ifeanyi A, Velusamy M, et al. Knowledge and attitude towards pharmacological management of acute agitation: a survey of psychiatrists, psychiatry residents, and psychiatric nurses. Acad Psychiatry 2017;41(3):333–6.

[8] Nordstrom K, Zun LS, Wilson MP, et al. Medical evaluation and triage of the agitated patient: consensus statement of the american association for emergency psychiatry project Beta medical evaluation workgroup. West J Emerg Med 2012;13(1):3–10.

[9] Stiebel VG. Safety and security in psychiatric emergency services and emergency departments. In: Glick RL, Zeller SL, Berlin JS, editors. Emergency psychiatry: principles and practice. 2nd edition. Philadelphia: Wolters Kluwer; 2021. p. 81–8.

[10] Richmond JS, Berlin JS, Fishkind AB, et al. Verbal de-escalation of the agitated patient: consensus statement of the american association for emergency psychiatry project BETA de-escalation workgroup. West J Emerg Med 2012;13(1):17–25.

[11] Lavelle M, Stewart D, James K, et al. Predictors of effective de-escalation in acute inpatient psychiatric settings. J Clin Nurs 2016;25(15–16):2180–8.

[12] Price O, Baker J, Bee P, et al. The support-control continuum: An investigation of staff perspectives on factors influencing the success or failure of de-escalation techniques for the management of violence and aggression in mental health settings. Int J Nurs Stud 2018;77:197–206.

[13] Price O, Baker J, Bee P, et al. Patient perspectives on barriers and enablers to the use and effectiveness of de-escalation techniques for the management of violence and aggression in mental health settings. J Adv Nurs 2018;74(3):614–25.

[14] Krull W, Gusenius TM, Germain D, et al. Staff perception of interprofessional simulation for verbal de-escalation and restraint application to mitigate violent patient behaviors in the emergency department. J Emerg Nurs 2019;45(1):24–30.

[15] Thompson SL, Zurmehly J, Bauldoff G, et al. De-escalation training as part of a workplace violence prevention program. J Nurs Adm 2022;52(4):222–7.

[16] Story AR, Harris R, Scott SD, et al. An evaluation of nurses' perception and confidence after implementing a workplace aggression and violence prevention training program. J Nurs Adm 2020;50(4):209–15.

[17] Somani R, Muntaner C, Hillan E, et al. A systematic review: effectiveness of interventions to de-escalate workplace violence against nurses in healthcare settings. Saf Health Work 2021;12(3):289–95.

[18] Gillam SW. Nonviolent crisis intervention training and the incidence of violent events in a large hospital emergency department: an observational quality improvement study. Adv Emerg Nurs J 2014;36(2):177–88.

[19] Beaulieu C, Wertheimer JC, Pickett L, et al. Behavior management on an acute brain injury unit: evaluating the effectiveness of an interdisciplinary training program. J Head Trauma Rehabil 2008;23(5):304–11.

[20] Crisis Prevention Institute. Nonviolent crisis intervention. 2022. Available at: https://www.crisisprevention.com/Our-Programs/Nonviolent-Crisis-Intervention. Accessed November 21, 2022.

[21] The Mandt System. Experts who know workplace dynamics. 2020. Available at: https://www.mandtsystem.com/our-approach/. Accessed November 21, 2022.

[22] Knox DK, Holloman GH Jr. Use and avoidance of seclusion and restraint: consensus statement of the american association for emergency psychiatry project Beta seclusion and restraint workgroup. West J Emerg Med 2012;13(1):35–40.

[23] SAMHSA's Trauma and Justice Strategic Initiative. SAMHSA's trauma-informed approach: key assumptions and principles. In: SAMHSA's Concept of Trauma and Guidance for a Trauma-Informed Approach. 2014. Available at: https://store.samhsa.gov/sites/default/files/d7/priv/sma14-4884.pdf. Accessed November 23, 2022.

[24] Kosman KA, Levy-Carrick NC. Positioning psychiatry as a leader in trauma-informed care (TIC): the need for psychiatry resident education. Acad Psychiatry 2019;43(4):429–34.

[25] Berlin JS, Zeller SL. Boarding of psychiatric patients in the emergency department: flow, throughput, and systemic change. In: Glick RL, Zeller SL, Berlin JS, editors. Emergency psychiatry: principles and practice. 2nd edition. Philadelphia: Wolters Kluwer; 2021. p. 16–29.

[26] ACGME. ACGME Program Requirements for Graduate Medical Education in Psychiatry. 2022. Available at: https://www.acgme.org/globalassets/pfassets/programrequirements/400_psychiatry_2022v2.pdf. Accessed November 19, 2022.

[27] Bennett JI, Dzara K, Mazhar MN, et al. A preliminary report on resident emergency psychiatry training from a survey of psychiatry chief residents. J Grad Med Educ 2011;3(1):21–5.

[28] Brasch J, Glick RL, Cobb TG, et al. Residency training in emergency psychiatry: a model curriculum developed by the education committee of the american association for emergency psychiatry. Acad Psychiatry 2004;28(2): 95–103.

[29] Fage B, Lofchy J. Education and training in the psychiatric emergency service. In: Glick RL, Zeller SL, Berlin JS, editors. Emergency psychiatry: principles and practice. 2nd edition. Philadelphia: Wolters Kluwer; 2021. p. 48–60.

[30] McIlwrick J, Lockyer J. Resident training in the psychiatric emergency service: duty hours tell only part of the story. J Grad Med Educ 2011;3(1):26–30.

[31] Bennett JI, Costin G, Khan M, et al. Postgraduate year-1 residency training in emergency psychiatry: an acute care psychiatric clinic at a community mental health center. J Grad Med Educ 2010;2(3):462–6.

[32] Kwok S, Ostermeyer B, Coverdale J. A systematic review of the prevalence of patient assaults against residents. J Grad Med Educ 2012;4(3):296–300.

[33] Antonius D, Fuchs L, Herbert F, et al. Psychiatric assessment of aggressive patients: a violent attack on a resident. Am J Psychiatry 2010;167(3):253–9.

[34] Dvir Y, Moniwa E, Crisp-Han H, et al. Survey of threats and assaults by patients on psychiatry residents. Acad Psychiatry 2012;36(1):39–42.

[35] Saheed M. Management of agitation and violence. In: Chanmugam A, Triplett P, Kelen G, editors. Emergency psychiatry. New York: Cambridge University Press; 2013. p. 25–40.

[36] Teo AR, Holley SR, Leary M, et al. The relationship between level of training and accuracy of violence risk assessment. Psychiatr Serv 2012;63(11):1089–94.

[37] Wong L, Morgan A, Wilkie T, et al. Quality of resident violence risk assessments in psychiatric emergency settings. Can J Psychiatry 2012;57(6):375–80.

[38] Zigman D, Young M, Chalk C. Using simulation to train junior psychiatry residents to work with agitated patients: a pilot study. Acad Psychiatry 2013;37(1):38–41.

Neurosciences

Advances in Psychiatry and Behavioral Health 3 (2023) 239–253

ADVANCES IN PSYCHIATRY AND BEHAVIORAL HEALTH

Neuropsychiatric Manifestations of Multiple Sclerosis and the Effects of Modern Disease-Modifying Therapies

Mohona Reza, MD, Jonathan F. Cahill, MD, Emily Federo Hungria, MD, Laura Stanton, MD, Michael Kritselis, DO, John E. Donahue, Victoria Sanborn, PhD, Chuang-Kuo Wu, MD, PhD*

Rhode Island Hospital, The Warren Alpert Medical School of Brown University, 593 Eddy Street, APC-7, Providence, RI 02903, USA

KEYWORDS
• Disease-modifying therapy • Multiple sclerosis • Alzheimer disease • Cognitive impairment
• Clinically isolated syndrome

INTRODUCTION

Multiple sclerosis (MS) is the most common immune-mediated inflammatory demyelinating disease of the central nervous system (CNS). MS is characterized pathologically by multifocal areas of demyelination with the loss of oligodendrocytes and astroglial scarring. Since 1993 when the first disease-modifying therapy (DMT)—interferon beta-1b—was approved for MS, the hopes that this relentlessly debilitating neurologic disorder will finally be controllable in long term have brought great excitement. In the subsequent 3 decades, more than a dozen DMTs have received Food and Drug Administration (FDA)-approval for MS. These medications are particularly effective in reducing MS relapse rate and MRI activity. Among the complicated symptoms in patients with long-standing MS, cognitive impairment (CI) and psychiatric disorders are most challenging because there are no effective therapies for treatment, no standardized diagnostic tests for consensus diagnosis and no protocols for standard of care. Moreover, although patients with MS can now have a prolonged life span, many of them will develop age-related comorbidities. In recent medical literature, late-onset (equal to or older than 65 years of age) Alzheimer disease (AD) has been reported more often in patients with MS [1]. Due to modern advancement in diagnostic tools for AD, more cases of young-onset (younger than 65 years) AD can be diagnosed with confidence. Yet, in patients with MS, young-onset AD (YOAD) would rarely be considered as a comorbid disease, because patients with MS in this age range can present CI and psychiatric symptoms mimicking those of patients with YOAD.

In this article, the authors plan to review and update the cognitive and psychiatric manifestations of MS that can be differentiated from concomitant AD in patients with MS. We will also examine the potential role of modern DMTs in mitigating or modifying the cognitive and psychiatric symptoms of MS.

Note: Mohona Reza, Emily Federo Hungria, Michael Kritselis, and Victoria Sanborn contributed equally to this article; they were all mentored by the senior authors Jonathan F. Cahill, Laura Stanton, John E. Donahue, and Chuang-Kuo Wu for this project.

*Corresponding author. Rhode Island Hospital, #593 Eddy Street, APC-7th Floor, Providence RI 02903. E-mail address: cwu6@lifespan.org

https://doi.org/10.1016/j.ypsc.2023.04.001
2667-3827/23/   © 2023 Elsevier Inc. All rights reserved.

COGNITIVE IMPAIRMENT

Historic Conceptualization of Cognition in Multiple Sclerosis

As he astutely characterized psychiatric features of MS, Charcot observed CI in his patients, describing patients with MS as showing "marked enfeeblement of the memory" and "conceptions that are formed slowly" [2]. Despite Charcot's early observations back in 1877, MS in clinical settings during the next several decades underemphasized cognition [3]. In fact, until the 1980s, estimates suggested CI was present in only 5% of MS [4]. Although prevalence of CI in MS was considered infrequent, the assessment of cognitive functions in MS began as early as in the 1920s. The 1950s saw greater pursuit of cognitive assessment in MS through the use of the Rorschach test, which showed that patients with MS performed more like persons with brain injury than healthy controls, a finding that was replicated through rigorous cognitive testing studies in the 1970s [5]. During the following 2 decades, how we characterize CI in MS would drastically change with the integration of neuropsychological assessment in longitudinal MS cohorts and the use of neuropathological detection methods and MRI.

Multiple Sclerosis as a Subcortical Dementia

For several decades, MS has been considered a "subcortical dementia" disorder because its demyelinating process primarily occurs in the white matter (WM) of the human brain [6]. This idea was supported by neuropathological studies using standard histochemical myelin stains to identify lesions (plaques) as well as early T2 MRI approaches, both of which emphasized disease processes in the WM. The characterization of MS as a subcortical dementia was also supported by clinical presentation in comparisons with other subcortical dementia disorders. Rao and colleagues in 1990 provided a comprehensive overview comparing MS to subcortical dementias such as Huntington disease and Parkinson disease (PD) and emphasized their neuropsychological similarities including slowed processing, secondary memory difficulty, impaired psychomotor skills, and conceptual reasoning [6]. In addition, MS, unlike "cortical" dementias, did not present CI associated with the gray matter (GM), such as primary memory, visuospatial skills, and language. Although the characterization of MS as a subcortical dementia involved a focus on CI in processing speed specifically, even early advocates for this characterization recognized that focal lesions of MS were variable in their locations in the brain and could lead to heterogenous presentations of symptoms beyond just subcortical.

Multiple Sclerosis Affects More than Just Subcortical White Matter

Recent sophisticated approaches to studying MS brain have demonstrated pathologic changes in GM. On average, 15% of the neocortex of MS brains is affected by demyelinating lesions, with some cases even showing lesions up to 70% [7]. Beyond lesion loads of WM and GM, long-standing MS causes atrophy of both subcortical and cortical brain structures [8]. As early as the 2000s, with advanced neuroimaging tools, specific regional atrophy in the MS brain was increasingly identified and found to be significantly associated with impairments demonstrated on neuropsychological testing. Some studies reported that MS can have greater volume loss in deep gray matter structures than persons with PD or amnestic-type of mild cognitive impairment (MCI). Patients with MS can also present greater thalamic atrophy than that of patients with AD. Some brain regions are more commonly impacted than others in MS, including hippocampi, the cerebellum, and the spinal cord; however, it seems that all structures of the brain are at risk of atrophy subsequent to MS. The thalamus, in particular, may be a key structure impacted very early in MS, even in clinically isolated syndrome (CIS) [9,10]. As the thalamus plays an imperative role in the connections between subcortical and neocortical functions, insult to this structure has a significant impact on many cognitive functions and neuronal pathways. Similarly, other deep GM structures important for connectivity throughout the brain, such as the cingulate cortex, are also damaged in MS and variably preceded by damage to nearby WM.

Increased recognition of the early damage to cognitively crucial deep gray matter structures of the brain in MS has altered our view of why this disease can involve heterogenous cognitive dysfunction.

Multiple Sclerosis-Specific Neuropsychological Evaluation

Improved neuropsychological assessment of patients with MS and detailed investigation of MS brains have gradually led to changes in how we characterize cognitive dysfunction in the disease course of MS. Dating back to 1975, office cognitive tests used for dementia were insensitive to CI in MS. As such, in the 1990s, neuropsychological batteries specific to CI of MS were developed, focusing on learning/memory and processing speed [5,6,11]. One example was the Minimal Assessment of Cognitive Function in MS. Recent studies show that aspects of processing speed, attention, and memory (as observed by Charcot) are indeed the most commonly impaired cognitive domains in MS. The cognitive tests, including *Symbol Digit Modalities Test, Paced Auditory Serial Addition Test, Selective Reminding Test, California Verbal Learning Test,* and *Brief Visuospatial Memory Test—Revised,* are most commonly used to identify neurocognitive profile specific to MS. Although less frequently studied, visuospatial/visuoperceptual impairment may also occur in up to 12% to 19% of patients with MS; this can be detected by Facial Recognition Test or Judgment of Line Orientation Test. In addition, a significant portion of patients with MS experience problem with executive function through the disease course. The Wisconsin Card Sorting Test and tasks of inhibition (ie, Stroop paradigm interference) and productivity (ie, letter fluency) are good identifiers of executive dysfunction in MS.

Investigation of Multiple Sclerosis Cognitive Subtypes

Given the heterogeneity of neuroanatomical and neuropsychological presentations of MS, investigators have attempted to impart more order and predictability by identifying subtypes of the CI [12]. For example, investigators have sought to determine whether cognitive outcomes differ among the 4 MS disease phenotypes, namely CIS, relapsing remitting MS (RRMS), secondary progressive MS (SPMS), and primary progressive MS (PPMS), each of which manifest different clinical presentations, and time course. CI has even been demonstrated in people with radiologically isolated syndrome, that is, individuals presenting without overt clinical symptoms but with MRI findings highly suggestive of MS [13]. In general, more severe lesion burden and chronic progression of MS are associated with worse cognitive functioning overall [14]. Deficits in processing speed, executive function, and episodic memory are typically more significant in RRMS than CIS. Severe irreversible deficits in most cognitive domains are observed in SPMS. PPMS are relatively rapidly advancing into severe impairment across all cognitive domains.

Other cognitive syndromes may also emerge in MS with some researchers proposing distinct cognitive phenotypes. A recent multicenter study in Italy with a total of 1212 patients with MS found that 19.4% of their sample did not show impaired performance on cognitive tests. Although 29.9% showed mild degree of impairment in verbal memory/semantic fluency, 19.5% presented mild degree of multidomain impairment and 13.8% exhibited severe executive/attention dysfunction. The rest, 17.5%, was noted to have severe degree of impairment in multiple cognitive domains. Detailed

analysis of the brain MRI features of patients with MS can explain these clinical phenotypes of CI [12]. Earlier, researchers had proposed 3 possible cognitive phenotypes of MS—isolated memory impairment group, isolated information processing speed impairment group, and combined deficits in processing speed and memory group [15]. Although this classification might help conceptualize patterns of CI and facilitate development of cognitive therapies in MS, usefulness of these cognitive phenotypes in clinical setting remains to be determined.

Changes in Cognitive Impairment in Multiple Sclerosis with the Introduction of Disease-Modifying Therapies

In recent years, DMTs have changed the presentation and progression of CI in MS. Interferon beta was introduced for the treatment of MS in the early 1990s followed by immunomodulatory treatments in the early 2000s, both of which slow MS progression [16]. Both platform therapies and escalation therapies have been found to improve cognitive functions in MS, with the most commonly evaluated and reported improvements noted for processing speed. To a less extent, improvement in verbal memory, visual memory, executive functions, and visuoperceptional abilities has also been reported. DMTs decrease relapses, thus halting the demyelinating process of CNS and preserving its functions; therefore, DMTs ameliorate aspects of CI due to MS.

PSYCHIATRIC ASPECTS

History of Neuropsychiatric Symptoms in Multiple Sclerosis

Since the nineteenth century, neuropsychiatrists have made associations between psychiatric disorders present in the context of the neurologic disorder—MS. During the years, our understanding of neuropsychiatric symptoms has evolved; for example, in the early nineteenth century, studies frequently found more than 50% of patients with MS had pathologic euphoria; however, more recent studies have found euphoria and pseudobulbar affect to be much less common [17].

The cause of neuropsychiatric symptoms has been a matter of interest. It has long been debated whether the symptoms are caused by a direct effect of the brain lesions themselves, or rather are due to the psychosocial stress of living with MS. More recent advances in neuroimaging have brought support to the idea that lesions in certain brain regions contribute at least in part to the various neuropsychiatric signs and symptoms accompanying MS. Since the advent of DMT in the 1990s, there has also been research into the effect of DMT itself on neuropsychiatric symptoms, harkening back to the first interferon beta trial where treatment groups had suicide attempts and the placebo groups did not [18]. Conversely, there has also been investigation into whether DMT can ameliorate neuropsychiatric symptoms.

Current Understanding of Neuropsychiatric Symptoms

Although neuropsychiatric symptoms more often develop as the disease progresses, they can also be present at the onset of neurologic symptoms, or can even sometimes be the sole initial complaint of patients ultimately diagnosed with MS. They are important to address because they have significant impacts not only in the quality of the patient's life but also in treatment of MS, including delays in diagnosis, and poor adherence to DMT. Although up to 60% of patients with MS experience neuropsychiatric symptoms, these are frequently underdiagnosed and undertreated [19]. Contributing to this challenge is the heterogeneity of the presentation of neuropsychiatric symptoms in people with MS. Among the more common conditions studied in MS there are major depressive disorder (MDD), bipolar disorder, anxiety, psychosis, and pseudobulbar affect, which we will focus on for the purposes of this article.

Depression

MDD is the most common neuropsychiatric disorder in patients with MS. MDD in MS has an estimated annual prevalence of 15%. Almost 50% of patients with MS experience depression during their life-long disease course [20]. Moreover, MDD often goes unrecognized and undertreated in patients with MS.

This may, in part, be because patients with MS with MDD tend to present with a different pattern of symptoms than depressed patients without MS. Depressed patients with MS are more likely to present with irritability than those without MS [20]. Additionally, depressed patients with MS are less likely to experience social withdrawal, low self-esteem, and excessive guilt. Compounding the difficulty in accurately identifying a major depressive episode in patients with MS is the overlap of and the potential for confounding the neurovegetative symptoms of MDD (ie, lack of appetite, low energy, diminished concentration) with the biological symptoms that can occur in the absence of depression in patients with MS. Considering this challenge, co-occurring symptoms that may help clinicians identify a major depressive episode in the MS population include low mood, anhedonia, suicidal ideation,

negative thought patterns, and impairment in functioning out of proportion to one's physical symptoms.

Although no doubt the psychosocial stressors of living with MS (ie, adjusting to illness and disability, living with the uncertainty of the disease course) contribute in part to depression, there has also been emerging evidence regarding the role of biological factors in causing major depression. A 2021 review article noted that most imaging studies reported a correlation between depressive symptoms and T1W and T2W lesions, particularly in the frontal and temporal lobe. They also found that brain atrophy, especially when involving the temporal gray matter and hippocampus, has been frequently associated with depression in MS [20]. Studies based on diffusion tensor imaging and functional MRI have also suggested a disconnection mechanism may contribute to depression [20]. In addition to brain lesions contributing to depressive symptoms in MS, abnormalities in the hypothalamic-pituitary-adrenal axis function have been found in patients with MS with MDD, and these changes have been associated with MS lesions [21].

Several medications used in the management of MDD in MS have side effects of depression, including steroids, baclofen, dantrolene, and tizanidine. There has been mixed evidence on DMT impact on major depression. Although studies found interferon beta to be associated with depression, subsequent studies have failed to find an association, although it remains common clinical practice to counsel on this potential effect [22]. Conversely, several studies have looked into whether DMT can alleviate depressive symptoms. A 2018 review found that natalizumab and fingolimod have some evidence of improvement in depression with this treatment, although this was not found to be statistically significant with natalizumab [23].

Suicide

Identification of MDD is crucial because it has been shown to be the greatest risk factor for suicidal ideation in patients with MS. Although some studies have not found a greater risk of completed suicide in MS, many studies have found a greater risk compared with the general population [24]. Investigating this, a recent meta-analysis that included 16 studies did find a statistically significant suicide rate ratio of 1.72 (95% CI 1.43–2.00) [24]. In addition to MDD being a risk factor for suicide, other risk factors include social isolation and substance use.

Concerns that DMT could have a side effect of suicidal ideation can be traced back to the studies in 1990s, when the original report of interferon beta trial in RRMS showed several suicide attempts in the treatment groups but none in the placebo group [18]. Although subsequent studies have failed to find an association, it remains common practice to warn about this potential adverse effect.

Bipolar Disorder

Bipolar disorder is much more common in patients in MS than in the general population, with prevalence estimated between 0.3% and 2.4%, or about twice as common than in people without MS. Regarding the reason behind this association, there has been evidence of a genetic linkage between MS and bipolar disorder. There have been few imaging studies for bipolar disorder in patients with MS but existing studies suggest that a higher lesion load is associated with manic episodes [25]. Although corticosteroids are well known to precipitate manic episodes, baclofen, dantrolene, and tizanidine have also been associated with manic episodes.

Anxiety

There has been much less research on anxiety disorders in MS than mood disorders, despite its high comorbidity in MS [26]. A 2017 meta-analysis study reported the prevalence of clinically significant anxiety symptoms was 34%, and that the prevalence of anxiety disorders was 10% [26]. Generalized anxiety disorder is the most common comorbid anxiety disorder at 18.6%, followed by panic disorder (10%), and then obsessive compulsive disorder (8.6%). MS treatment itself may induce anxiety. Many DMTs require self-injection, and a phenomenon of self-injection anxiety, likened to a specific phobia in diagnostic and statistical manual of mental disorders, 5th edition (DSM-5), has been described [27]. Glatiramer acetate's side effects include anxiety, as well as palpitations, tachycardia, and shortness of breath.

Psychosis

Psychotic symptoms are less common, compared with other neuropsychiatric manifestations of MS. Only a small number of studies investigated the prevalence of psychosis in patients with MS; few distinguish psychotic disorders from psychotic symptoms. Although several population-based studies have found schizophrenia to be more common in patients with MS than in the general population, few studies have found the opposite [28]. A 2015 systematic review noted that the prevalence of psychosis was 0.41% to 7.46%, and the prevalence of schizophrenia was 0% to 7.4% [28]. Brief psychotic disorder and bipolar disorder with psychotic features are thought to be the most common varieties of psychotic

disorders in MS. Regarding types of psychotic symptoms reported, studies reported the most common were delusions (81%), followed by auditory hallucinations (59%) and visual hallucinations (50%) [29–31].

Regarding the cause of psychotic symptoms in patients with MS, studies have identified several possible mechanisms, including brain lesions, inflammation, and medication side effects. Lesions in the periventricular WM, in particular in the frontal and temporal regions, are found to be associated with psychotic symptoms. There is also evidence for a neuroimmune imbalance in psychotic disorders such as schizophrenia, similar to patients with MS. Regarding the impact of medications, psychotic symptoms are known side effects of corticosteroids and beta interferon.

Interestingly, however, different from the general population where psychosis can often develop or worsen in response to steroids, there are reports of psychosis in patients with MS being ameliorated by steroids. A recent review article recorded that while patients with MS presenting psychosis were frequently resistant to antipsychotic treatment (75% of cases), many had significant improvement of both psychiatric and neurologic symptoms with corticosteroid treatment (95% of cases) [29–31].

Pseudobulbar Affect

Pseudobulbar affect, also known as "pathologic laughing and crying," or "emotional incontinence," or "emotional lability," is another neuropsychiatric manifestation of MS. It is an affective disorder of emotional expression, with patients experiencing a disparity between their expression of emotions and their internal emotional experience. It is not unique to MS and has been described in several other neurologic conditions, including amyotrophic lateral sclerosis, AD, PD, stroke, and traumatic brain injury. In MS, it is estimated to have a prevalence of about 11% [32]. It occurs more often in later stage of the disease course—in patients with greater disability. The exact cause is unknown but it is hypothesized to be due to a disruption in pathways responsible for appropriate social and cognitive regulation, such as the cortico–pontine–cerebellar circuit.

Treatment of Multiple Sclerosis and its Effect on Neuropsychiatric Symptoms

Although there is no cure for MS, DMTs can prevent permanent damage. Permanent damage to the CNS can occur early in the disease, thus it is important for prompt treatment once there is confirmed diagnosis of MS. DMTs can be categorized by route of administration (oral, injectables, and intravenous) [Table 1]. Most of

TABLE 1
Disease Modifying Therapies[a] for Multiple Sclerosis

Drug or Drug Class	Usual Dosing Schedule(s)	Mechanism of Action	Potential Neuropsychiatric Effects
Injection			
Interferon beta (mult. formulations)	SC every other day SC 3 × weekly IM once weekly SC every other week	Increases anti-inflammatory agents, downregulates expression of proinflammatory cytokines	Depression, suicidal thoughts have been reported Modest reduction of brain atrophy
Glatiramer acetate	SC 3 × weekly	Inhibits T cell response to several myelin antigens	Modest reduction of brain atrophy
Ofatumumab	SC once monthly	Anti-CD20 mab (B-cell)	Significant brain atrophy reduction
Oral			
S1P-receptor modulators (mult. formulations)	PO daily	Prevents lymphocyte egress from lymphoid tissues	Significant brain atrophy reduction Possible improvement in depression
Teriflunomide	PO daily	Inhibits pyrimidine synthesis	Reduction of brain atrophy
Fumarates (mult. formulations)	PO twice daily	Enhances Nrf2 transcriptional pathway, which regulates enzymes to counter act oxidative stress	Modest reduction of brain atrophy
Cladribine	Two 1-wk cycles (4–10 tabs PO per cycle) annually × 2 y	Inhibits DNA repair enzymes including DNA polymerase and ribonucleotide reductase	Significant brain atrophy reduction
Intravenous			
Natalizumab	IV every 28 d	Anti-alpha4 integrin mab	Significant brain atrophy reduction Possible improvement in depression
Mitoxantrone	IV every 3 mo with lifetime max	DNA intercalating agent	
Alemtuzumab	IV × 5 d in year 1 and × 3 d in year 2	Anti-CD52 mab	Significant brain atrophy reduction
Ocrelizumab	IV every 6 mo	Anti-CD20 mab (B-cell)	Potential improvements in MS-related quality of life, which includes cognitive and mood measures Significant brain atrophy reduction
Rituximab	IV every 6 mo typically (not FDA approved)	Anti-CD20 mab (B-cell)	

[a] All except rituximab are FDA-approved for relapsing forms of MS, including active secondary progressive MS. Mitoxantrone is also FDA-approved for (chronic) secondary progressive MS. Ocrelizumab is also approved for primary progressive MS. *multi, multiple. *mab, monoclonal antibody.

the earliest DMTs were small molecules administered by subcutaneous and intramuscular injection. These DMTs were modestly effective and had generally mild side effects. During the past 30 years, the development of more effective therapies has revolutionized the field. Now, monoclonal antibodies and other more potent immunosuppressants can arrest MS in many patients [33]. The concept of "no evidence of disease activity", which indicates no new MS relapses, no new MRI lesions, and no progression of disability is increasingly the goal of treatment.

Less is known about the specific effects of DMTs on cognitive, behavioral, and mood symptoms of MS. Although some of the older, low-efficacy DMTs, particularly interferon, have been associated with cognitive and mood side effects, in general, poorer adherence to treatment is correlated to a higher prevalence of neuropsychiatric symptoms. This may be due to direct effects of DMT treatment on reducing symptoms and thereby improving quality of life or may be related to a reduction in brain atrophy with the use of most DMTs [34]. The degree of whole brain atrophy and thalamic atrophy is correlated to worsening cognitive function in MS. In today's MS clinics, the treatment of MS with high-efficacy DMTs from the onset of disease is the most effective strategy for long-term control of symptoms and slowing disability progression [35]. In this section, we will discuss frequently used DMTs and what is known about their effects on neuropsychiatric symptoms.

Ocrelizumab, rituximab, and ofatumumab are monoclonal antibodies against the CD20 molecule on the surface of B cells. These DMTs are highly effective in preventing clinical relapses, the appearance of new MRI lesions, and progression of disability in MS. By reducing inflammatory damage to specific brain areas, these DMTs may also reduce worsening of mood and cognitive symptoms. One study reported significant improvements on health-related quality of life at 12 months in individuals that were treated with ocrelizumab [33]. There were improvements in the Neuro-QoL (quality of Life), which measured 11 domains including ability to participate in social roles and activities, anxiety, cognitive function, depression, emotional and behavioral dyscontrol, fatigue, lower extremity function, positive effect and well-being, satisfaction with social roles and activities, stigma, and upper extremity function [33]. Natalizumab is a humanized monoclonal antibody that is an inhibitor of the α4β1 integrin. This integrin is an adhesion molecule that is expressed on the surface of lymphocytes and is involved in the migration across the endothelia in the CNS. Ten studies found that

depression symptoms improved following natalizumab treatment, although this was not statistically significant [23].

Fingolimod was the first oral therapy approved for RRMS. It is an S1P inhibitor that prevents the release of lymphocytes from secondary lymphoid organs. It is typically well tolerated with no neuropsychiatric side effects. Eight publications showed that depression improved with the initiation of fingolimod [36]. One study examined changes in anxiety symptoms and showed a nonsignificant improvement [23]. Dimethyl fumarate is another oral medication that is generally well tolerated and effective against RRMS. It exerts its anti-inflammatory and cytoprotective effects by enabling nuclear factor (erythroid-derived 2)-like 2 (Nrf2) pathway and Nrf2-independent pathways. In animal studies, dimethyl fumarate improved depression and anxiety by reducing brain catalase levels in mice [37]. Teriflunomide, an active metabolite of leflunomide, is an oral medication that inhibits dihydroorotate dehydrogenase, an enzyme involved in pyrimidine synthesis. This prevents the proliferation of activated lymphocytes. Studies have shown teriflunomide improving cognition largely through its effect on brain volume loss [38].

Interferon beta is a class I interferon that downregulates the expression of MHC molecules on antigen-presenting cells. This decreases proinflammatory and increases anti-inflammatory cytokines. It ultimately inhibits T-cell proliferation, and blocks trafficking of inflammatory cells to the CNS. Possible serious side effects include depression, suicidal thoughts, hallucinations, or other behavioral health problems. However, depression data collected from individual clinical trials have failed to identify a consistent association [39].

Glatiramer acetate is composed of 4 amino acids. Its mechanism of action possibly involves altering the balance between proinflammatory and regulatory cytokines. Along with interferon beta, glatiramer acetate has relatively low efficacy in MS. This medication has no known mood-related side effects, and there are limited data on any benefits from glatiramer acetate on neuropsychiatric symptoms [39].

There is a high rate of neuropsychiatric symptoms such as depression, behavioral dysregulation, and CI in patients with MS. The prompt initiation of DMT is crucial to prevent ongoing CNS inflammatory injury. By reducing CNS inflammation and slowing brain atrophy in MS, DMTs may also reduce the burden of these neuropsychiatric symptoms in the disease.

CONCOMITANT ALZHEIMER DISEASE

"Typical" MS Cognitive Profile in Aging

Previous research concerning cognitive symptoms associated with MS in aging is somewhat limited. Because of longer life expectancy and more effective DMTs, recent research has begun to exert greater focus on aging-related CI in MS. Compared with age and education matched healthy controls, a study found that older adults with MS show slower processing speed and verbal fluency (common deficits in MS), suggesting that the MS cognitive profile may remain largely consistent with age [40]. Another study noted that older adult patients with MS showed higher prevalence of CI than younger patients with MS; moreover, regarding all cognitive domains, the prevalence of impairment in each cognitive domain was the same across age groups (processing speed 70%, verbal learning 50%, executive function 48%, and visuospatial learning 27%) [41]. These data support the notion that cognitive presentation in MS remains the same during the aging process. The interaction of aging and MS diagnosis accounts for the greatest variation in performance on tasks assessing processing speed and executive function. These findings indicate that cognitive functions could likely worsen with aging in MS, although the general cognitive profile may hold over time. This provides a crucial piece of information for differentiating MS from other cognitive disorders common in aging.

Differences between CI in multiple Sclerosis and Alzheimer Disease

Recent review of the literature identified several studies that compared cognitive performance in older adults with MS with cognitive function of older adults with amnesic-type MCI or suspected AD. In general, older adults with MS showed (1) worse processing speed; (2) better category fluency, confrontation naming, and executive functions; and (3) preserved autobiographical and semantic memory when compared with persons with suspected AD. These cognitive differences, paired with biological markers, may help delineate the 2 degenerative diseases in older adults, namely cognitive disorder of older patients with MS versus neurocognitive profile suggestive of underlying AD in older adults with a history of MS. However, heterogenous presentations of both conditions as well as the possibility of comorbidity may become an increasingly encountered challenge.

Comorbid Multiple Sclerosis and Alzheimer Disease

As patients with MS lives longer, it is expected that a greater number of older adults with MS will develop aging-related neurodegenerative disorders. In their recent systematic review, Luczynski and colleagues described case studies and case series concerning 24 patients with evidence of comorbid MS and AD [42]. Clinical presentations and age of onset of the diseases varied. The study applied postmortem autopsy and found that severe MS demyelinating pathologic condition, even when inactive, was associated with greater amounts of amyloid and tau in the brain. Authors suggested that this may be due to overlapping mechanisms of the diseases, including mitochondrial dysfunction, inflammation, and poor immune functioning. Their review also demonstrated a variety of clinical presentations of patients with MS-AD comorbidity. For example, one of the earliest cases described was that of a 63-year-old woman with history of progressive dementia who, postmortem, showed chronic foci of MS lesions, encephalitis, AD plaques, tau, and degeneration with atrophy of the temporal lobes and enlarged ventricles. Before her death, she showed near-complete loss of vocabulary and marked confusion, symptoms atypical for MS. Another case was that of a 73-year-old man with a 2-year history of memory impairment identified as having probable AD. During reevaluation 15 months later, he showed notable declines in orientation, memory, and concentration and was found postmortem to have only 2 separate MS demyelinating lesions but many neuritic plaques and neurofibrillary tangles distributed in the brain. For both cases, autopsy was critical for identifying presence of MS, which would have gone undetected when considering only their cognitive symptoms and associated time course.

Although discriminating MS from other neurodegenerative disorders in older adults is difficult, it has been even more challenging when these pathologic conditions present in patients aged younger than 65 years. Flanagan, Knopman, and Keegan in 2014 reported 3 patients in their 50s who were later determined to have comorbid MS and AD [43]. The first case was a 56-year-old woman with no prior history of typical MS attacks who initially showed short-term memory impairment, dyscalculia, and limb apraxia followed by progressively worsening dementia during the next 7 years. She later showed aphasia and severe CIs. Autopsy revealed chronic MS pathologic condition and severe AD pathologic condition. The second case was a 53-year-old woman who had developed positional vertigo, was later developing upper extremity weakness and gait imbalance, and then experienced short-term memory impairment 1 year later. She went on to develop progressive dementia and, 4 years after onset of initial symptoms, exhibited constructional apraxia, dyscalculia, executive dysfunction, inattention, and impaired working memory. Neuroimaging studies revealed typical MS demyelinating lesions and significant parietal lobe atrophy as well as a glucose hypometabolism pattern characteristic of AD. Cerebro-spinal fluid (CSF) analysis showed markers of both MS and AD. The third case, a 53-year-old man, developed bilateral upper extremity paresthesia attributed to MS and then began experiencing progressive dementia 9 years later. On testing, he showed global CI. Brain MRI studies showed both MS demyelinating plaques and mesial temporal lobe atrophy. Brain PET revealed findings of hypometabolism suggestive of AD; the CSF assays found positive results of MS biomarkers.

In the medical literature, recently more case reports describe AD as the comorbidity in the patients with MS of equal to or older than 65 years, based on the presentation of progressive CI more than expected in the disease course of MS. Rarely the comorbidity reported concerns with psychiatric symptoms in these patients. In MS, the mean age of onset ranges from 20 to 30 years of age. Patients with MS with age onset later than 40 years are considered as late-onset MS (LOMS). By contrast, YOAD, occurring in patients aged younger than 65 years, represents only about 10% of all AD cases. Due to advanced MRI, improved detection of demyelinating lesions in the brain and spine has allowed more confident diagnosis of RRMS in LOMS. It is extremely rare to encounter YOAD clinically in patients with LOMS.

Tips for Differentiating Multiple Sclerosis or Identifying Comorbidities

MS is a degenerative condition with several identifying neuropsychiatric features. However, the disease is also heterogenous in its cognitive and psychiatric presentations and early attempts to classify it as a kind of "subcortical dementia" have proven increasingly simplistic. This is further complicated by the limited research conducted on its progression and changes during the aging process. Regardless, the culmination of research across the decades suggests that a combination of careful analysis of neurologic, psychiatric, and cognitive symptoms, considered together with biomarkers as well neuroimaging techniques—all considered in the context of time course—is needed to differentiate MS from other neurodegenerative disorders, such as AD. The neuropsychological assessment of processing speed, verbal fluency, and memory will likely continue to be the most useful tool in differentiating MS from AD. Given our updated understanding of heterogeneous cognitive symptoms in MS, using comprehensive

batteries when clinically indicated is most important. Psychiatric symptoms, such as depression and anxiety, would likely be present much earlier in the course of the disease for MS than in AD. The behavioral symptoms such as executive dysfunction, apathy, and disinhibition may be present in MS as well. Early neurologic symptoms common in MS, such as balance and vision changes, should not be overlooked in persons middle-aged to older-aged because their occurrences may signal undetected or late onset MS, which could otherwise be misdiagnosed. Furthermore, for persons presenting with a mixture of neurologic and psychiatric symptoms, application of CSF markers and neuroimaging tools should all be considered for differential diagnosis. An important caveat is that the presence of atrophy due to MS has been increasingly recognized; yet, this also can be the hallmarks of AD on neuroimaging studies, that is, diffuse cortical atrophy and hippocampal atrophy. Finally, reported cases in the postmortem autopsy studies of MS and AD are ultimately educational and enlightening for further research in the near future.

AN ILLUSTRATIVE CASE REPORT

A 55-year-old left-handed Caucasian man, who had 16 years of education and studied few years to pursue a master's degree, was working and specialized in graphic design with computer software programs for years. At age 29, he had first experienced episodes of numbness in fingers and pain with fleeting electrical sensations. At age 42, he developed sudden onset of diplopia due to right eye's ophthalmoparesis; the brain MRI study findings established the diagnosis with multiple sclerosis (Fig. 1). In addition, he had a history of well-controlled bipolar disorder treated with lamotrigine 1 year before his MS diagnosis was made. He had also received selective serotonin reuptake inhibitor (SSRI)/antidepressants for anxiety and depression during the following years. Subsequently he had a relapse with hemisensory loss with a new enhancing lesion in brain stem on MRI at age 45. In the following years for follow-up, brain MRI studies revealed few new MRI lesions without clinically significant relapse. He had received disease–modifying treatments—namely first with an interferon beta 1a injectable medicine and then switching to an oral agent—fingolimod.

By age 52, he had experienced CI for several years and could not keep up with his job. Then, a neuropsychological test demonstrated CI involving mental processing/executive function, memory, and visuospatial

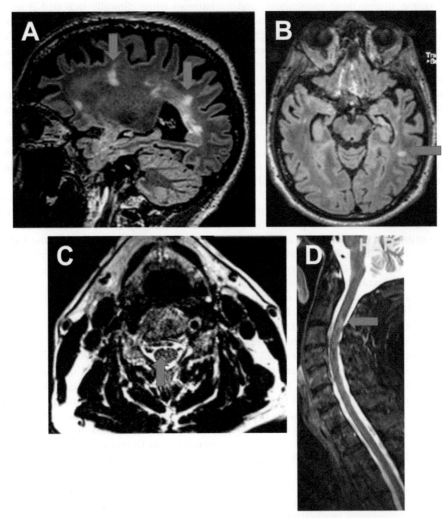

FIG. 1 MRI studies of demyelinating lesions (plaques). (A) Lesions within corpus callosum by FLAIR sagittal sequence (Dawson's fingers). (B) A subcortical WM demyelinating lesion (*blue arrows*) of left temporal lobe. (C) A demyelinating lesion of the posterior column of cervical spinal cord (cross-sectional view). (D) A demyelinating lesion of the cervical spinal cord (sagittal view). FLAIR, fluid-attenunated inversion recovery.

skills. At age 53, he started ocrelizumab for the diagnosis of SPMS. Regarding his cognitive symptoms, later on, he exhibited difficulty speaking and doing self-care tasks. His last brain MRI study at age 54 revealed bilateral temporal lobe atrophy with hippocampal atrophy compared with his previous study done 3 years ago (Fig. 2). Meanwhile, he also experienced intensive mood symptoms and behavioral issues. He eventually needed inpatient psychiatric care for treating excessive anxiety with paranoia, obsessive behavior/pacing, and insomnia with monitored

antipsychotic treatment. He had a rather stable course RRMS with an Expanded Disability Status Scale score of 3.5 when he received ocrelizumab at age 53. Afterward, he unexpectedly presented a progressive course of CI and outstanding psychiatric presentation. Clinical impressions suggested an underlying concomitant neurodegenerative process in addition to the secondary progressive course of MS. At age 55, he received the hospice care at home and died of COVID-19 pneumonia. A postmortem brain autopsy was requested.

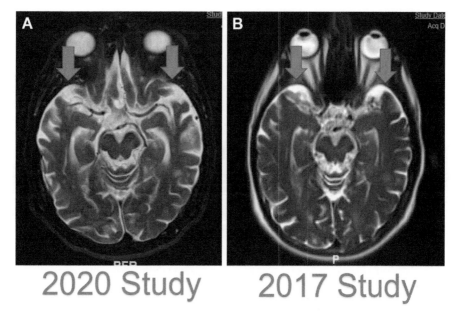

FIG. 2 Compared with the brain MRI of 2017 study, cerebral cortical atrophy with hippocampal atrophy of bilateral temporal lobes (*blue arrows*) is evidently seen in the 2020 study.

Neuropathologic Findings

External examination of the brain after fixation in 20% formalin was remarkable for the presence of mild-to-moderate cerebral atrophy involving the bilateral frontal lobes, anterior parietal lobes, and superior temporal lobes (Fig. 3A). Serial coronal sectioning revealed possible demyelinating lesions, characterized by areas of tan discoloration, scattered throughout the cerebral WM, involving the left inferior frontal gyrus, right middle frontal gyrus, and left posterior occipital WM (Fig. 3B). Representative sections were taken for microscopic examination, including sections of the suspected demyelinating lesions as well as standard sections for the evaluation of neurodegenerative diseases.

Examination of paraffin-embedded, hematoxylin and eosin/Luxol fast blue (H&E/LFB)-stained sections revealed spongiosis and reactive gliosis involving the cerebral cortex with sparing of the occipital cortex, consistent with the atrophic changes seen grossly. Scattered areas of demyelination, highlighted by pallor of the LFB, were evident involving the left inferior frontal WM as well as periventricular WM (Fig. 4A). None of

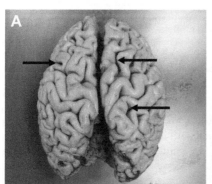
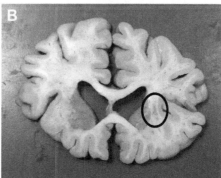

FIG. 3 External examination of the patient's brain following fixation was remarkable for the presence of cerebral atrophy (*arrows*) involving the bilateral frontal lobes, anterior parietal lobes, and superior temporal lobes. Coronal sections revealed scattered areas of suspected demyelination (*circle*) scattered throughout the cerebral WM.

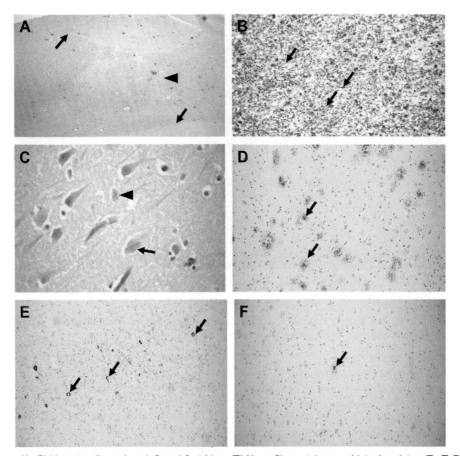

FIG. 4 (**A, C**) Hematoxylin and eosin/Luxol fast blue. (**B**) Neurofilament immunohistochemistry. (**D, F**) Beta-amyloid immunohistochemistry. (**E**) Phosphorylated tau (AT8) immunohistochemistry. (**A**) Microscopic examination revealed scattered areas of demyelination, shown as areas of pallor on Luxol fast blue staining (*arrowhead*), within the cerebral WM. Note the adjacent normal gray matter structures (Caudate nucleus, insular cortex; *arrows*) above and below the area of demyelination, respectively (2× magnification). (**B**) Staining for neurofilament highlights preserved axons (*arrows*) within the area of demyelination (40× magnification). (**C**) Both granulovacuolar degeneration (*arrowhead*) and Hirano bodies (*arrow*) are seen within the hippocampal formation (40× magnification). (**D**) Staining for beta-amyloid revealed numerous diffuse and mature plaques (*arrows*) within the prefrontal cortex (20× magnification). (**E**) Staining for phosphorylated tau highlights numerous neurofibrillary tangles (*arrows*) and threads within the occipital cortex, including the line of Gennari (20× magnification). (**F**) Staining for beta-amyloid highlights scattered diffuse plaques (*arrow*) within the pons (40× magnification).

the areas observed were completely devoid of myelin, and no inflammation was apparent. Bielschowsky silver stain and immunohistochemical staining for neurofilament highlighted the relative preservation of axons within the areas of demyelination (Fig. 4B). The overall findings were consistent with demyelinating plaques in the setting of long-standing immunomodulatory treatment. It was noted that the number of plaques seen on neuropathologic examination was less than what

was appreciated on radiologic examination, and no spinal cord lesions could be appreciated.

Regarding microscopic examination for neurodegenerative disease, granulovacuolar degeneration and Hirano bodies were noted within the hippocampal formation (Fig. 4C). Bielschowsky silver stain revealed numerous neurofibrillary tangles and neuritic plaques with the prefrontal cortex, entorhinal cortex, transentorhinal cortex, and amygdala. Sparse neurofibrillary tangles and neuritic plaques within area CA1 of the hippocampus and subiculum, and rare neurofibrillary tangles within areas CA3 and CA4 were observed. These findings were confirmed on immunohistochemical staining for phosphorylated tau (AT8), which also revealed neurofibrillary tangles and neurites within the calcarine cortex, including the line of Gennari (Fig. 4E). Immunohistochemical staining for beta-amyloid highlighted numerous diffuse plaques within the prefrontal cortex (Fig. 4D), entorhinal cortex, and transentorhinal cortex. Moderate diffuse plaques within the molecular layer of the dentate gyrus, and scattered diffuse plaques within the caudate, putamen, insular cortex, thalamus, and pons (Fig. 4F). These overall findings indicated severe AD neuropathologic change, graded using the Montine Criteria are A3/B3/C3 [44], which was consistent with a high probability of clinical diagnosis of AD and the likely explanation of the patient's dementia. It should be noted that the manifesting of AD before the age of 65 years is defined as early-onset AD (or alternatively called "young-onset AD"—YOAD) [45].

DISCUSSION

This is a unique case presenting a disease course of MS with few uncomplicated relapses in the initial 10 years after his diagnosis of RRMS was made at age 42. At the time, he received DTMs, including interferon beta and fingolimod. Meanwhile, he was treated for mood symptoms with a diagnosis of bipolar disorder in a stable condition. However, after he was 52 years of age, CI occurred and affected his ability to maintain his job and independent daily living. Meanwhile, he experienced outstanding psychiatric and behavioral issues before he died at 55, despite a new treatment—ocrelizumab for SPMS. This case has puzzled the clinicians in 3 aspects: (1) The disease course seems to progress rapidly despite less occurrence of relapses and adequate treatment; (2) Most patients with MS develop aging-related AD after age 65; and (3) The outstanding psychotic symptoms are unusual in progression of SPMS. The postmortem brain autopsy demonstrates less degree of the MS demyelinating pathologic condition, on one hand, and severe degree of Alzheimer pathologic condition, on the other hand. These findings indicate the likelihood that the MS demyelinating process has been mitigated by the DMTs; yet the early-onset AD has progressively emerged as the driving cause of deterioration. Recent studies on comparison of inflammation in MS and AD suggest that stably controlled patients with MS aged older than 65 years would develop less β-amyloid deposition defined by the β-amyloid tracer-brain PET scan because the MS-related inflammation can reduce β-amyloid deposition [46]. This case reported in

this article implies that early-onset AD in patients with MS aged younger than 65 years has a different disease course; despite the MS inflammation can be under control with DMTs, the AD pathologic condition, if developing, is not attenuated by the inflammatory demyelination. In patients with MS aged younger than 65 years who develop progressive CI with psychiatric symptoms, YOAD should be considered for differential diagnosis.

SUMMARY

In sum, the recent advance in DMTs continues to improve the quality of life in patients with MS by controlling CNS inflammation and preventing neurodegeneration. Although DMTs have reduced the burden of neuropsychiatric symptoms in MS, persistent CI of MS can still affect daily living. As patients with MS get older and reach the expected lifespan beyond 70 and 80 years of age, understandably they thus have an increased risk of developing late onset AD. With newly developed diagnostic tools and biomarkers in AD, they can benefit from early diagnosis and proper treatment to mitigate the cognitive symptoms. For the patients with MS who are aged younger than 65 years and has unusual presentation of progressive CI and complicated psychiatric symptoms, YOAD should also be considered for differential diagnosis by using advanced diagnostic tools of AD in order to confirm the comorbidity. Therefore, proper intervention and therapies can be provided by the specialists; the concerning caregivers will be informed in time of the complicated comorbidity situation so that they can prepare for the care plan.

FUNDING

Dr Victoria Sanborn is supported by the neuropsychology fellowship of psychiatry department of Rhode Island Hospital and Brown University. Dr Mohona Reza is supported by a Clinical Care Fellowship from the National Multiple Sclerosis Society, United States.

CLINICS CARE POINTS

- Neuropsychiatric symptoms and cognitive Impairment are common in the patients with multiple sclerosis of different stages.
- There are useful diagnostic tools that can assist clinicians to detect and to monitor cognitive impairment and psychiatric symptoms.

- Disease-modifying treatments of multiple sclerosis are crucial to reduce inflammation and burden of neuropsychiatric symptoms.
- Concomitant Alzheimer's Disease is difficult to be differentiated from the cognitive impairment occurring in the progressive course of multiple sclerosis. Clinicans have to pay attention to this situation.
- Recent advances in developing biomarkers of Alzheimer's disease could facilitate the diagnostic process.
- It is crucial to request psychiatry services to manage the neuropsychiatric symptoms of patients with multiple sclerosis.

DISCLOSURE

Dr Cahill receives research funding from F. Hoffman-La Roche. The other authors have nothing to disclose.

ACKNOWLEDGMENT

We thank the assistance provided by Theresa Fogerty, who obtained further medical history for the case report.

REFERENCES

[1] Luczynski P, Laule C, Hsiung G-Y-R, et al. Coexistence of multiple sclerosis and alzheimer's disease: a review. Multiple Sclerosis and Related Disorders 2019;27: 232–8.

[2] Charcot JM. Lectures on the diseases of the nervous system delivered at La Salpetriere. London: New Sydenham Society; 1877.

[3] Benedict RH, DeLuca J, Enzinger C, et al. Neuropsychology of multiple sclerosis: looking back and moving forward. JINS 2017;23(9–10):832–42.

[4] Kurtz JF. Neurologic impairment in multiple sclerosis and the Disability Status Scale. Acta Neurol Scand 1970;46:493–512.

[5] Peyser JM, Poser CM. Chapter 14. Neuropsychological correlates of multiple sclerosis. In: Filskov SB, Boll TJ, editors. Handbook of clinical neuropsychology volume 2. New York: John Wiley & Sons. Inc.; 1986. p. 364.

[6] Rao SM. Chapter 12. Multiple sclerosis. In: Cummings JL, editor. Subcortical dementia. 1st edition. Oxford, New York: Oxford Press University; 1990. p. 164.

[7] Kutzelnigg A, Lucchinetti CF, Stadelmann C, et al. Cortical demyelination and diffuse white matter injury in multiple sclerosis. Brain 2005;128:2705–12.

[8] Amato MP, Bartolozzi ML, Zipoli V, et al. Neocortical volume decrease in relapsing-remitting MS patients with mild cognitive impairment. Neurology 2004;63: 89–93.

[9] Magliozi R, Fadda G, Brown RA, et al. Ependymal-in gradient of thalamic damage in progressive multiple sclerosis. Ann Neurol 2022;92:670–85.

[10] Steenwijk MD, Geurts JJ, Daams M, et al. Cortical atrophy patterns in multiple sclerosis are non-random and clinically relevant. Brain 2016;139(1):115–26.

[11] Hansen S, Lautenbacher S. Neuropsychological assessment in multiple sclerosis. Z für Neuropsychol 2017. https://doi.org/10.1024/1016-264X/a000197.

[12] De Meo E, Portaccio E, Giorgio A, et al. Identifying the distinct cognitive phenotypes in multiple sclerosis. JAMA Neurol 2021;78(4):414–25.

[13] Labiano-Fontcuberta A, Martinez-Gines M, Aladro Y, et al. A comparison study of cognitive deficits in radiologically and clinically isolated syndromes. Mult Scler 2016;22:250–3.

[14] Brochet B, Ruet A. Cognitive impairment in multiple sclerosis with regards to disease duration and clinical phenotypes. Front Neurol 2019;10:261.

[15] Leavitt VM, tosto G, Riley CS. Cognitive phenotypes in multiple sclerosis. J Neurol 2018;263:562–6.

[16] Landmeyer NC, Burkner P-C, Wiendl H. Disease-modifying treatments and cognition in relapsing-remitting multiple sclerosis. Neurology 2020;22:e2373–83.

[17] Duncan A, Malcolm-Smith S, Ameen O, et al. The Incidence of Euphoria in Multiple Sclerosis: Artefact of Measure. Mult Scler Int 2016;2016:5738425.

[18] Interferon beta-1b in the treatment of multiple sclerosis: final outcome of the randomized controlled trial. The IFNB Multiple Sclerosis Study Group and The University of British Columbia MS/MRI Analysis Group. Neurology 1995;45(7):1277–85.

[19] Marrie RA, Horwitz R, Cutter G, et al. The burden of mental comorbidity in multiple sclerosis: frequent, underdiagnosed, and undertreated. Mult Scler 2009; 15(3):385–92.

[20] Masuccio FG, Gamberini G, Calabrese M, et al. Imaging and depression in multiple sclerosis: a historical perspective. Neurol Sci 2021;42(3):835–45.

[21] Fassbender K, Schmidt R, Mössner R, et al. Mood disorders and dysfunction of the hypothalamic-pituitary-adrenal axis in multiple sclerosis: association with cerebral inflammation. Arch Neurol 1998;55(1): 66–72.

[22] Rickards H. Depression in neurological disorders: Parkinson's disease, multiple sclerosis, and stroke. J Neurol Neurosurg Psychiatry 2005;76(Suppl 1):i48–52.

[23] Gasim M, Bernstein CN, Graff LA, et al. Adverse psychiatric effects of disease-modifying therapies in multiple Sclerosis: A systematic review. Mult Scler Relat Disord 2018;26:124–56.

[24] Shen Q, Lu H, Xie D, et al. Association between suicide and multiple sclerosis: An updated meta-analysis. Mult Scler Relat Disord 2019;34:83–90.

[25] Feinstein A, du Boulay G, Ron MA. Psychotic illness in multiple sclerosis. A clinical and magnetic resonance imaging study. Br J Psychiatry 1992;161:680–5.

[26] Boeschoten RE, Braamse AMJ, Beekman ATF, et al. Prevalence of depression and anxiety in Multiple Sclerosis: A systematic review and meta-analysis. J Neurol Sci 2017; 372:331–41.

[27] Mohr DC, Cox D, Merluzzi N. Self-injection anxiety training: a treatment for patients unable to self-inject injectable medications. Mult Scler 2005;11(2):182–5.

[28] Marrie RA, Reingold S, Cohen J, et al. The incidence and prevalence of psychiatric disorders in multiple sclerosis: a systematic review. Mult Scler 2015;21(3):305–17.

[29] Sabe M, Sentissi O. Psychotic symptoms prior or concomitant to diagnosis of multiple sclerosis: a systematic review of case reports and case series. Int J Psychiatry Clin Pract 2022;26(3):287–93.

[30] Silveira C, Guedes R, Maia D, et al. Neuropsychiatric Symptoms of Multiple Sclerosis: State of the Art. Psychiatry Investig 2019;16(12):877–88.

[31] Johansson V, Lundholm C, Hillert J, et al. Multiple sclerosis and psychiatric disorders: comorbidity and sibling risk in a nationwide Swedish cohort. Mult Scler 2014; 20(14):1881–91.

[32] Fitzgerald KC, Salter A, Tyry T, et al. Pseudobulbar affect: Prevalence and association with symptoms in multiple sclerosis. Neurol Clin Pract. 2018;8(6):472–81.

[33] Glanz BI, Zurawski J, Casady EC, et al. The impact of ocrelizumab on health-related quality of life in individuals with multiple sclerosis. Mult Scler J Exp Transl Clin 2021; 1–10.

[34] DeLuca GC, Yates RL, Beale H, et al. Cognitive impairment in multiple sclerosis: clinical, radiologic and pathologic insights. Brain Pathol 2015;25(1):79–98.

[35] Politte LC, Huffman JC, Stern TA. Neuropsychiatric manifestations of multiple sclerosis. Prim Care Companion J Clin Psychiatry 2008;10(4):318–24.

[36] Bayas A, Schuh K, Baier M, et al, REGAIN Study Group. Combination treatment of fingolimod with antidepressants in relapsing-remitting multiple sclerosis patients with depression: a multicentre, open-label study - REGAIN. Ther Adv Neurol Disord 2016;9(5):378–88.

[37] Iniaghe LO, Ilondu CA, Eseka EO, et al. Dimethyl Fumarate Improves Depression and Anxiety by Reducing Brain Catalase Levels in Mice. Faseb J 2017;31:989.8.

[38] Sprenger T, Kappos L, Sormani MP, et al. Effects of teriflunomide treatment on cognitive performance and brain volume in patients with relapsing multiple sclerosis: Post hoc analysis of the TEMSO core and extension studies. Mult Scler 2022;28(11):1719–28.

[39] Hauser SL, Cree BAC. Treatment of Multiple Sclerosis: A Review. Am J Med 2020;133(12):1380–90.

[40] Branco M, Ruano L, Portaccio E, et al. Aging with multiple sclerosis: prevalence and profile of cognitive impairment. Neurol Sci 2019;40:1651–7.

[41] Jakimovski D, Weinstock-Guttman B, Roy S, et al. Cognitive profiles of aging in multiple sclerosis. Front Aging Neurosci 2017;11:105.

[42] Luczynski P, Laule C, Hsiung G-Y, et al. Coexistence of multiple sclerosis and Alzheimer's disease: a review. Mult. Scler. Relat. Disord 2019;27:232–8.

[43] Flanagan EP, Knopman DS, Keegan BM. Dementia in MS complicated by coexistent Alzheimer disease: diagnosis premortem and postmortem. Neurol Clin Pract 2014; 4(3):226–30.

[44] Montine TJ, Phelps CH, Beach TG, et al. National Institute on Aging-Alzheimer's Association guidelines for the neuropathologic assessment of Alzheimer's disease: a practical approach. Acta Neuropathol 2012;123:1–11.

[45] Cacace R, Sleegers K, Van Broeckhoven C. Molecular genetics of early-onset Alzheimer's disease revisited. Alzheimers Dement 2016;12(6):733–48.

[46] Zeydan B, Lowe VJ, Reichard RR, et al. Imaging biomarkers of Alzheimer's disease in multiple sclerosis. Ann Neurol 2020;87:556–67.

Printed and bound by CPI Group (UK) Ltd, Croydon, CR0 4YY

08/05/2025

01864749-0010